CAMBRIDGE GEOGRAPHICAL STUDIES

---

14 SPATIAL DIFFUSION

An Historical Geography of Epidemics in an Island Community

CAMBRIDGE GEOGRAPHICAL STUDIES

1 *Urban Analysis,* B. T. Robson
2 *The Urban Mosaic,* D. W. G. Timms
3 *Hillslope Form and Process,* M. A. Carson and M. J. Kirkby
4 *Freight Flows and Spatial Aspects of the British Economy,* M. Chisholm and P. O'Sullivan
5 *The Agricultural Systems of the World: An Evolutionary Approach,* D. B. Grigg
6 *Elements of Spatial Struture: A Quantitative Approach,* A. D. Cliff, P. Haggett, J. K. Ord, K. A. Bassett and R. B. Davies
7 *Housing and the Spatial Structure of the City: Residential Mobility and the Housing market in an English City since the Industrial Revolution,* R. M. Pritchard
8 *Models of Spatial Processes. An Approach to the Study of Point, Line and Area Patterns,* A. Getis and B. N. Boots
9 *Tropical Soils and Soil Survey,* Anthony Young
10 *Water Management in England and Wales,* Elizabeth Porter
11 *Geographical Change and Industrial Revolution,* John Langton
12 *Population and Metropolis: The Demography of London 1580–1650,* Roger Finlay
13 *Population Growth and Agrarian Change: An Historical Perspective*, D. B. Grigg

Spatial Diffusion

An Historical Geography of Epidemics in an Island Community

A. D. CLIFF

Fellow of Christ's College, Cambridge;
University Lecturer in Geography, University of Cambridge

P. HAGGETT

Professor of Urban and Regional Geography, University of Bristol

J. K. ORD

Reader in Statistics, University of Warwick

G. R. VERSEY

Formerly Senior Technical Officer,
Department of Geography, University of Cambridge

CAMBRIDGE UNIVERSITY PRESS

Cambridge
London New York New Rochelle
Melbourne Sydney

Published by the Press Syndicate of the University of Cambridge
The Pitt Building, Trumpington Street, Cambridge CB2 1RP
32 East 57th Street, New York, NY 10022, USA
296 Beaconsfield Parade, Middle Park, Melbourne 3206, Australia

First published 1981

Text set in 10/12 pt Linotron 202 Times, printed and bound
in Great Britain at The Pitman Press, Bath

British Library cataloguing in publication data

Spatial diffusion. – (Cambridge geographical studies).
1. Epidemiology – Case studies
2. Medical geography – Case studies
3. Epidemiology – Iceland
4. Medical geography – Iceland
I. Cliff, Andrew David II. Series
614.5′23′094912 RA650.6.I2 80–41329

ISBN 0 521 22840 9

Contents

Preface

If the scientific analysis of the peculiar problems which islands pose for spatial diffusion studies needs an origin, then it may well be found in Charles Darwin's notebooks for 1835. His period on the Galápagos Islands led him to write that the biology of island groups 'will be well worth examination'. And so it has proved to be. This book, which explores the historical geography of spatial diffusion through an island setting, sets out both to demonstrate general principles and to dissect a specific case. It brings together the work of two geographers (A. D. C. and P. H.), a statistician (J. K. O.) and an historical illustrator (G. R. V.), from three universities in a common concern to track down the particular geography by which a phenomenon – in our case study, a childhood disease – is passed through a human population. We do this to indicate the possibilities and difficulties which lie within this form of analysis. We do not expect that our models will last for long without changes in the furnace of empirical trials in other places, but we do expect them to contribute to the future development of stronger and more resilient models of a process which is both intrinsically fascinating and of no little importance.

The work described in this book has been funded from two sources. We have been supported since 1975 on a Social Sciences Research Council grant (SSRC, #HR 3534), 'Geographical Modelling and Forecasting for Epidemiological and Population Data'. The book forms part of the final report for this project, and our thanks are due to SSRC for their financial assistance. We are also grateful to the Nuffield Foundation for a grant from their Social Sciences Small Grants Scheme which enabled us to carry out library work on unpublished material in Reykjavík. Without this, our data sources and historical information would have been limited indeed.

We wish to acknowledge the efforts of four graduate students whose work has made an important contribution to parts of chapters 5, 6 and 7 of this book. F. Ball (now of the Statistics Department, University of Sussex), C. Goodall (now of the Statistics Department, Harvard University) and A. Sutherland were supervised by one of us (A.D.C.) as students working on field projects as part of the postgraduate Diploma in Mathematical Statistics at Cambridge University. Similarly, R. C. Souza (now of the Pontifícia Universidade Católica do Rio de Janeiro) carried out research on Bayesian forecasting methods for epidemics under the direction of J.K.O. while a PhD student supervised by Professor P. J. Harrison of the Statistics Department, Warwick

University. Our indebtedness to all four is made clear in the appropriate sections of the chapters concerned.

Since much of the substantive part of this work was carried out in Iceland itself, we wish to express our special appreciation of the help provided by the appropriate Icelandic authorities. At the Statistical Bureau of Iceland (Hagstofa Íslands), the director, Klemens Tryggvason, and his senior demographer, Guðni Baldursson, went to exceptional lengths to provide archival data, guidance on translation and helpful working conditions. Without their interest, this book could not have been written. In Reykjavík, Dr Finnbogi Guðmundsson placed the resources of the National Library of Iceland (Landsbókasafn Íslands) at our disposal. Miss Rosemary Graham of Trinity College Library, Cambridge, translated substantial sections of the Icelandic archival material with immense care and concern for geographical accuracy; the bond maps in chapter 4 are based directly on her work.

Although the responsibility for errors is the authors' alone, we appreciate the help of those who kindly read and commented on parts of the final manuscript. We would like to acknowledge in Iceland, in addition to those already listed, the help of Dr Julius Sigurjónsson, Professor of Medicine, and Dr Sigúrður Þórarinsson, Professor of Geology and Geography, of the University of Iceland (Háskoli Íslands), and also Dr Ólafur Ólafsson, Director General of Public Health in Iceland (Landlæknir). In England, Dr. D. A. J. Tyrrell, FRS, Deputy Director of the Clinical Research Centre, Harrow, and Head of the Division of Communicable Diseases, and Dr P. E. M. Fine of the London School of Hygiene and Tropical Medicine, read parts of the manuscript from the critical viewpoint of the epidemiologist. Professor W. R. Mead of the Department of Geography at University College, London, brought his experience of the Nordic countries and their geography to bear, and, together with Mr Brian Holt of the British Embassy in Reykjavík, provided guidance on Icelandic sources of information.

The final preparation of the manuscript involved help by some of the secretarial and technical staff at both Bristol and Cambridge Universities, and we acknowledge their assistance.

The Icelandic form of spelling has been retained for all Icelandic proper names and place names in this monograph. These frequently include letters peculiar to the Icelandic language and alphabet, viz.:

Þ , þ pronounced as *th* in theatre,
Ð, ð pronounced as *th* in breathe,
Æ , æ pronounced as *i* in time,
Ö , ö pronounced as *u* in sun.

Note on names of medical districts

The Icelandic for medical district is *læknishérað* (plural: *læknishéruð*). Names of medical districts are derived from the seat of the doctor (e.g., Laugaráslæknishérað), the area comprising the district (e.g., Mýralæknishérað) or the population in that area (e.g., Svarfdalalæknishérað). Throughout this book *læknishérað* is omitted to save repetition, and names of medical districts appear as either the stem (e.g., Laugarás) or the genitive case (e.g., Mýra) of the origin. As further examples, Reykjavík, Akureyri and Ísafjörður refer to places, while Reykjavíkur, Akureyrar and Ísafjarðar refer to the medical districts based on these centres.

1 Introduction

1.1 The problem

A stone is tossed into a pond. The consequent splash forms a large wave immediately around the entry point. Within a second, waves are starting to move out in a circular pattern across the surface of the water. Some seconds later, very small ripples are disturbing the weeds on the far side of the pond.

Information is tossed into a communication system. An American president is killed by a sniper's bullet at 12.31 p.m. on 22 November 1963 on a Dallas road. Information is beamed out on radio and television around the world, is passed by word of mouth from one listener to the rest of his family, or is told by the garage man to the motorist stopping for petrol.

A virus is tossed into a susceptible population. Passengers arriving at an Icelandic port from Copenhagen in the early summer of 1907 include a few known to be suffering from measles infection. One escapes the quarantine procedures, and joins the local population, some of whom are off to the capital city, Reykjavík, to form the crowds gathering for a visit by the King of Denmark. The virus is transmitted between some neighbours in the crowd. Within 16 months, an epidemic has spread through the whole island infecting over 7,000 people and killing 354.

Although the stone, the assassination and the epidemic are, in most respects, wholly dissimilar phenomena, one being trivial, the other two historic, they do share something in common: they all involve waves moving outward through a medium away from a single centre. In the case of the stone, the wave pattern is simple and circular; in the others, the waves move through many pathways at different velocities and in an intensely complex pattern. What they share is the property of spatial diffusion; that is, the ability to spread outwards or to disperse from one or more limited centres to a wider geographical area.

It is the spatial aspect of this spread process that has particularly attracted geographers to the study of diffusion (see chapter 2), and this book focusses on the geographer's approach to spatial diffusion. It is concerned with the velocity of diffusion waves, the channels that such waves follow, the forms they take, the regularity with which they can be speeded up (or slowed down), and so on. In other words, it is concerned with the discovery of spatial order within diffusion processes.

In examining these issues, it may be useful for readers both inside and outside the geographical profession to note that contemporary research and inquiry within geography are in a state of flux. The last two decades have seen considerable theoretical and conceptual advances, not least in the examination of those spatial processes of which spatial diffusion forms a significant part. But there has been a failure to weld these gains on different fronts into a common philosophical perspective. As a result, researchers in geography are often faced with either/or choices between positions which are sometimes argued antagonistically. Thus, quantitative work may be linked to a logical positivist framework, or behavioural studies to a hermeneutic viewpoint.

In this book, we have tried, as far as is possible, to draw on all the geographical traditions which seem capable of contributing to our central problem. We use the term *historical geography* to indicate our concern with archival source materials spread over an 80-year time period, but combine this with quantitative modelling less frequently associated with historical studies. In each instance, we have tried to be catholic in relating the method to the central diffusion issues addressed, and we have not followed a narrow sectarian path.

1.2 Previous studies of spatial diffusion

Spatial diffusion studies have been reported in geographical journals for all decades of this century. Much of the work has been concerned with understanding the spread of cultural traits, the diffusion of agricultural innovations, and the factors which affect the propensity to adopt an item. The research has been predominantly descriptive and idiographic, and any formulation of general models of the diffusion processes involved has been slow. We would argue, however, that the development of such models should be a prime goal of geographical research in this area.

If we consider the mathematical theory of epidemics, we find a different tradition. It was about 75 years ago that the field initially became established through the work of William Hamer and Ronald Ross. Although this field has as long a history of diffusion studies as has geography, the emphasis has been upon models of disease development with relatively little large-scale empirical testing. The epidemiological literature is rich in potentially useful models if the modelling and empirical emphases of mathematical epidemic theory and geography can be brought together. Part of the challenge of this task lies in the difficulty of developing realistic models which incorporate spatial components. Thus, Bailey (1957, p. 135) has commented: 'The complexity of this type of work is formidable, especially when an attempt is made to allow for geographical spread as well.' Indeed, it is this complexity which has meant that most epidemic models are aspatial and are concerned with projecting the ultimate size of epidemics rather than their spatial characteristics. One purpose of this book is to attempt an integration of the modelling and empirical strands referred to above by applying spatial developments of various epidemic models to the diffusion of one infectious disease (measles) in an isolated island community (Iceland). To help in an evaluation of the models developed, we also apply more conventional regression methods to the data collected.

There are obvious humanitarian reasons why the spread of epidemic diseases should be studied. Adequate modelling of the diffusion process should ultimately permit probability forecasts to be made both of the likely *times* and the likely *places* of recurrence; this should, in turn, enable more effective control programmes to be instituted. In this context, Bailey's (1957, p. 1) introduction to his classic book, *The Mathematical Theory of Epidemics* is worth recalling:

> The fearful toll of human life and happiness exacted through the ages by widespread disease and pestilence affords a spectacle that is both fascinating and repellent. A recital of the astronomical numbers of casualties suffered in this way by the human race is almost stupefying in its effect, and makes the consequences of all past wars seem almost trivial in comparison. Thus in Europe in the 14th century there were some 25 million deaths out of a population of perhaps 100 million from the Black Death alone. In 1520 the Aztecs lost about half of their population of $3\frac{1}{2}$ million from smallpox . . . It has been estimated that Russia suffered about 25 million cases of typhus in the years from 1918 to 1921 with a death rate of approximately 10 per cent. In the world pandemic of influenza in 1919 the total number of deaths is thought to have been in the region of 20 million over twelve months.

Against this background, even small advances in control strategies are arguably worthwhile. The need to predict likely places of occurrence is an integral part of efficient control and provides the geographer with an important opportunity to apply his particular spatial skills to the problem.

Models of the spread of infectious disease should also be useful generally in the analysis of innovation and cultural diffusion patterns. Simple infectious diseases like measles rely for their transmission on close contact between infected individuals and those at risk. A basic assumption of most innovation studies is that person-to-person contact is essential for information spread. Resistance to 'infection' and lengths of transmission periods are generally better understood for infectious diseases than for innovations; it therefore seems sensible to use the more accurately defined disease-spread mechanisms to identify a class of workable models for spatial diffusion problems which operate through personal contact. Because of the public health aspect, a wealth of data pours forth each week and month on the detailed pattern of disease distribution around the world. This vast data bank stands in stark contrast to the limited information available on innovation and cultural diffusion, and makes the modelling of disease spread a more viable proposition. Again, epidemics frequently repeat themselves in time and space in a way that cultural events usually do not. This makes model development and verification for disease spread simpler than is the case for innovations, and their use in forecasting more likely.

The fascination of studies concerned with the spread of disease has meant that many researchers have been attracted from a variety of disciplines to try to sieve the data records to find those persistences in spatial and temporal behaviour which might throw light on the progress of disease, or which might allow some early-warning system to be developed. Frequently, the results have been disappointing, but always with a sufficient hint of regularity to attract a later generation of workers back to the same problem. The perennial questions remain: Does the distribution map throw light on the origin or progress of an epidemic?

Does the epidemic spread in recognisable ways? Can we learn anything from the maps that would help to indicate or to delay its impact? In this book, we look at these questions, and try to determine whether, despite its many limitations, analysis on an aggregated geographical scale is capable of yielding information on the evolution of epidemic maps which is not apparent from work at the detailed clinical level.

1.3 Organisation of the book

In this book, our treatment of diffusion processes moves from the general to the specific, and then back to the general again. We start with an overview of some of the phenomena that have been analysed by geographers within a diffusion framework. In the main part of the book, we examine the spatial regularities observable in the recurrent epidemic waves formed by a specific infectious disease – measles – in a particular region setting, Iceland. Various models of the patterns are proposed and tested. Finally, we move back to the general by considering future research trends and some of the questions outlined above.

1.3.1 General issues: the question of diffusion

In chapter 2, we define the term 'spatial diffusion', and review some case studies of phenomena examined as spread processes. These phenomena range from agricultural innovations to bush fires, disease, settlement patterns, wage and price inflation, and agrarian riots. The studies show that certain elements in the spread patterns repeat themselves from item to item. These regularities are concerned with (1) the spatial spread: the extent to which diffusion is wave-like as opposed to being guided through specific channels, and (2) the temporal build-up of the process. Some Monte Carlo models which incorporate these elements are described and illustrated.

1.3.2 Case study: measles in Iceland

In chapters 3–7, we select the specific disease of measles from the variety of diffusion phenomena discussed and examine its epidemic history in an island context. In chapter 3, we justify our choice of measles as an indicator of a spread process and point out the features of the disease which make it particularly suitable for the development and testing of spatial diffusion models. We also indicate why we regard Iceland as one of the best areal settings for this work.

We have been able to collect detailed information on 16 major measles epidemic waves which passed through Iceland in the period from 1896 to 1975. Data have been obtained for some 50 medical districts on a monthly basis for that entire period. The time–space data matrix is reproduced in the Appendix to the book. Medical reports are available to support the numerical information, and our approach in chapters 4 and 5 is to use this historical record to reconstruct the main features of the disease waves. In chapter 4, these reports are analysed and a qualitative model of the spread process involving both contagious and hierarchical components is proposed. The documentary evidence is much less detailed for the period 1946–75 than for 1896–1945, and so, in chapter 5, we supplement the reports using a variety of statistical methods. We establish the relationship between patterns of spread and factors such as the school system, changing methods of transport, and Iceland's decreasing internal and external isolation.

In chapters 6 and 7, formal models of the epidemic waves are proposed and tested. We concentrate upon the period between 1945 and 1970, and, where appropriate, use the patterns defined empirically in chapters 4 and 5 to structure the models. Both single- and multi-region models are defined, and both fixed and time-varying parameter versions are examined. In chapter 6, time series methods are used, where the nature of the process at any point in time is related directly to its immediate past history in other areas within a regression framework. However, explicitly process-based epidemic models do exist, such as those developed by Hamer (1906), Soper (1929), Reed and Frost (see Abbey, 1952). In these, the sizes of the populations with the disease and those at risk are considered, and geographical patterns of mixing between them are established to handle spatial spread. These models are considered in chapter 7. Generally, the models proposed are calibrated on between one and three of the immediately post-war measles waves, and the models are then used to provide *ex post* forecasts of cases for some of the more recent waves. Model evaluation is undertaken.

1.3.3 General issues: conclusions and future research

The concluding chapter of the book discusses the implications of the work undertaken in earlier chapters for both disease control and, more generally, spatial diffusion studies. We set out with great expectations that we would be able to provide reasonable forecasts of both epidemic recurrences and magnitudes. This has not proved possible; we eventually sacrificed ability to predict epidemic size in order to provide better estimates of the likely times and places of occurrence of epidemics. This is justified on the grounds that 'where?' and 'when?' are more important for disease control. We doubt whether it will ever be possible to forecast these processes with great accuracy but, by emphasising our ability to identify high-risk zones of infection, we hope that epidemics and pandemics, like the poor, will not always be with us.

2 The study of spatial diffusion

2.1 Introduction

The *Oxford English Dictionary* defines *diffuse* as 'to disperse or be dispersed from a centre; to spread widely, disseminate'. However, in the geographical literature, the term, diffusion, has two distinct usages. *Expansion diffusion* is the process whereby information, a material or a disease, for example, spreads from one place to another. In this expansion process, the item being diffused remains, and often intensifies, in the originating region, but new areas are also occupied by the item in subsequent time periods (Figure 2.1A). A typical example would be the diffusion of improved rice grains in India (Farmer, 1977). *Relocation diffusion* is also a spatial spread process, but the items being diffused leave the areas where they originated as they move to new areas. The migration of the black population of the United States from the rural South to the northern cities in the twentieth century could be viewed as a relocation process, where members of a population at time t_1 change their location between t_1 and t_2 (Figure 2.1B). Figure 2.1C shows how the two processes of expansion and relocation may be combined.

Two examples of the above processes are shown in Figure 2.2. Figure 2.2A shows the spread of a bush fire near Hobart, Tasmania, in the afternoon of 7 February 1967. The expansion diffusion element is represented by the fire edge, while the spot fire showers represent relocation diffusion. The distance between the origin and the coast along the main axis of the fire's advance is about 14 km (9 miles). Figure 2.2B shows the spread of one of the world's great cholera pandemics – the El Tor strain – between 1960 and 1971. The El Tor strain of cholera was first identified in the bodies of six Muslim pilgrims at the El Tor quarantine station outside Mecca in 1905. In the 1930s, the same strain was recognised as endemic in the Celebes, which have a largely Muslim population. For another 30 years, there was little news of El Tor until, in 1961, it began to spread with devastating speed out from the Celebes. By 1964, it had reached India, replacing the normal cholera strain which

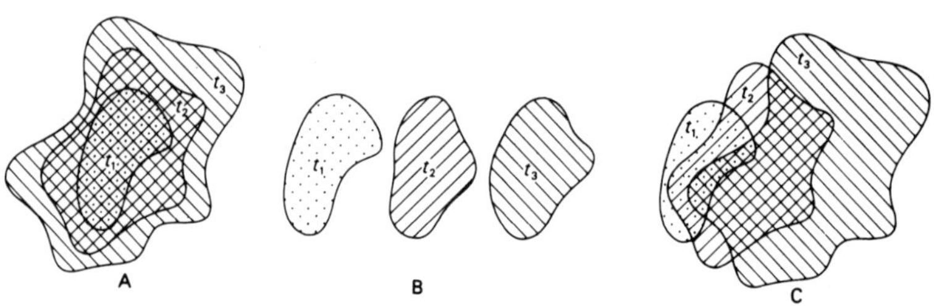

Fig. 2.1 Types of spatial diffusion. (A) Expansion diffusion. (B) Relocation diffusion. (C) Combined expansion and relocation processes. The term t_i denotes the time period. *Source:* Haggett (1979, p. 300).

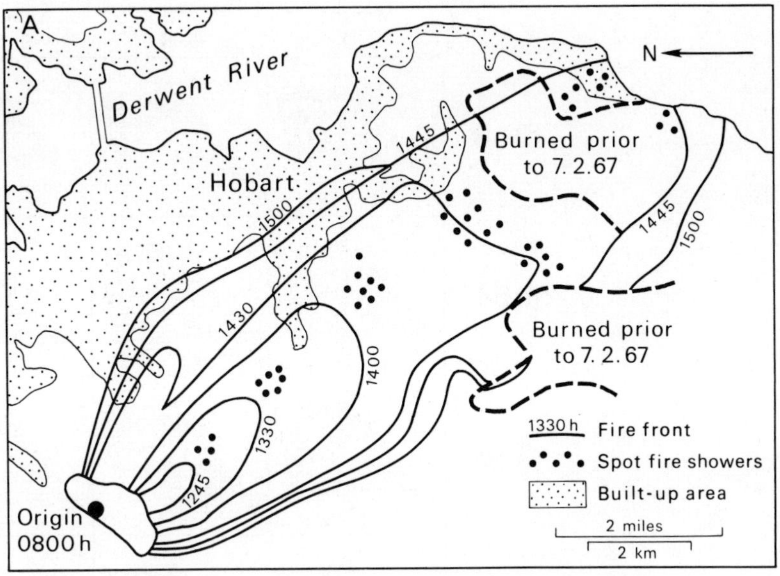

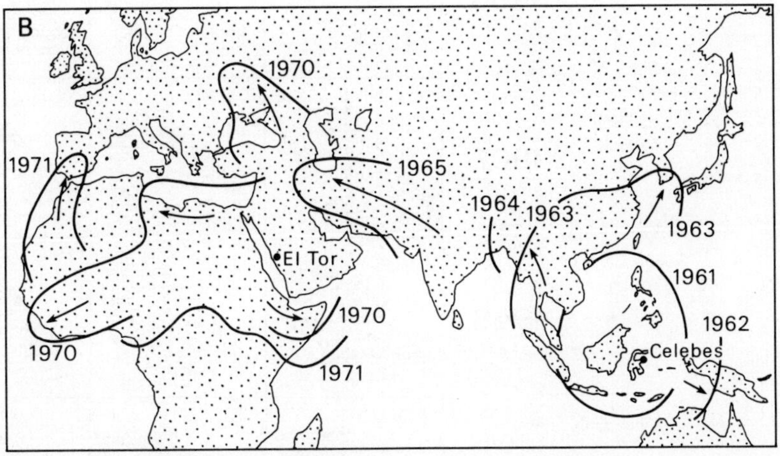

Fig. 2.2 Examples of combined expansion and relocation diffusion. (A) The spread of a bush fire near Hobart, Tasmania, 7 February 1967. (B) Spread of the El Tor cholera pandemic, 1960–71. *Sources:* (A) data from A. G. Arthur in Edgell (1973, p. 7). (B) data from W. H. O. Bulletins.

had been endemic in the Ganges delta for centuries, and by the early 1970s, it was pushing south into central Africa and west into Russia and Europe. The El Tor outbreak is also an example of diffusion by relocation and expansion. The strain diffuses by relocation through some areas (as in Spain, where small isolated outbreaks were recorded in 1971), but it also diffuses by expansion because it remains endemic in the Celebes.

Expansion diffusion occurs in two ways. *Contagious* spread depends on direct contact. It is in this way that infectious diseases like measles pass through a population, from person to person. This process is strongly influenced by distance because nearby individuals or regions have a much higher probability of contact than remote individuals or regions. Therefore, contagious spread tends to occur in a centrifugal manner from the source region outward. An example of this process is shown in Figure 2.3. A wildlife rabies epidemic has been progressing

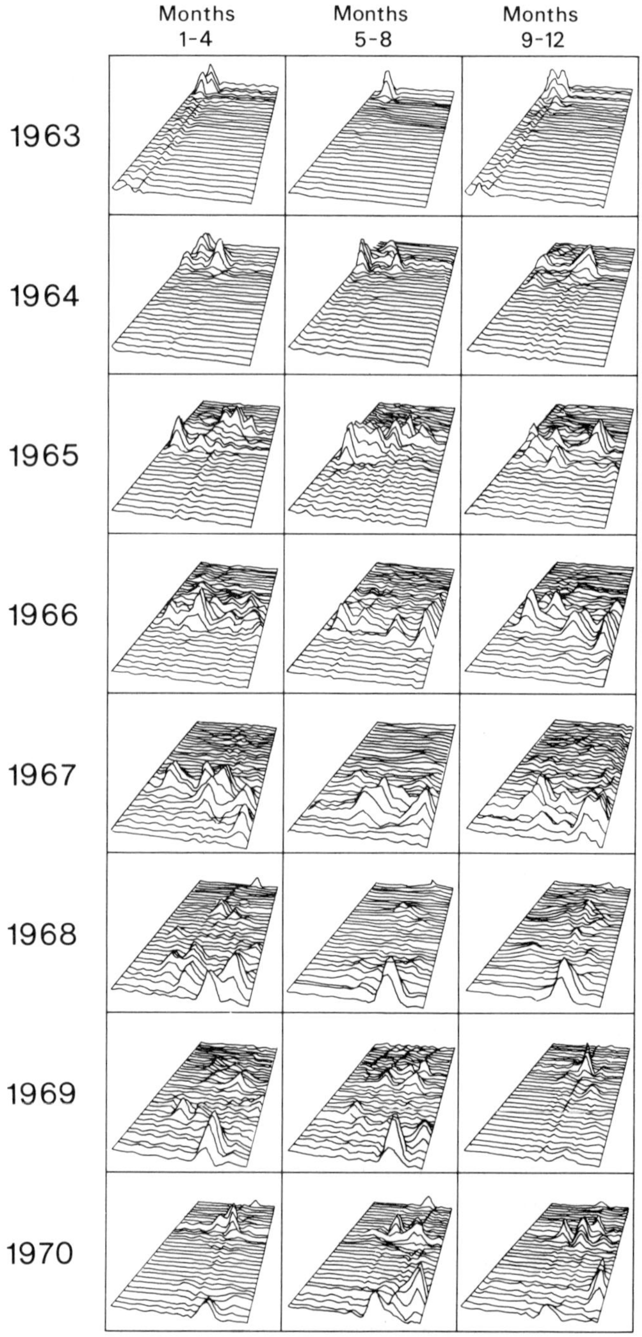

Fig. 2.3 Plots of case occurrences of rabies in Central Europe by four-monthly periods, 1963–70. *Source:* Mc. A. Sayers, Mansourian, Tan and Bögel (1977, p. 17).

steadily across central Europe over recent years. Mc. A. Sayers, Mansourian, Tan and Bögel (1977) have collected data on the number of rabid animals reported in a $133 \times 133\,\text{km}^2$ area of Süd Württemberg, Stockach and Uberlingen, and Figure 2.3 is a plot of case occurrences for four-monthly intervals in the study area, 1963–70. Note the steady southwards advance of the epidemic wave throughout the period and, from 1968 onwards, a recurrent wave behind the main front.

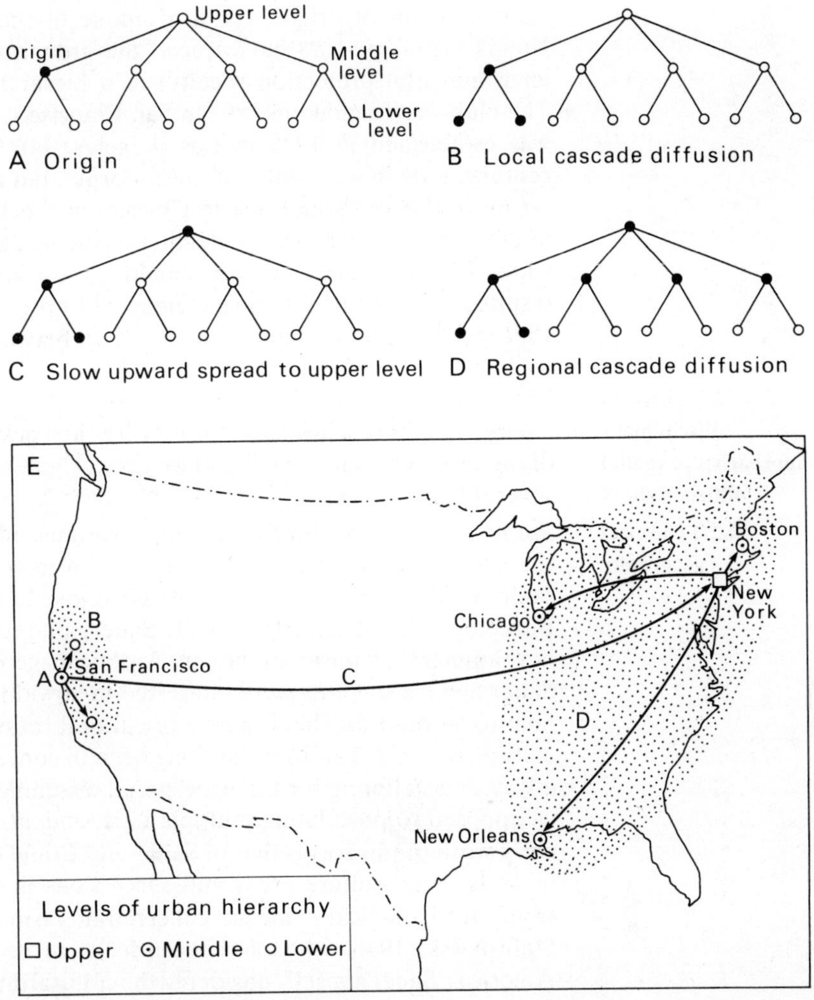

Fig. 2.4 Hierarchical diffusion. These diagrams show the spread of an innovation through a hierarchy. The innovation begins at a middle level (A) in a small county town, and spreads rapidly down to a lower level (B) by local cascade diffusion to villages in its vicinity. Spread to an upper level such as a regional capital (C) is much slower. Once there, rapid downward spread over the entire area occurs (D) by a regional cascade process. (E) Hypothetical spread process involving elements (A)–(D) for an innovation introduced on the Western Seaboard of the United States (cf. Sierra Club). Stipple shows extent of spread. *Source:* Haggett (1979, p. 301).

Expansion diffusion may, however, occur in a very different fashion, namely by hierarchical spread. This describes transmission through an ordered sequence of classes or places. The process is typified by the diffusion of innovations (such as new styles in women's fashions or new consumer goods, for example television) from large metropolitan centres to remote villages. Within socially structured populations, innovations may be adopted first on the upper level of the social hierarchy and then trickle down to the lower levels. *Cascade diffusion* is a term reserved for processes which are always assumed to be downwards from larger to smaller centres. When specifying a movement that may be either up or down the hierarchy, geographers generally prefer the term *hierarchical diffusion.* Figure 2.4 shows how diffusion may begin at a lower point in a hierarchy, move slowly upward, and then expand rapidly. We might think of this as a 'Beatles' pattern': a musical style beginning in a provincial city (Liverpool) moves to the national capital (London), and then on to other capitals throughout the world. Finally, it reaches the local music shop in small towns thousands of miles from its point of origin. As an example of these ideas, Nystuen and Kolars (1974, p. 129) have traced the growth of the Sierra Club (an environmental protection society) as a hierarchical diffusion process. The club was founded in 1892 in San Francisco, and a separate chapter was established in 1906 in Los Angeles. For the next quarter of a century, growth was confined to California, but a New York centre was set up in the 1930s and one in Chicago in the 1950s. With the leap in interest in environmental protection in the last two decades, the Sierra Club has flourished. As we should expect from Figure 2.4D, this resulted in many new branches being set up in smaller cities. Around Chicago, seven new chapters were set up between 1963 and 1973.

2.2 Different disciplinary approaches to spatial diffusion study

Spatial diffusion studies have not been the province of any single discipline. Approaches have varied with the backgrounds and traditions of the researchers involved, and we review here some sample work from several fields.

2.2.1 Cultural geography

Studies concerned with the spread of various cultural phenomena over the Earth's surface have accounted for an important portion of geographical research effort in the last 60 years. In the United States, the Berkeley School, led by Carl O. Sauer, played a central role in the development of these studies in American geography (Clark, 1954). Sauer and his students were interested in how diffusion processes might help to account for the dispersal of cultural traits from given origins or cultural hearths. This topic has long been of concern to archaeologists as a way of accounting for the widespread dissemination of cultural traits, as opposed to postulating multiple independent origins. Typical of the early work of this sort is that of Sauer and Brand (1930), who attempted to deduce the culture areas and successions in south-eastern Arizona from archaeological evidence collected at various Pueblo sites, and of Stanislawski (1946), who traced the diffusion of the grid-pattern town in the Americas. Sauer himself considered the cultural diffusion idea at the world scale in *Agricultural Origins and Dispersals* (Sauer, 1952). A more recent example is that of Crowley (1978), who studied the spread of Amish settlement in the United States since 1717. His findings are illustrated in Figure 2.5.

It was in the United States, too, that the historian, Frederick Jackson Turner, developed his great theme of the frontier in American history, and it has proved to be one of the key ideas of cultural diffusion studies. In geometric terms at least, Turner's (1920) frontier thesis was a simple one. He saw the tide of innovations moving remorselessly outwards from the Eastern Seaboard: '. . . stand at the Cumberland Gap and watch the procession of civilization, marching single file – the buffalo following the trail to the salt springs, the Indian, the fur trader and hunter, the cattle raiser, the pioneer farmer – and the frontier has passed by. Stand at South Pass in the Rockies a century later and see the same procession with wider intervals between' (Turner, 1920, p. 12).

Turner's work was taken up by Webb in his classic regional study of the central grasslands in the United States, *The Great Plains* (1927), while Gulley (1959) and Mikesell (1960) have shown how Turner's ideas

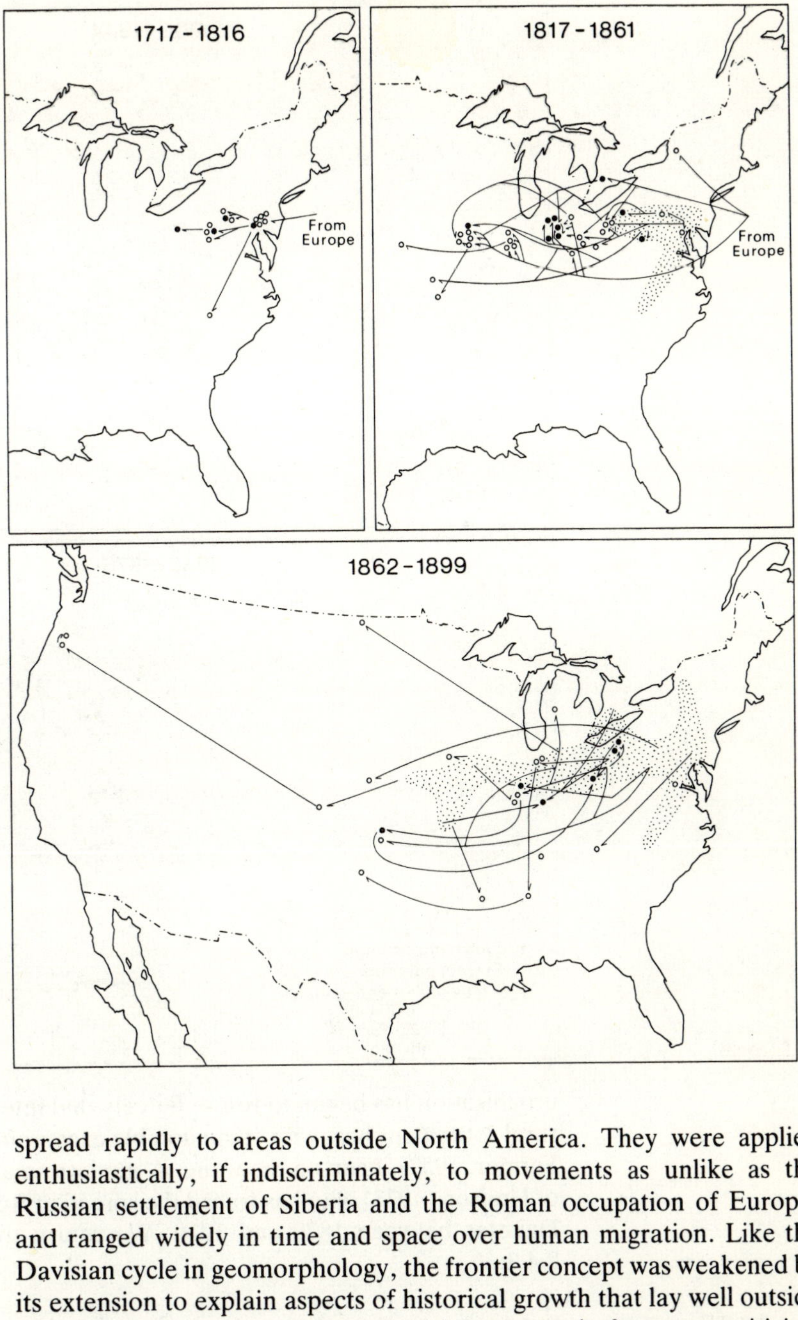

Fig. 2.5 Spread of Amish settlement in the conterminous United States, 1717–1976. Arrows indicate known links between parent settlements and new colonies. *Source:* Crowley (1978, pp. 252–9).

spread rapidly to areas outside North America. They were applied enthusiastically, if indiscriminately, to movements as unlike as the Russian settlement of Siberia and the Roman occupation of Europe, and ranged widely in time and space over human migration. Like the Davisian cycle in geomorphology, the frontier concept was weakened by its extension to explain aspects of historical growth that lay well outside its competence and, in recent years, it has come in for severe criticism from historians. Nevertheless, it played an important part in the development of human geography in the inter-war years. Isaiah Bowman led a vigorous school in the United States concerned with the frontiers of settlement in various parts of the world, and the findings, published by the American Geographical Society as *The Pioneer Fringe* (Bowman, 1931) and *Pioneer Settlement: Co-operative Studies* (Joerg, 1932), have become classics of that period. Since 1945, the tide of

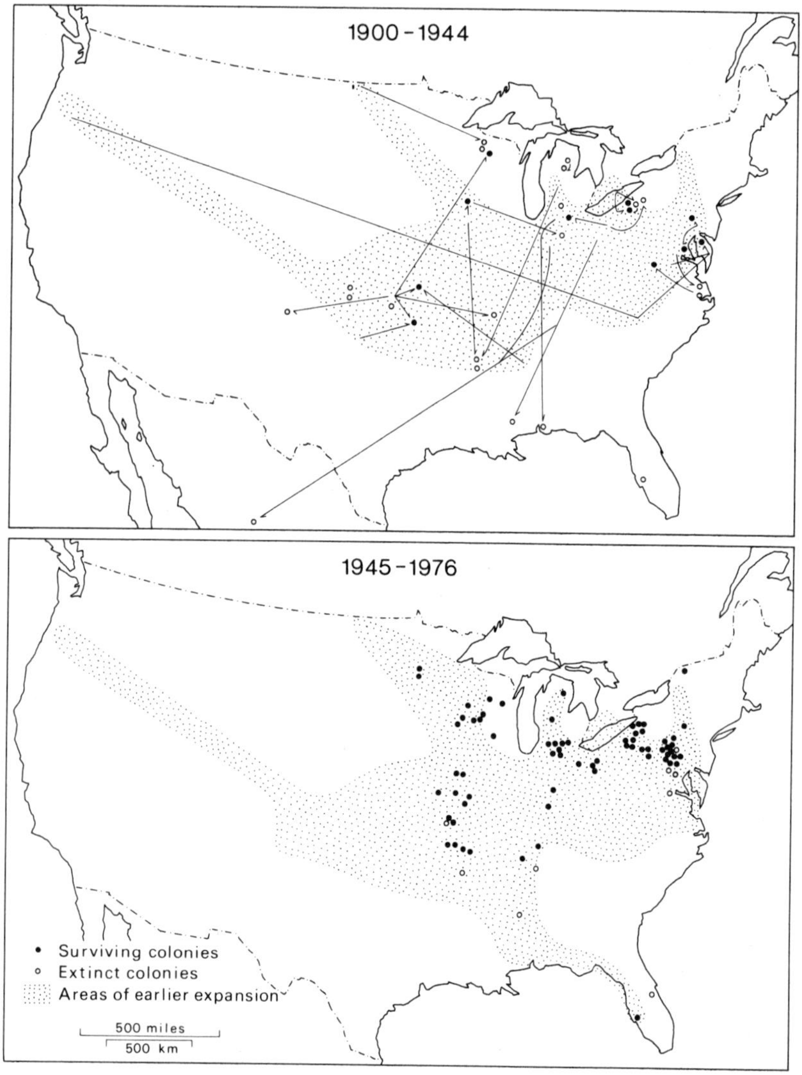

Fig. 2.5 (contd)

urbanisation has begun to run so fiercely that interest in the extension of rural settlement has, with some notable exceptions (e.g., Parsons, 1949; Farmer, 1957), been on the wane. A modern small-scale example is that of Hudson (1973) who has traced the spread of frontier settlement in the Dakotas between 1870 and 1910. We return to this study in section 2.4.1.

2.2.2 Economics Purely economic phenomena have similarly been studied within a diffusion framework. Of particular current interest is the spread of wage rises and price inflation. The outstanding early work is that of Lösch (1940, translated 1954, chapter 17) on price changes in space. As an example, we have redrawn from his data the spread of the business depression of 1929–31 in the United States through the state of Iowa. Note the steady east-to-west movement of the depression shown in Figure 2.6. More recently, Curry (1976) has developed Lösch's theme

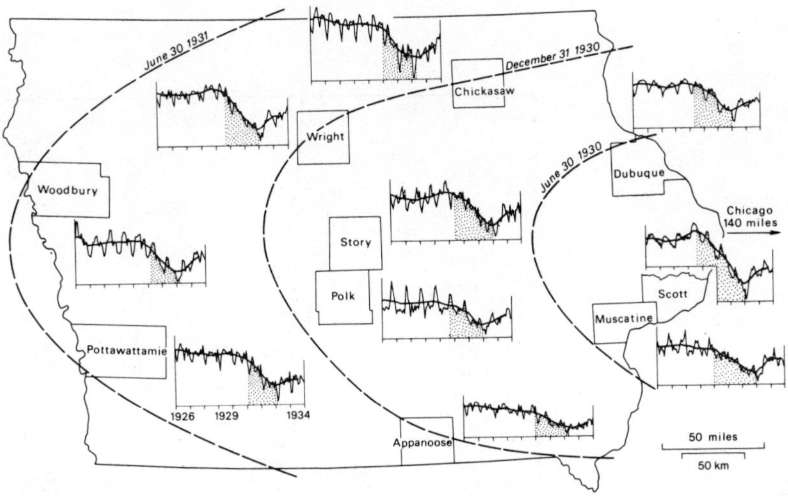

Fig. 2.6 Spread of the business depression of 1929–31 through the state of Iowa, central United States. Graphs show indices of business activity and their running means for ten counties in the state. Stipple indicates period of consistent fall in the running mean. Time contours indicate time of arrival of depression front at various places in the state. Note the ripple-like spread from Chicago, the nearest focus of disturbance, along the main transport arteries, here oriented east–west. *Sources:* Lösch (1954, p. 407); Iowa State Planning Board, second report (1935, p. 194).

by analysing the spread of inflation in a random spatial economy. The inter-regional transmission of unemployment and wage rates has also been treated as a diffusion process (King and Forster, 1973; Stokes, Jones and Neuburger, 1975; Weissbrod, 1976).

2.2.3 Sociology

A further line of approach to diffusion study has come from the field of sociology. Here, the concern has been with the spread of concepts through a society, the role of leaders in starting innovations, and the problem of resistance to change. Rogers (1962) has reviewed some hundreds of such studies, largely concerned with the innovation of new techniques in the farming communities of the United States, but ranging back to include Neolithic diffusion rates (Edmondson, 1961). Work in this field has concentrated particularly on the factors which influence the propensity to adopt innovations and the speed of take-up. Clearly, factors such as age, sex and income of the recipient individuals are important, as is the nature of the innovation.

2.2.4 Epidemiology

The analysis of disease transmission as a spatial spread process has been a major interest of epidemiologists since the work of Hamer at the turn of the century, and it continues to be an important concern. The spread of El Tor cholera and rabies have already been considered in Figures 2.2 and 2.3 as processes with an element of contagious expansion diffusion. An example of relocation diffusion is shown in Figure 2.7. Each influenza epidemic is characterised by a virus of a different type, and the 1957 strain reached pandemic proportions. On a world scale, the virus appeared to reach the world outside China by two pathways: westwards via the Trans-Siberian railway into European Russia, and by sea from Hong Kong to Singapore and Japan (Stuart-Harris, 1965, p. 102). The spread around the rest of the world is shown by plotting on Figure 2.7A the month in which the infection was first recorded. Figure 2.7B shows the assumed spread of the same viral infection in northern England as

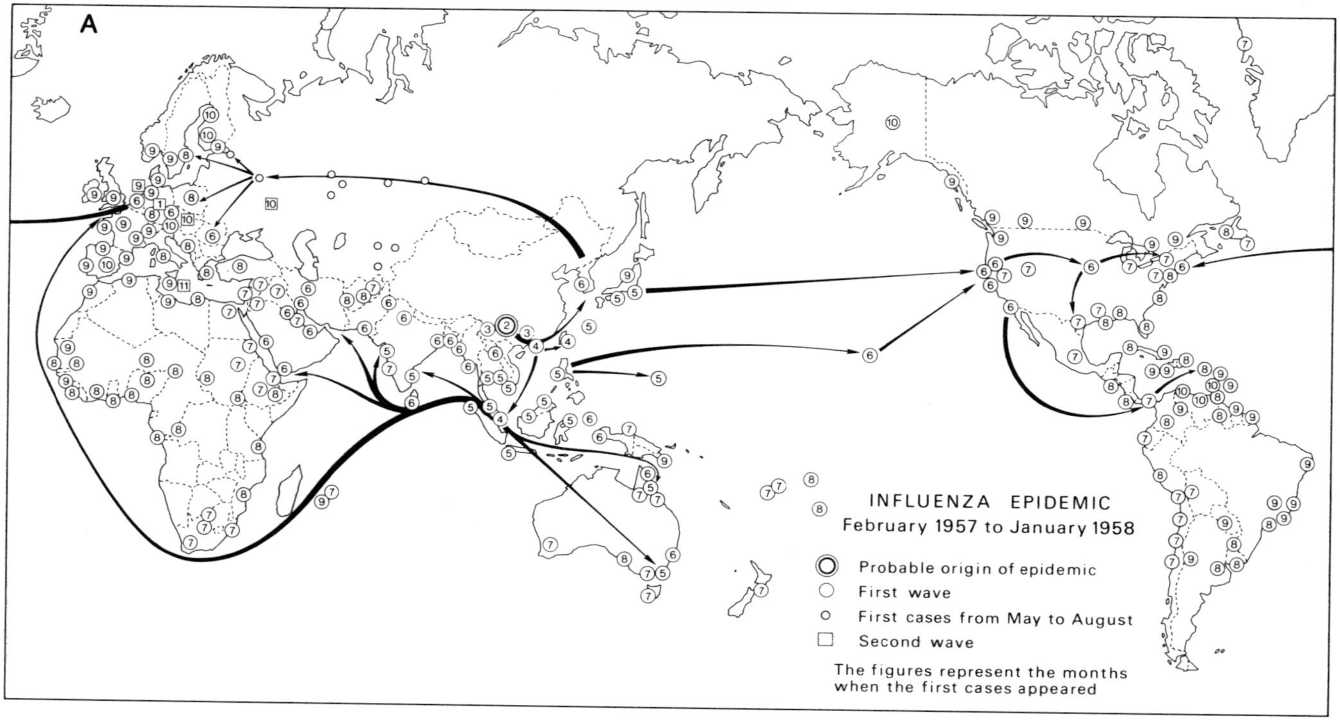

Fig. 2.7(A) Spread of the world influenza epidemic, 1957–8. *Source:* Stuart-Harris (1965, p. 103). (B) Diffusion of same epidemic on a local scale in northern England. *Source:* Hunter and Young (1971, p. 647).

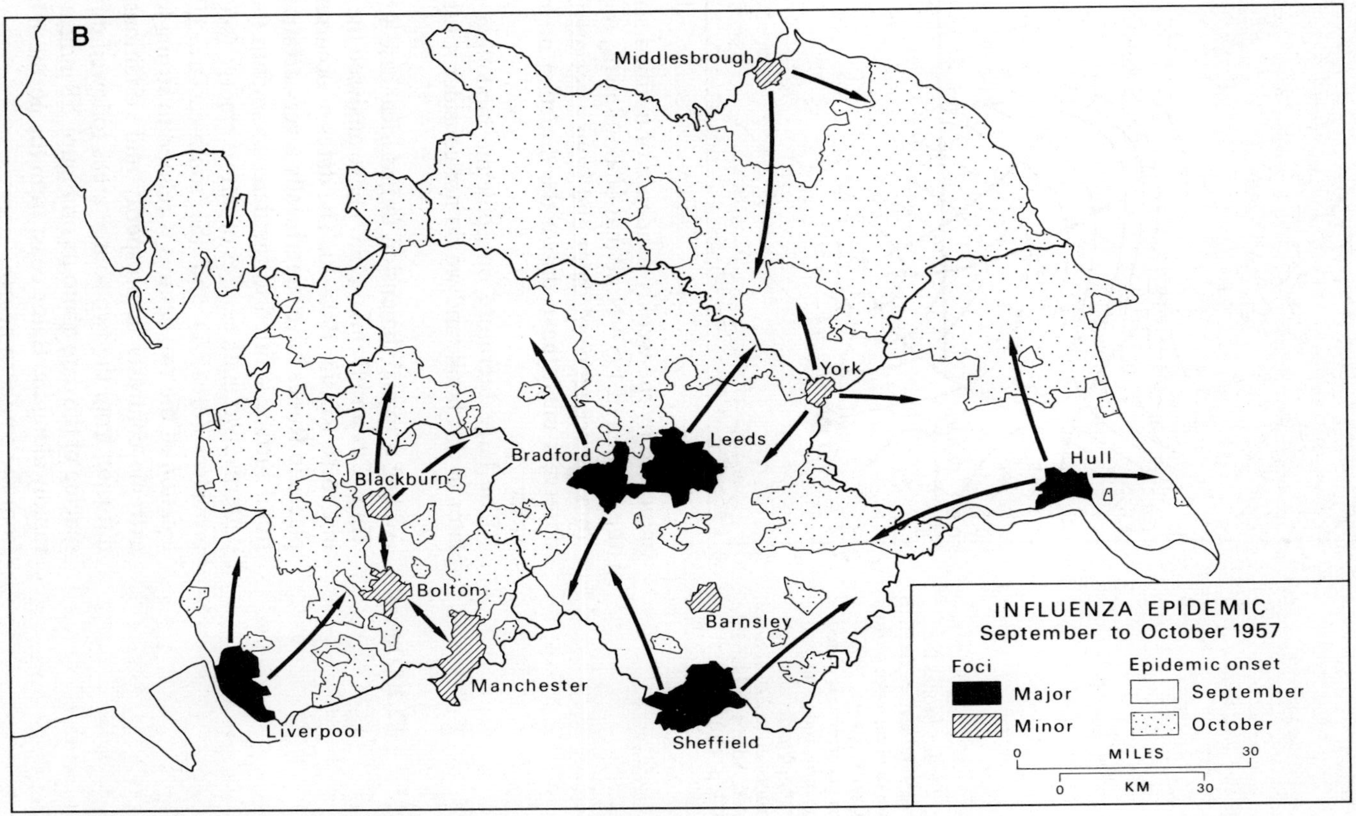
B
Middlesbrough
York
Leeds
Bradford
Hull
Blackburn
Bolton
Barnsley
Manchester
Liverpool
Sheffield
INFLUENZA EPIDEMIC
September to October 1957
Foci
Major
Minor
Epidemic onset
September
October
0
MILES
30
0
KM
30

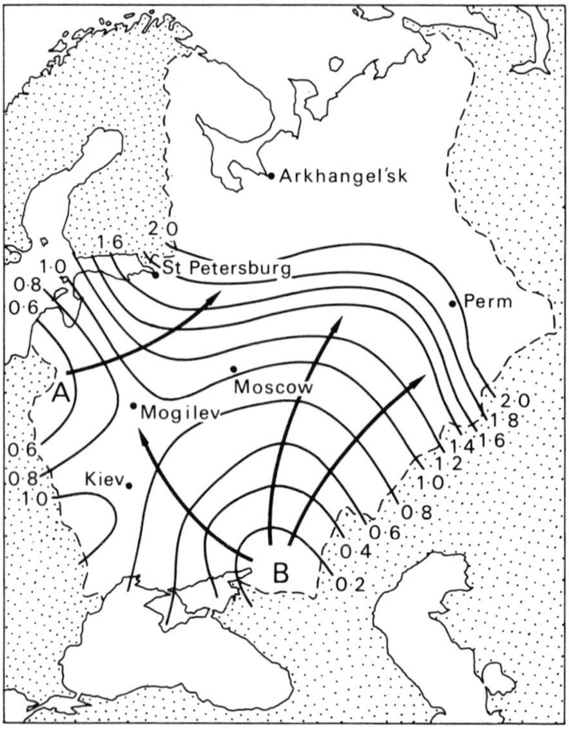

Fig. 2.8 Isochrones for cubic trend surface fitted to dates of occurrence of riots in Czarist Russia, 1905–7. First occurrence is coded year zero, and other years are coded in decimal divisions up to 2.0. *Source:* Abler, Adams and Gould (1972, p. 430).

indicated by the weekly incidence of notified acute pneumonia cases in the autumn of 1957. Note that on both maps, the flow lines are inferred from the sequence of dates and from associated clinical reports. Other observers might have drawn the direction arrows in slightly different ways.

The large literature on epidemic modelling is reviewed in context later in this book, and we do not consider it further here.

2.2.5 Others

Adding a spatial dimension to historical case studies is also important. Thus, Cox and Demko (1967) have analysed the spread of agrarian riots in Czarist Russia, 1905–10. The dates of occurrence of riots at different places in Russia have superficially a very erratic pattern. If, however, a trend surface is fitted to the dates to smooth them into broad regional patterns, two main centres of unrest emerge (see Figure 2.8): the Baltic provinces (area A) and the south-eastern Ukraine (area B). The location of the two centres is related to strong local tensions caused by extreme contrasts in prosperity and conditions of tenancy. Outward diffusion from the two source areas followed different patterns. As the spacing of the date contours on Figure 2.8 indicates, rioting spread more rapidly along the Baltic coast from the northern hearth and more slowly from the southern hearth.

It is evident from the above discussion that many topics in many disciplines have been looked upon as diffusion phenomena. Brown (1968) and Brown and Moore (1969) have provided extensive bibliographies on the various research strands, and these authors have also

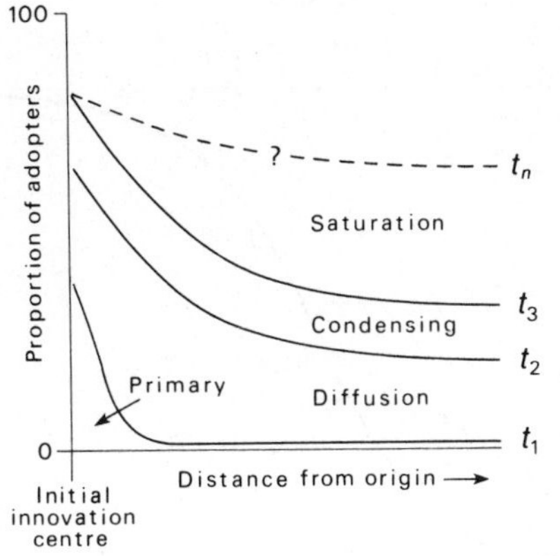

Fig. 2.9 Hypothetical profiles for diffusion waves. *Source:* Hägerstrand (1952, p 13).

attempted to synthesise the various approaches within a common conceptual framework. In the remainder of this chapter, a smaller canvas is painted: our emphasis is upon the stochastic models for diffusion processes used within geography and their applications.

2.3 Geographical models of the spatial diffusion process

2.3.1 Wave profiles

Much of the geographical interest in diffusion studies stems from the work of the Swedish geographer, Torsten Hägerstrand, and his colleagues at the Univerity of Lund. Hägerstrand's *Innovation Diffusion as a Spatial Process,* originally published in 1953, was concerned with the acceptance by farmers of several agricultural innovations, such as the control of bovine tuberculosis by vaccination and subsidies for the improvement of grazing, in an area of central Sweden. This book was the precursor of various similar practical studies, particularly in the United States.

In one of his early studies of a contagious diffusion process, Hägerstrand (1952) described a four-stage model for the passage of what he termed *innovation waves* (*innovationsförloppet*), but which are more generally called diffusion waves. From maps of the diffusion of various innovations in Sweden, ranging from bus routes to agricultural methods, Hägerstrand drew a series of cross-sections to show the profile of the wave form at different points in time. He suggested that diffusion profiles can be broken into four types, each of which describes a distinct stage in the passage of an innovation through an area. Consider Figure 2.9, which shows the relationship between the proportion of adopters of an innovation against distance from the original centre of innovation. The *primary stage* marks the beginning of the diffusion process. A centre of adoption is established at the origin. There is a strong contrast in the level of adoption between this centre and remote areas which is reflected in the steep decline of the level of adoption curve beyond the origin. The *diffusion stage* signals the start of the actual spread process; there is a powerful centrifugal effect, resulting in the rapid growth of acceptance in areas distant from the origin and by a reduction in the strong regional contrasts typical of the primary stage. This results in a flattening of the slope of the proportion of adopters curve. In the *condensing stage*, the relative increase in the numbers accepting an item

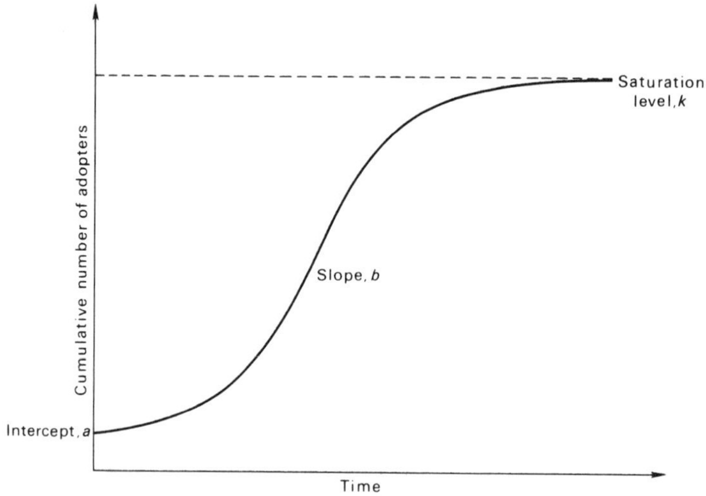

Fig. 2.10 A logistic curve.

is equal in all locations, regardless of their distance from the original innovation centre; the acceptance curve moves in a parallel fashion. The final, *saturation, stage* is marked by a slowing and eventual cessation of the diffusion process, which produces a further flattening of the acceptance curve. In this final stage, the item being diffused has been adopted throughout the country, so that there is very little regional variation.

Since Hägerstrand's original work, other Swedish geographers have carried out similar studies to test the validity of this four-stage process. For instance, Tornqvist (1967) has traced the spread of televisions in Sweden by observing the growth of television ownership from 1956 to 1965. Using information obtained from 4,000 Swedish post office districts, he demonstrated that television was introduced into Sweden relatively late, yet, within nine years, about 70 per cent of the country's households had bought their first set. Tornqvist's results broadly confirm Hägerstrand's analysis. The diffusion process slowed down, thus indicating the beginning of the saturation phase, at the end of the study period.

The shape of the profile in both time and space has been formally modelled. We consider first the temporal build-up in the number of adopters of an innovation. If the total susceptible population at the start ($t = 0$) of the process is known, then the cumulative number of that total who will have become adopters at $t = 1, 2, \ldots$ commonly follows an S-shaped curve when plotted against t (see Figure 2.10). We use y_t to denote the cumulative number of adopters in the total population at risk. Figure 2.10 implies that acceptance of an innovation is rather slow at first. This is followed by a rapid build-up as the innovation 'takes off'. Ultimately, there is a levelling out as saturation of the susceptible population is approached. The model most commonly fitted to profiles of the form of Figure 2.10 is the logistic. See, for example, Griliches (1957), Mansfield (1961), Casetti (1969), Casetti and Semple (1969) and

Cliff and Ord (1975a) for detailed applications. The logistic model is given by

$$p_t = (1 + e^{a-bt})^{-1}, \tag{2.1}$$

or

$$y_t = k(1 + e^{a-bt})^{-1}, \tag{2.2}$$

where p_t is the proportion of adopters in the population at t, y_t is defined above, and a, b and k are parameters. The model is readily fitted by ordinary least squares, since both equations (2.1) and (2.2) reduce to simple regressions on taking the appropriate transformation. The parameter, k, is usually interpreted as the maximum possible number of adopters (the saturation level), a is the intercept, and b is the slope coefficient.

The structure of equation (2.1) is made clearer by looking at the first derivative, or the rate of change, r_t, in p_t with respect to time, where, from Cliff and Ord (1975b),

$$r_t = \frac{dp_t}{dt} = bp_t(1 - p_t). \tag{2.3}$$

Since p_t is the proportion of the susceptible population which has actually adopted by time t, $(1 - p_t)$ is the proportion still at risk. The quantity, $p_t(1 - p_t)$, then represents the probability that a random meeting between two individuals is between an adopter and a potential adopter, while the parameter b represents the rate at which meetings take place (the rate of mixing). Note that b is the same *whatever the distance between the adopter and the potential adopter*; that is, equation (2.1) implies spatially homogeneous mixing between adopters and potential adopters. This assumption is apparently in conflict with the contagious diffusion idea discussed earlier. Cliff and Ord (1975b) have suggested the following extension of the logistic model which allows homogeneous mixing within n regions ($i = 1, 2, \ldots, n$), but less mixing between regions (cf. Rapoport's (1951) distance-biassed net or 'island' model):

$$r_{it} = (1 - p_{it})\Big(b_i p_{it} + \sum_{j \neq i} c_{ij} p_{jt}\Big). \tag{2.4}$$

Here, c_{ij} is the rate of mixing between the ith and jth regions in addition to previous notation. Equation (2.4) reduces to (2.3) for each i when all $c_{ij} = 0$. Casetti and Semple (1969) have also considered extensions of the logistic model to handle inhomogeneous mixing as a function of the distance between adopters and potential adopters. Their models may be applied provided that a diffusion pole (that is, the original centre from which the diffusion process started) can be specified. Model (2.4) does not demand this *a priori* specification. Cliff and Ord (1975a) have applied a model of the form of (2.4) to data on the adoption of tractors in the central farming region of the United States, and have shown how the model may be structured to test hypotheses about the existence of diffusion poles.

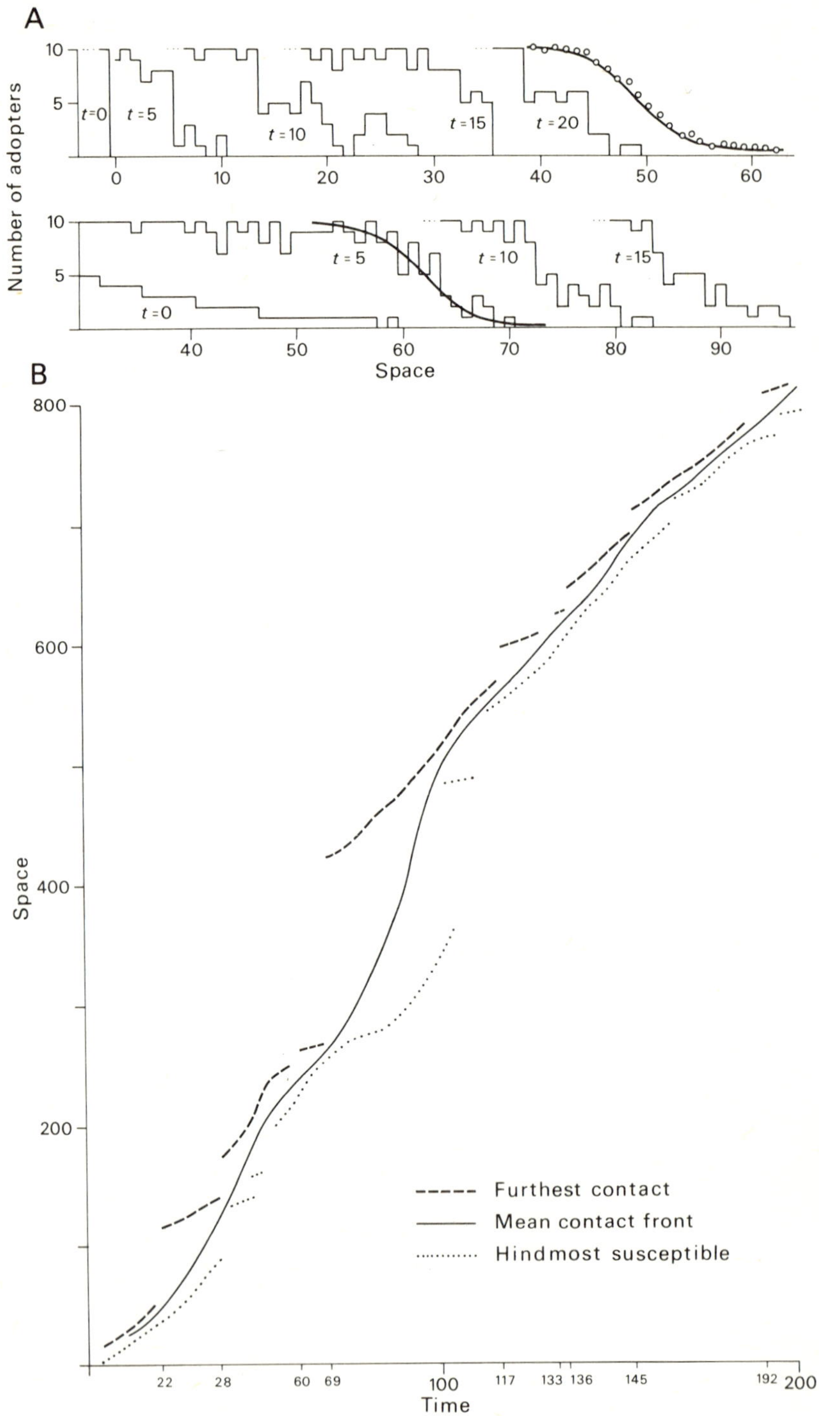

Fig. 2.11(A) Diffusion process along a line with exponentially bounded contact probabilities. Number of adopters at various times, t, is shown. Open circles indicate average shape of the wavefront between $t = 105$ and $t = 200$ with logistic fitted. In the upper diagram, initial adopters at $t = 0$ are all concentrated at the origin; in the lower diagram, they are spread along the line. (B) Location of furthest contact from the origin, mean contact and hindmost susceptible for a diffusion process along a line with non-exponentially bounded contact probabilities. Discontinuities in the pecked and dotted curves indicate break-up of the wavefront. *Source:* Mollison (1977, pp. 307–8).

0·0096	0·0140	0·0168	0·0140	0·0096
0·0140	0·0301	0·0547	0·0301	0·0140
0·0168	0·0547	0·4431	0·0547	0·0168
0·0140	0·0301	0·0547	0·0301	0·0140
0·0096	0·0140	0·0168	0·0140	0·0096

Fig. 2.12 Hägerstrand's mean information field (MIF). Each grid cell is 5×5 km^2.

The wavefront of adoption formed in space by an innovation may also be described by a logistic. Whether or not this is possible depends upon the probability of contact between the carrier of the innovation and recipients. In general, this contact probability is likely to fall with increasing distance between the carrier and the recipient. Mollison (1977) has shown that if the contact probability falls off with increasing distance at least as rapidly as an exponential decay curve, then the diffusion wavefront will migrate steadily across space, and may be approximated by a logistic curve (see Figure 2.11A and compare with the profiles in Figures 2.9 and 2.10). If, however, the contact probability is not bounded exponentially, the wavefront will disintegrate into a series of spatially erratic contacts (Figure 2.11B). The purely contagious spread which occurs with exponentially bounded contact probabilities has already been illustrated in section 2.1 and Figure 2.3; it is commonly referred to as the *neighbourhood effect.*

2.3.2 Hägerstrand's Monte Carlo diffusion model

The first major attempt within geography to formulate a model of the *process* of spatial diffusion was that of Hägerstrand (1953). In developing the model in the context of innovation diffusion, Hägerstrand assumed that the decision of a potential adopter to accept an innovation was based solely upon information received orally at face-to-face meetings between the potential adopter and adopters. He further assumed that the contact probabilities between tellers and receivers conformed to the neighbourhood effect. Hägerstrand's model was stochastic and was based upon the following rules:

(1) The input numbers and spatial locations of adopters in the model were the actual configurations at the start of the diffusion process. The study area was divided up by a lattice of 5×5 km^2 cells.

(2) A potential adopter was assumed to accept the innovation as soon as he was told by an adopter.

(3) In each iteration of the model, every adopter was allowed to contact one other person, adopter or non-adopter. The probability, P_i, that a carrier would contact an individual located in the ith cell of the study lattice is shown in Figure 2.12. Each cell in this floating grid, which Hägerstrand called a *mean information field* (MIF) is 5×5 km^2,

and outside the grid, $P_i = 0$. These probabilities were estimated from an analysis of migration and telephone traffic data. The floating grid was placed over each existing adopter in turn, so that the adopter was located in the central cell of the MIF. What Figure 2.12 tells us is that an adopter located in the centre of the central cell of the MIF has approximately a 44 per cent chance of contacting someone within (about) 0–2.5 km of himself, and that this contact probability decays over space to less than one per cent at a distance of about 14 km (along diagonals) from the adopter and to zero beyond 14–18 km. Since the probability is taken as zero beyond 18 km, it is clear that the MIF is exponentially bounded.

The location of each carrier's contact was determined in two steps. First, a random number, r, $0 \leqslant r \leqslant 1$, from a rectangular distribution, located the cell i according to the rule,

$$\sum_{m=1}^{i-1} Q_m < r \leqslant \sum_{m=1}^{i} Q_m, \tag{2.5}$$

where Q_m, the probability of a contact in cell m with population n_m, is

$$Q_m = \frac{P_m n_m}{\sum_{m=1}^{25} P_m n_m}. \tag{2.6}$$

A second random number from a rectangular distribution on $[1, n_m]$ was drawn to locate the receiver in the cell. If the receiver was a potential adopter, he immediately became an adopter by rule (2); if the receiver was an existing adopter, the message was lost; if the receiver was identical with the carrier, a new address was sampled.

(4) To take into account the reduction in interpersonal communication likely to be caused by physical features such as rivers and forests, two simplified types of barrier were introduced into the model plane, namely zero- and half-contact barriers. When an address crossed a half-contact barrier, the telling was cancelled with probability 0.5. However, two half-contact barriers in combination were considered equal to one zero-contact barrier.

Using this model, Hägerstrand performed a series of computer runs to simulate the spatial pattern of acceptance of a subsidy for the improvement of pasture on small farms in the Asby district of central Sweden. Hägerstrand (1967, pp. 23–5) gives the results from three runs of the model, and we reproduce in Figure 2.13 one of these outcomes. Note the spatially highly contagious build-up of adopters produced by the model which we would expect from Mollison's findings discussed above.

2.3.3 Modifications of the Hägerstrand model

(1) Barriers and corridors

Although in rule (4) of the model, a very simplified system of resistance to communication was proposed by Hägerstrand, barriers to diffusion waves are likely to be much more complex in reality. The effect of barriers has been looked at by Yuill (1965). His study area comprised a 30 × 18 regular lattice of cells, and his MIF was 3 × 3 rather than the

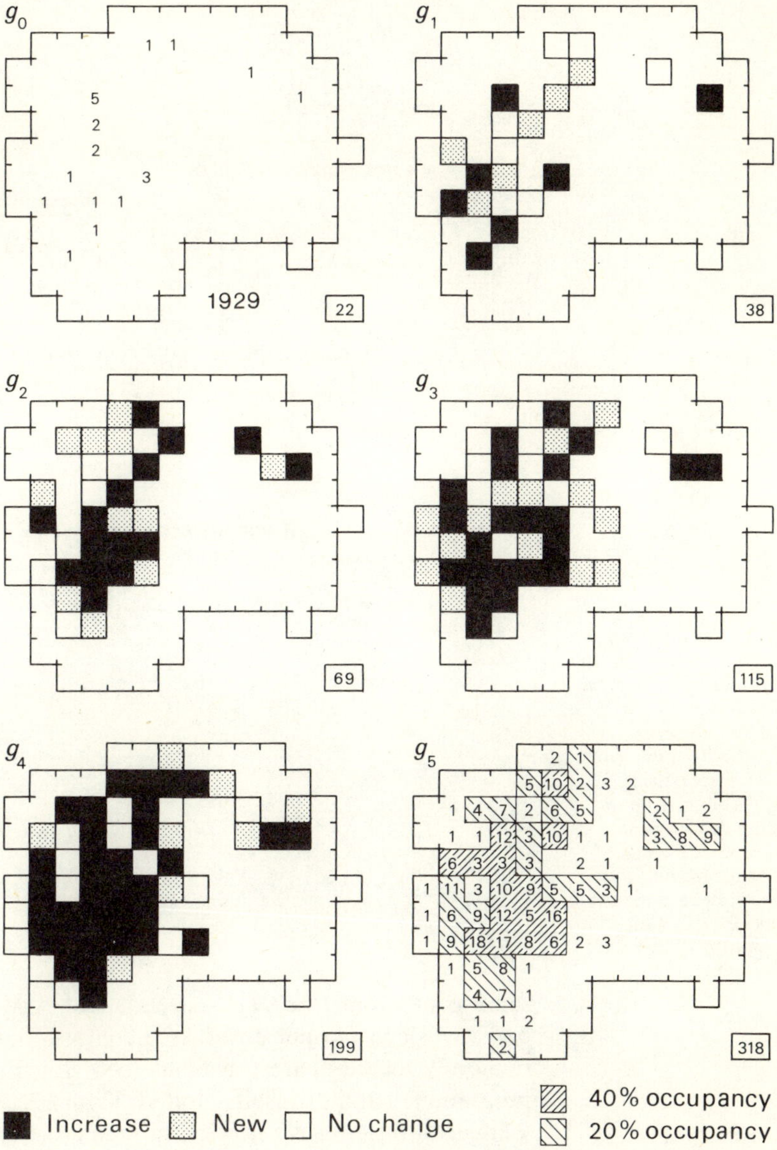

Fig. 2.13 Spatial pattern of acceptance of the improved pasture subsidy in central Sweden at the end of each iteration, g_1–g_5, for one realisation of the Hägerstrand model. Map g_0 gives the actual configuration of adopters in 1929 used to start the model. In generations g_1–g_4, squares were coded black if adopters continued to build up in already 'infected' cells. Squares occupied by adopters for the first time in a particular generation are stippled. For g_5, the numbers of adopters are given, and cells are shaded if 20 per cent or 40 per cent of the total population of potential adopters in them had accepted the subsidy. Numbers in rectangles at map corners give the total number of adopters on each map. *Source:* Hägerstrand (1967, p. 23).

5 × 5 grid used by Hägerstrand. Figure 2.14A gives the MIF, and we assume that two initial adopters (the solid circles) have been located in the central cell. Imagine further that centring the grid over those two adopters has caused two cells of the MIF to be occupied by barriers (the stippled cells). The location of each carrier's contact in the next generation of the model (cf. Hägerstrand's Monte Carlo experiment) is shown by the arrows. Yuill envisaged four types of barrier cell in decreasing order of blocking effectiveness: type I, *super absorbing*, which absorbed the new contacts and destroyed the transmitters; type II, the *absorbing* barrier, which absorbed new contacts but did not affect the transmitters; type III, the *reflecting* barrier, which absorbed the new contacts, but the transmitters were allowed to make a new contact in the

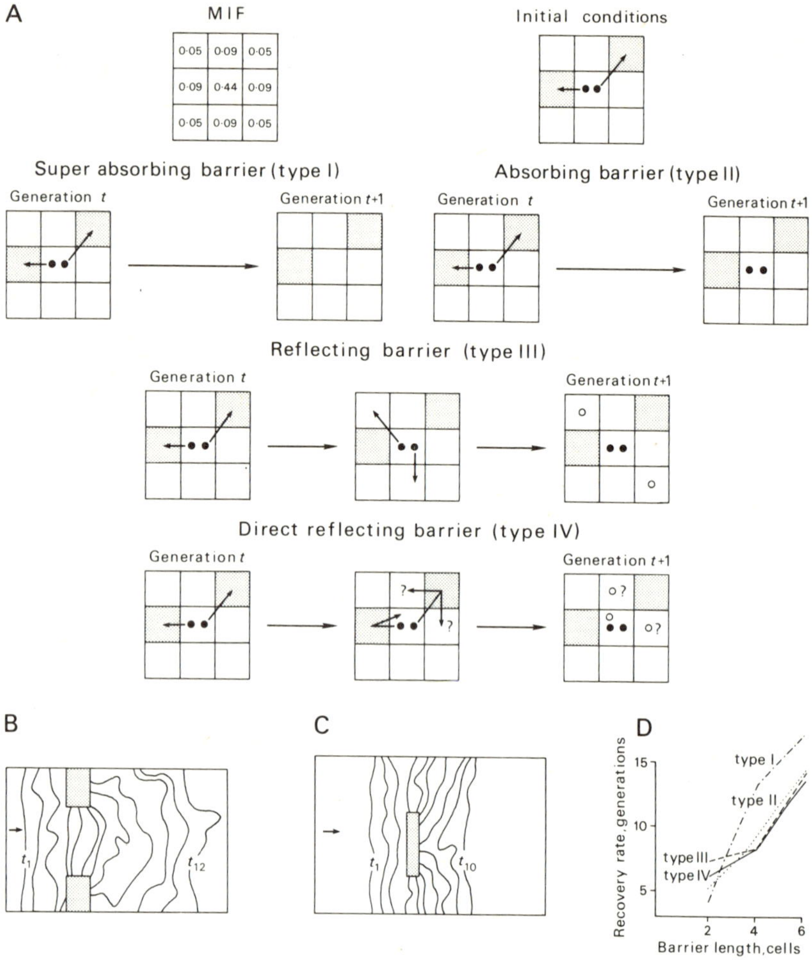

Fig. 2.14 Barrier effects on diffusion waves. (A) MIF and the four types of barriers used by Yuill. (B) Diffusion wave passing through opening in an absorbing barrier. (C) Diffusion wave passing around a bar barrier. (D) Recovery rates around bar barriers. *Source:* Yuill (1965, pp. 19, 25, 29).

same generation (the open circles); and type IV the *direct reflecting* barrier, which did not absorb the contacts but instead reflected them randomly to the nearest available cell. Each situation was separately programmed and its results plotted. Figure 2.14B shows the advance of a linear diffusion wave ($t = 1$) through an opening in an absorbing bar barrier. The wavefront becomes distorted in its passage through the opening because of the loss of contacts at the barrier edge (a frictional drag effect), but it re-forms by about the twelfth generation. Yuill has referred to the number of generations required for the wave to return to its original form after first encountering the barrier as the *recovery rate.* An alternative version of the bar barrier is shown in Figure 2.14C where the diffusion wave passes around a bar and re-forms after about nine generations. Here the recovery rate is directly related both to the barrier length and to the kind of barrier, with the curve for the type I (super absorbing) barrier showing strong contrasts to those of the other three types (Figure 2.14D).

Although Yuill's results were limited by the range of postulates he tried and by computer capacity, the approach is of direct interest to,

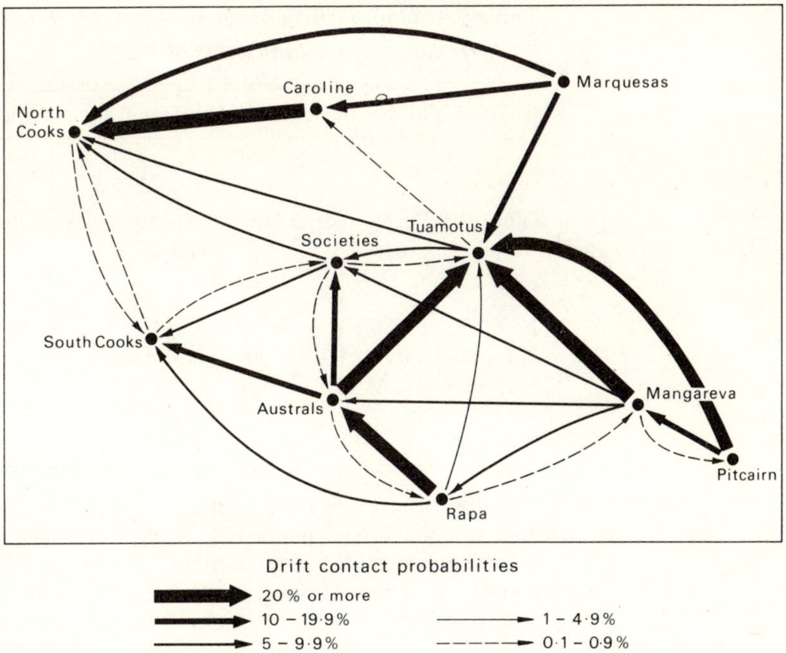

Fig. 2.15 Drift contact probabilities among the Polynesian islands. *Source:* Levison, Ward and Webb (1973, p. 51).

among others, historical geographers. The exact impact of the Appalachians, the Blue Mountains, or the Serra do Mar in holding back the inland spread of settlement from the American, Australian and Brazilian coastlines has long been argued (cf. Turner's frontier hypothesis of section 2.2.1). By using more complex MIFs and environmental weightings for the barriers, different models may be evolved. These can be assessed in a hypothesis-testing sense. As a further example, the technique might be applied to Pyle's (1969) tracks for cholera epidemics in the United States in the nineteenth century, which progressed inland from the Eastern Seaboard and across the Appalachians. Pyle's work is discussed later in this section.

Yuill's work, by viewing the spread of an innovation as a wave phenomenon, also ties back to Hägerstrand's studies discussed in section 2.3.1. The idea of diffusion waves has been developed further by Morrill (1968, 1970). Morrill has applied various polynomial, sine and cosine waves to innovation phenomena, and he has considered what happens when waves from different centres meet for the cases of complementary and opposing innovations.

The obverse of a barrier is a corridor of movement, and the identification of such corridors is the theme of a study by Levison, Ward and Webb (1973). These authors constructed a Monte Carlo model to simulate the pattern of settlement of Polynesia by raft voyagers. The drift tracks of the rafts, from a variety of starting points, were determined by sampling from ancillary probability distributions describing factors such as wind frequency, direction and force, ocean currents and survival rates. Voyages were terminated by either (a) 'contact' with another island or (b) expiry of the voyage as determined by the survival

Table 2.1. *Comparison of the speed of different diffusion processes for the Christaller* $k = 3$ *landscape of Figure 2.16*

	Number of settlements affected by each period*		
Time periods	Purely hierarchical process	Purely neighbourhood effect	Combined hierarchical and neighbourhood process
1	1(33%)	1(33%)	1(33%)
2	3(56%)	7(41%)	9(63%)
3	9(78%)	13(58%)	27(100%)
4	27(100%)	19(85%)	—
5	—	26(98%)	—
6	—	27(100%)	—

* Figures in brackets indicate the proportion of population contacted by each time period, where population and hierarchical ranks are related in the following manner: A settlements = 27 population units; B settlements = 9 population units; C settlements = 3 population units; D settlements = 1 population unit.

rate probabilities. Mapping of the distribution of voyage-termination points in Polynesia permitted estimates to be made of the probability of reaching the various Polynesian islands from the different starting points (see Figure 2.15).

(2) Central place diffusion

As we noted in the discussion of Figure 2.4, for certain kinds of innovations such as fashions, we might expect there to be a strong central place hierarchy effect in the adoption regime, as opposed to a simple neighbourhood effect. Thus, Hägerstrand (1967) has stated:

> A closer analysis shows that the spread along the initial 'frontier' is led through the urban hierarchy. The point of introduction in a new country is its primate city, sometimes some other metropolis. Then centres next in rank follow. Soon, however, this order is broken up and replaced by one where the neighbourhood effect dominates over the pure size succession.

Notice, however, that Hägerstrand is arguing for a mixed central place/neighbourhood effect process, rather than either alone. Hudson (1969) rejects the idea of pure hierarchical diffusion (that is, no neighbourhood effect) on the grounds that the cumulative build-up of adopters with time will not follow the logistic curve, and he looks at a mixed hierarchical/spatially contagious process which does yield an S-shaped curve. Alves (1974) has disputed Hudson's suggestion that pure hierarchical diffusion will not produce a logistic build-up, and he proposes a hierarchical model which does. Hierarchical diffusion processes are also considered in Pedersen (1970), Berry (1972) and Hudson (1972).

In Figures 2.16A and B, we have constructed an artificial Christaller $k = 3$ landscape. Centre A is the highest order centre, and D is the lowest. An innovation is introduced in centre A and is allowed to diffuse

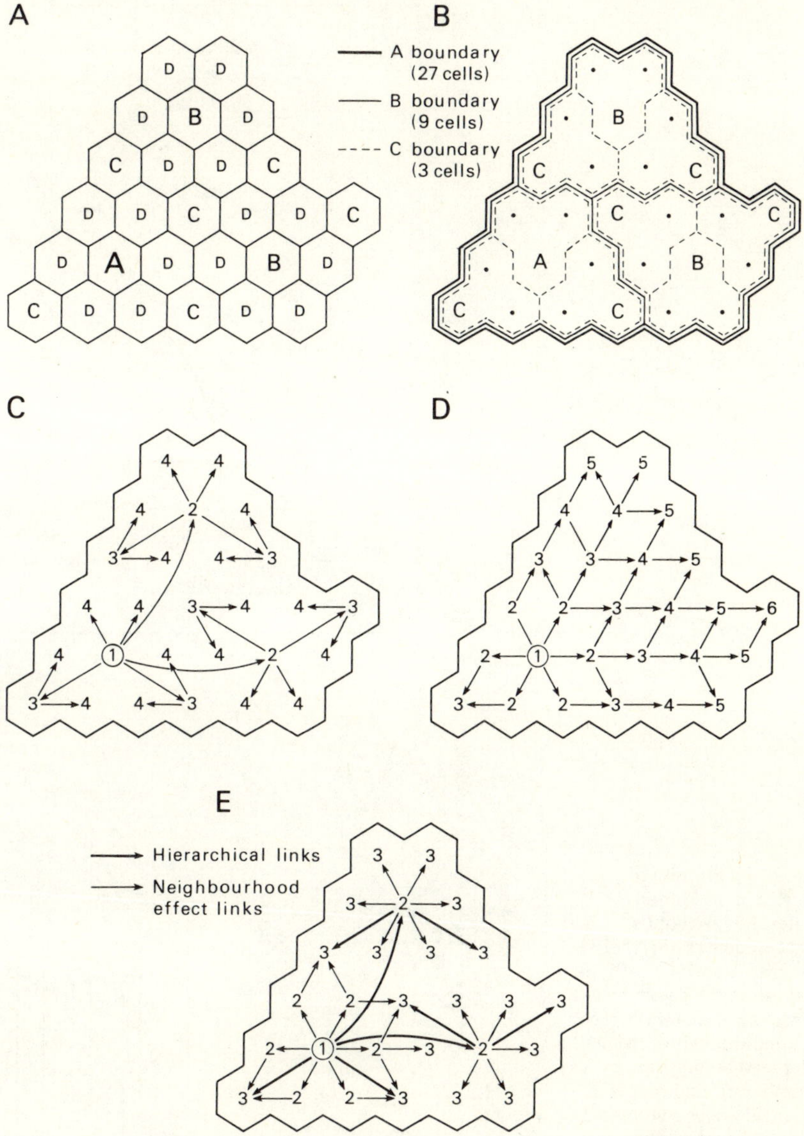

Fig. 2.16 Patterns of diffusion through a system of settlements. (A) Christaller $k = 3$ landscape with A to D level settlements. (B) Boundaries of trade areas of undivided settlements. (C) Purely hierarchical diffusion process from primate city A. (D) Purely neighbourhood diffusion from city A. (E) Combined hierarchical and neighbourhood diffusion processes. Numbers indicate time period innovation reaches the settlements. *Source:* Haggett, Cliff and Frey (1977, p. 241).

to other places by purely hierarchical spread (Figure 2.16C), purely contagious spread (2.16D) and by a mixed process (2.16E). It is evident from Table 2.1 that the mixed process produces the most rapid spread of the innovation, as we would expect, and it highlights the fact that purely contagious spread is a much slower process than purely hierarchical diffusion (cf. the polynuclear diffusion of Figure 2.8).

An example of a diffusion process operating through a central-place structure is provided by Pyle (1969), who studied the spread of cholera in the United States in the nineteenth century. By plotting the date of the first recorded outbreak of cholera in each affected city of the United States for the three great epidemics of 1832, 1848–9 and 1866, Pyle attempted to reconstruct the ways in which the cholera waves moved

A

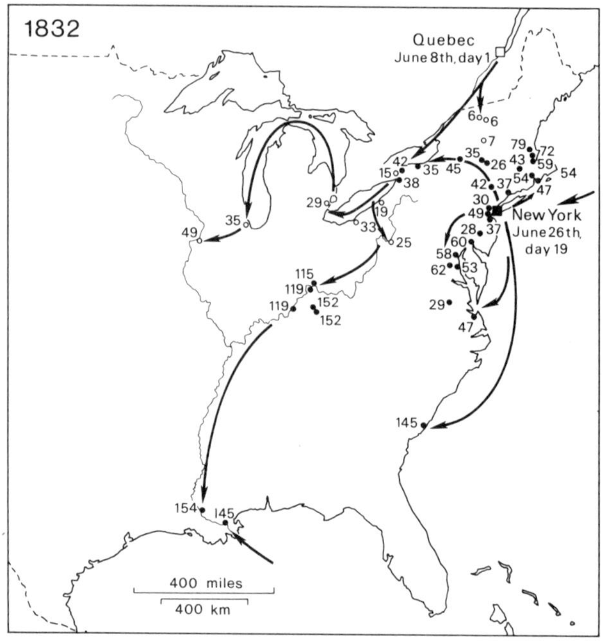

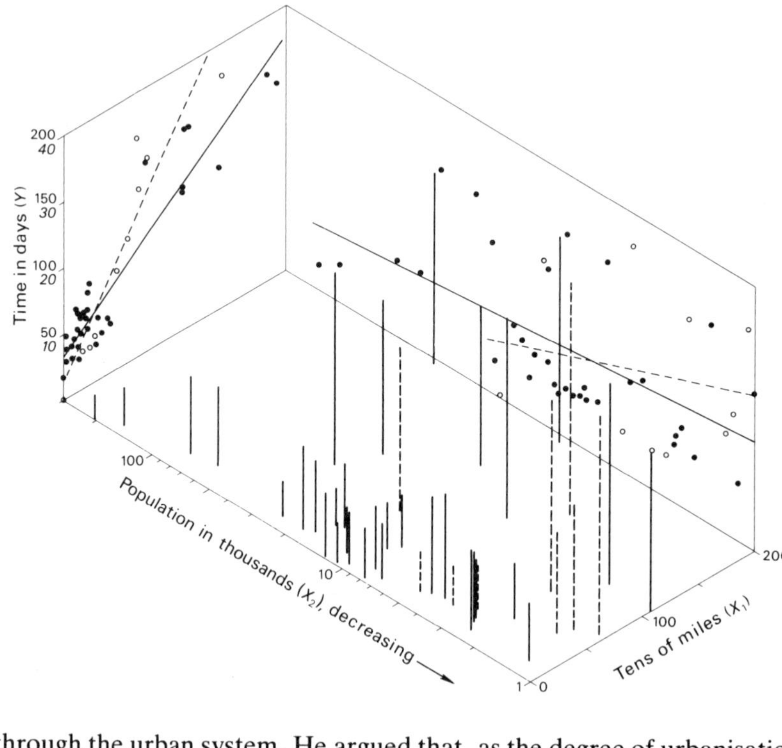

Fig. 2.17 Diffusion of cholera in the United States. For each of the great epidemics of (A) 1832, (B) 1848–9 and (C) 1866, the maps show the day of first reporting of cholera in each city and the main corridors of spread as suggested by Pyle (1969). End-planes of block diagrams give simple regressions of date of reporting (Y) against distance from origin (X_1), back-planes give regression of Y against population size (X_2); columns show combined relationship of $Y = f(X_1, X_2)$. For details, see text.

through the urban system. He argued that, as the degree of urbanisation in the United States increased throughout the nineteenth century, the transmission process changed from one dominated by distance from the point of introduction of the disease, with near places infected first (1832), to mixed hierarchical/contagious spread (1848–9), and finally to spread dominated by the urban-size hierarchy (1866).

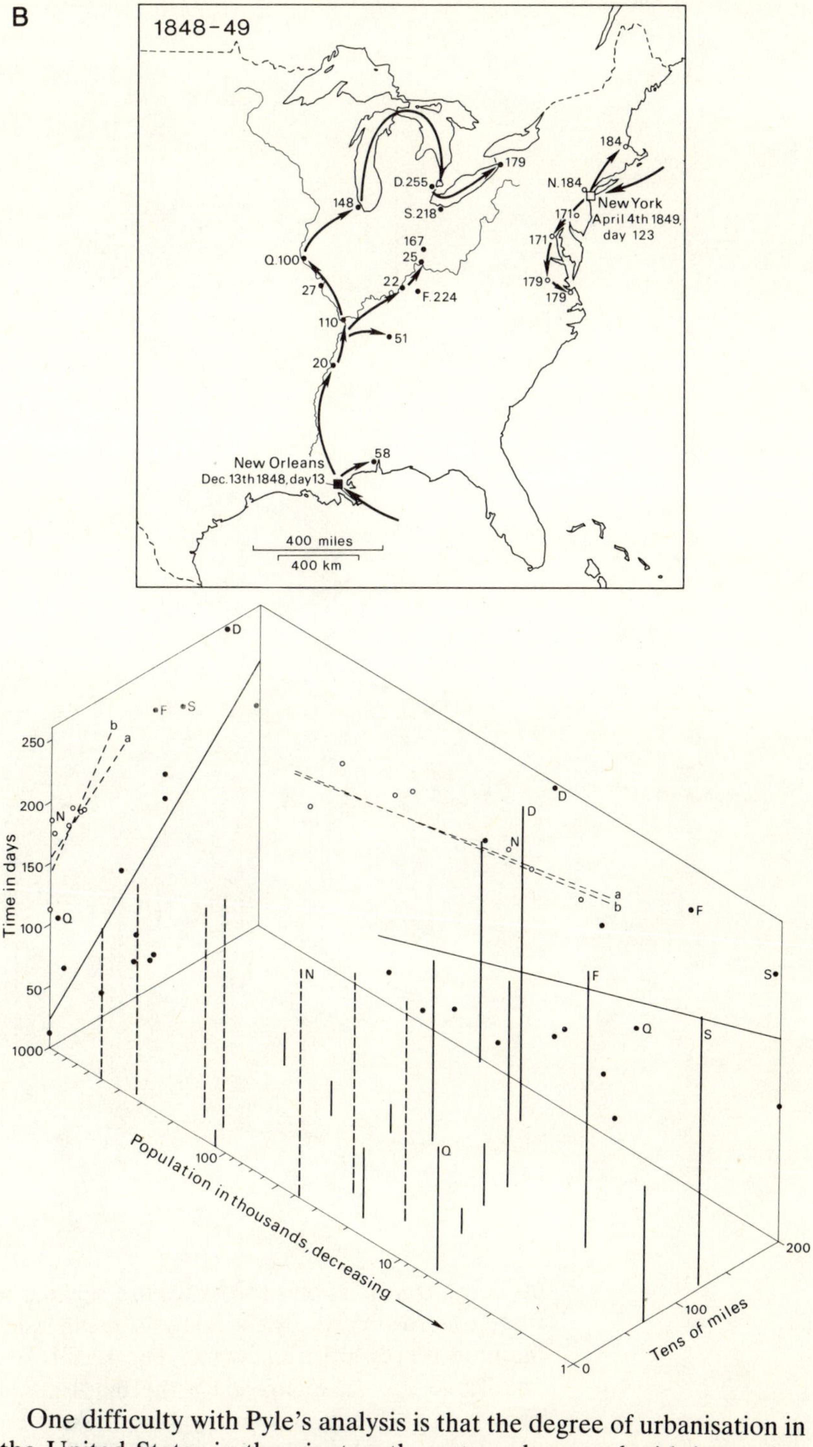

Fig. 2.17(B)

One difficulty with Pyle's analysis is that the degree of urbanisation in the United States in the nineteenth century decreased with increasing distance from the Eastern Seaboard, a point of introduction of cholera in all three epidemics. That is, there is a high level of correlation between the urban size and distance-from-origin variables whose effects

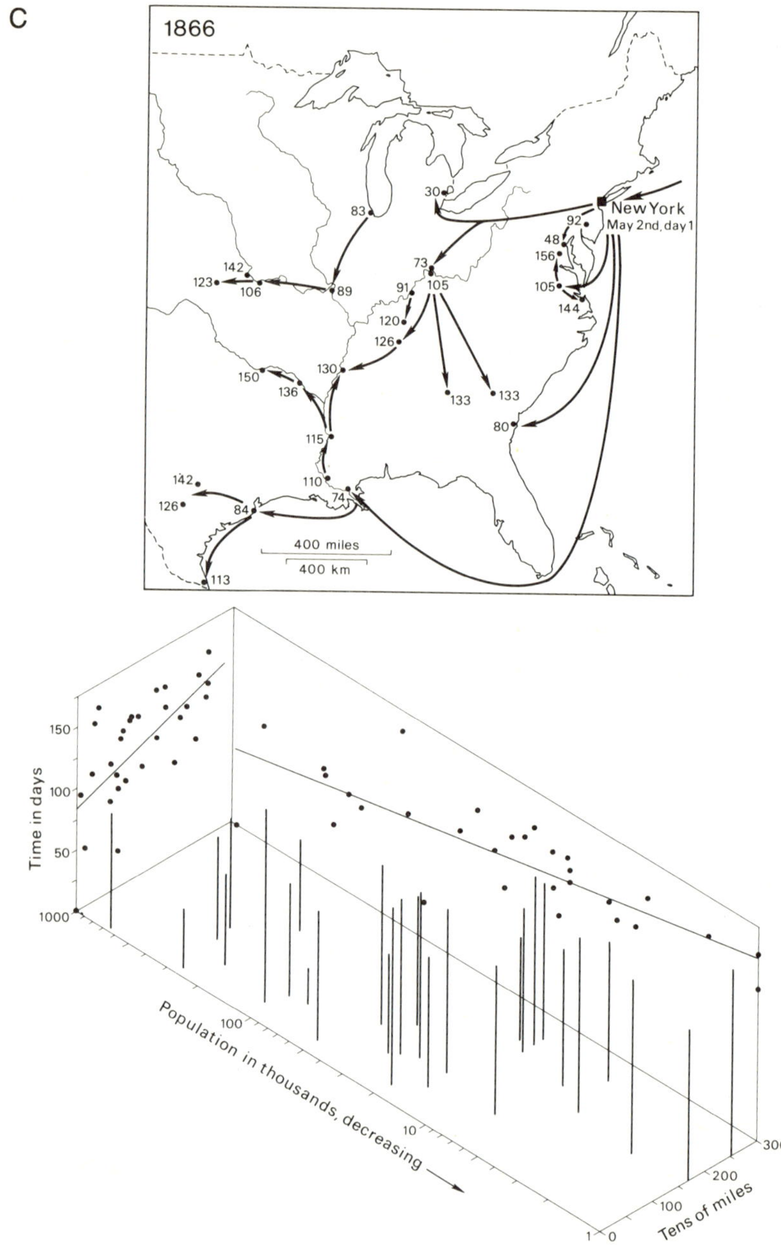

Fig. 2.17(C)

upon the transmission process we are seeking to disentangle. We have therefore reworked Pyle's analysis using the original data within a multiple regression framework. The results are shown in Figure 2.17 and Table 2.2. In Figure 2.17, the maps give the day of reporting of cholera in each city; the first reported case is coded day one, and other days are serially numbered thereafter. The arrows indicate the main directions of spread. The block diagrams all have the same form:

(1) the end-planes show various simple regressions of date of reporting (Y) against distance from the origin (X_1);

Table 2.2. *Results of stepwise multiple regression analysis of US cholera data for waves of 1832, 1848–9 and 1866*

			Coefficients					
Epidemic	n	Route	Constant	Distance	Population	R^2	$r_{P,D}$	Process
1832	34	New York	34.85	0.722 (0.068)		0.779		Predominantly wave spread
			44.29	0.712 (0.067)	−8.49 (5.89)	0.793	−0.11	
1832	10	Canadian origin	2.98	0.278 (0.047)		0.816		Predominantly wave spread
			6.27	0.266 (0.048)	−4.83 (4.52)	0.842	−0.25	
1848	15	New Orleans interior waterways	21.66	0.975 (0.328)		0.404		Mixed contagious/ hierarchical spread
			77.96	0.993 (0.277)	−50.13 (20.06)	0.608	0.03	
1848	7	New York origin	217.44		−24.00 (12.44)	0.427		Downwards hierarchical spread but substantial correlation between P and D
			204.76	0.293 (0.819)	−19.87 (17.92)	0.444	−0.65	
1848	6	New York origin (Newark omitted)	141.10	1.492 (0.556)		0.643		Time of reporting increases with increasing distance + *upwards* spread. But near collinearity between P and D
			−15.67	4.097 (1.349)	54.12 (26.65)	0.850	−0.95	
1866	30	–	148.51		−29.52 (6.34)	0.437		Downwards hierarchical spread, but substantial correlation between P and D
			154.91	−0.030 (0.085)	−31.38 (8.35)	0.439	−0.64	

Notes: Numbers in brackets are standard errors of regression coefficients. $r_{P,D}$ is Pearson correlation coefficient between the regressor variables, population and distance.

(2) the back-planes give the simple regressions of date of reporting (Y) against population size (X_2);

(3) the multiple regression relationship of date of reporting against distance from origin and population is indicated by the columns rising from the base-plane.

We now consider each epidemic in turn. The 1832 wave had two points of introduction, in Quebec City and New York City. The regressions for the Canadian origin wave appear as the open circles, italicised numbers and pecked lines in Figure 2.17A. The evidence of Table 2.2 clearly supports Pyle's interpretation of wave spread along the main corridors of movement, with places more distant from the origin affected later.

In 1848, spread was up the Mississippi system from New Orleans, and along the Eastern Seaboard from New York. The regressions for the New York origin wave have open circles and pecked lines on Figure 2.17B; (a) is based on $n=7$ places and (b) on $n=6$ places, omitting Newark, which, although only 10 miles from New York City, was equal last to report cholera. In Table 2.2, the results for the New Orleans route provide good evidence in support of Pyle's contention that the process now displays both hierarchical and contagious spread components. For the New York route, however, urban size alone seems to dominate when $n=7$. If Newark is omitted, spread occurs *up* the size hierarchy. For the New York route, the sample sizes are so small and the degree of correlation between population size and distance so great that it is difficult to have much confidence in the results. Finally, for the 1848 epidemic (New Orleans route), we have identified *Q*uincey, *S*andusky, *F*rankfort and *D*etroit which seem to have odd dates of reporting in terms of the other dates for the river system.

Turning now to the 1866 wave, Table 2.2 seems to indicate that urban size is much more important than distance from the origin as an explanatory variable. However, again there is high correlation between the size and distance variables, and we can see from Figure 2.17C that both simple regressions look perfectly reasonable. It is the collinearity between the two regressors which is confounding the interpretation.

We have re-examined Pyle's data, not to point out deficiencies in his analysis, – indeed, as far as one can tell, the results seem broadly to support his conclusions – but to indicate the difficulties caused by the high negative correlation between the population and distance-from-origin variables. We shall be faced again with exactly the same problems in chapter 5, where we try to disentangle the hierarchical and contagious diffusion elements in the transmission of measles epidemics through the Icelandic urban system.

2.4 Post-Hägerstrand models in geography

2.4.1 The perimeter model

The perimeter model is discussed in Bartholomew (1973). In this model, members of the population are immobile and can communicate only with their immediate neighbours. New adopters appear solely at the edges of existing areas of adoption, and the pattern of diffusion follows the density of the susceptible population. Bartholomew (1973, p. 332) argues that such models are of little geographical (spatial) interest:

> For this reason [growth restricted to the perimeter of existing areas of adoption only] the analysis cannot be expected to yield much of interest about the pattern [of spread]. We [are] instead . . . more concerned with the rate of growth of the total numbers in a situation where contacts are constrained by geography.

That is, there is a shift of emphasis in these models away from the spatial pattern of growth in numbers of adopters, which has been the main point of interest so far in this chapter, to a consideration of the temporal

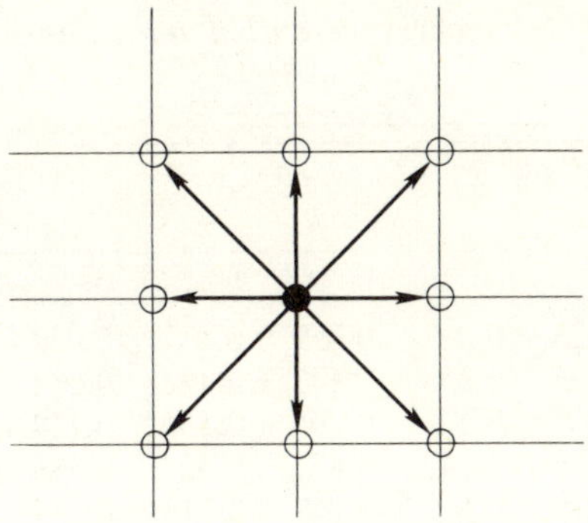

Fig. 2.18 Location of initial adopter (solid circle) and possible neighbouring contacts (open circles) for a simple perimeter model.

take-up. The spatial build-up is dictated very much by the structure of the network, as we have seen in Figure 2.16C for the case of a central-place system where higher order centres dominate lower order ones.

As an example of a perimeter model, Bartholomew (1973, p. 332) discusses a model developed by Bailey (1967). Consider a square lattice, and suppose that individuals are located at the vertices of the grid. At $t = 1$, a single adopter located in the centre of the lattice may contact any one of his eight immediate neighbours (see Figure 2.18), but no-one else. A pure birth process is assumed. The chance of a susceptible, or potential adopter, hearing from a neighbouring adopter is p, and all contacts are taken to be independent. In the first generation, the number of new adopters, r, will have the binomial distribution (Bartholomew, 1973, p. 332),

$$\binom{8}{r} p^r(1-p)^{8-r}, \quad r = 0, 1, 2, \ldots, 8. \tag{2.7}$$

In the next generation, all potential adopters who are neighbours of adopters may again be contacted, but no-one else. If a given potential adopter has a adopters as neighbours, the probability that he will become an adopter is $1 - (1 - p)^a$. In a study area of finite extent, this kind of model can produce the characteristic sigmoidal growth curve in the total number of adopters shown in Figure 2.10.

A geographical application of the model is to be found in Hudson (1973). Hudson considered the settlement of quarter-section areas in the Dakotas, 1870–1910. A square mile contains $s = 4$ 160-acre land parcels. All parcels are assumed to be equally attractive, and at any time, $N = 0, 1, \ldots, 4$ of these parcels will be taken. The probability that a claim is made to one of the parcels in the time interval, Δt, is thus taken to be proportional to the number of parcels available. Let λ denote the time homogeneous rate at which this process takes place. If the proportion of available parcels at $t = 0$ is denoted as q, then Hudson writes the probability that exactly i parcels are taken at $t = 0$ as

$$P_i(0) = \binom{s}{i} p^i q^{s-i}, \quad i = 0, 1, \ldots, s, \tag{2.8}$$

Table 2.3. *Proportion of sections in which* N *quarters were filed in the Sanborn County Township of Ravenna*

	Number of years since settlement began*											
	0		2		4		6		8		10	
N	o	b	o	b	o	b	o	b	o	b	o	b
0	0.824	0.811	0.382	0.260	0.088	0.067	0.059	0.031	0.000	0.004	0.000	0.001
1	0.147	0.174	0.235	0.416	0.265	0.258	0.147	0.172	0.054	0.047	0.000	0.016
2	0.024	0.014	0.265	0.250	0.265	0.375	0.265	0.356	0.118	0.211	0.059	0.119
3	0.000	0.001	0.088	0.067	0.353	0.242	0.471	0.327	0.588	0.422	0.559	0.389
4	0.000	0.000	0.029	0.007	0.029	0.059	0.059	0.113	0.235	0.316	0.382	0.475

* o = observed; b = binomial. *Source:* Hudson (1973, p. 450).

(cf. equation (2.7)) and the growth equation for the process as

$$P_N(t) = \binom{s}{N} [1 - q\exp(-\lambda t)]^N [qe^{-\lambda t}]^{s-N}, \quad N = 0, 1, 2, \ldots, s. \quad (2.9)$$

Hudson fitted this model to data from the eastern tier of four Sanborn townships, South Dakota. We give the results for Ravenna in Table 2.3. Here, as in other townships, the model overestimates the proportion of quarter-sections with two or four occupied quarters and underestimates those with three occupied quarters late in the period of settlement. Hudson suggests this indicates reluctance on the part of latecomers to file claims to the last quarter in a section. The proportion of sections with only one occupied quarter ($N = 1$) is overpredicted in the early stages, which Hudson explains by multiple claims, most of which were made in the early years.

2.4.2 Epidemic models

The continued development of epidemic models in the last two decades has spilled over into geography in the work of Cliff, Haggett, Ord, Bassett and Davies (1975) and Haggett (1975). These developments are discussed in detail in chapter 7.

2.5 Conclusion

In this chapter, we have defined the term *spatial diffusion* and have illustrated its application in studies as varied as those on the spread of diseases like rabies and cholera, the acceptance of agriculture innovations, the spatial transmission of economic impulses, and migration. Diffusion in the plane usually displays both contagious and hierarchical spread components. The more rapidly the probability of contact between a transmitter and a receiver of news, a disease, etc. falls off with increasing distance between them, the more wave-like will be the diffusion process. Temporally, the cumulative number of acceptors of an innovation, people infected with a disease, characteristically builds up in a way which can be described by the logistic distribution. The classic Hägerstrand model, which is based upon contagious spread, has been described and some results from it discussed.

One of the major problems associated with many of the studies considered in this chapter is that – in the nature of the item being diffused – they tend to be idiographic. Historical events rarely repeat themselves exactly, farmers can accept a given innovation only once, and so on. If we are to be able to model a diffusion process adequately, we need one data set upon which to calibrate it and another data set upon which to test it; thus, we need a process which repeats itself in time and space in a way that cultural events seldom do. In the next chapter, we identify the transmission of measles epidemics as a process which has the necessary time–space stability to make it an excellent vehicle for the development of diffusion models. Further, we argue there that Iceland is one of the best areas in which to test such models.

3 The choice of diffusion phenomenon

3.1 Introduction

A geographer attempting to build further on the spatial diffusion models reported in the preceding chapter is faced with a choice between two possible approaches. One is to pursue the theoretical exploration of relatively simple spatial situations on the lines developed by, for example, Hudson (1972), Bailey (1975), and Mollison (1977). The problem with this path is that, as we noted in section 1.2, small increments in spatial complexity rapidly lead to relatively large increases in mathematical sophistication and, eventually, to intractability.

The other approach, the one initially followed here, is to isolate a real-world example of a spatial diffusion process and to subject it to careful quantitative analysis. In chapters 4 and 5, we follow this second path, to find that it eventually rejoins the first (chapters 6 and 7), but at a point further along the trail. This gain is made from the insights into the spatial process obtained from the empirical study, and the fact that these insights enable us to specify a few appropriate spatial models from amongst the large number of possible formats. In this chapter, we outline the various real-world examples available and explain how we came to make our eventual choice.

3.2 Some initial requirements

To find a suitable spatial diffusion phenomenon and to find a part of the world in which it could be studied proved to be a frustrating task. It is worth recording the search in some detail. We began by setting up the ideal experimental conditions which we hoped to be able to fulfil. These ideal conditions embodied four basic requirements:

(1) *Replicability*. If we were to avoid reporting 'one-shot' phenomena, we would need to study a spatial process which repeated itself very frequently. If we term each separate diffusion episode a wave, then we require a multiple-wave rather than a single-wave phenomenon for model building.

(2) *Stability over time and space*. If we are looking at multiple waves, then it is essential to know that the waves which occur at different times or in different places are identical in all important respects. This stability requirement proved to be an even more severe constraint on suitable experimental material than did (1).

(3) *Observability*. The existence of a stable, multiple-wave diffusion process was not enough. In order to be able to study and to model the process, we need to ensure that the process is observable both in principle and in practice. Thus, to meet our third requirement, we need a diffusion phenomenon which yields accurate observations

at frequent intervals in both time and space. Clearly, an acceptable definition of 'frequent' will depend on the periodicity of the phenomenon in both domains. To analyse a multiple-wave phenomenon (requirement (1)) we need observations which occur sufficiently often in time, as compared with the periodicity of the process, to enable several individual waves to be distinguished.

(4) *Isolation.* Even if all the requirements (1)–(3) are met, a further essential prerequisite remains. The preceding chapter will have shown that diffusion processes are generally complex; if, therefore, we have multiple waves which overlap with one another in either time or space, the picture which emerges may be too complicated to be disentangled with existing methods. If each of the waves studied has a distinct starting point in both time and space and runs its course before the next wave (probably originating in a different location) begins, then the chance of learning more about its generating process is greatly increased.

There are, of course, many other constraints which we would have liked to impose upon our choice of diffusion phenomenon. Simplicity of transmission process, a high level of data accuracy, a close relevance to the human condition, could all be argued for. In practice, the four essential requirements proved so constraining that others could not be entertained; indeed we were sometimes pessimistic about our chance of finding any suitable material on which to begin work. Thus, while many human geographers have chosen to analyse innovations (and some of the more productive studies, such as that of Hägerstrand, have been on this theme), the single-wave character of most innovations ruled them out of consideration here. One potentially promising area was that of the inter-regional transmission of business cycles, and we had ourselves explored this topic in an earlier study (Bassett and Haggett, 1971; Cliff, Haggett, Ord, Bassett and Davies, 1975). Even though further study of this multiple-wave phenomenon seemed worthwhile, it had eventually to be rejected on the grounds that it failed to meet our stipulation on stability (requirement (2)). Recent research, such as that by Waterman (1972) on Australian business cycles, has stressed that each wave may have a quite different causal structure than that which preceded or followed it. Definitions of the starts, peaks and ends of business cycles (the classic 'turning-point' problem) also made them unattractive in terms of our fourth criterion.

At the end of our winnowing process, only two items remained from those initially examined. One was 'epidemics' and the other 'islands'. We turn now to look at the reasons for their retention, and the key role we see them playing in the further development of spatial diffusion theory.

3.3 The choice of epidemics as diffusion phenomena

We noted earlier in the book (sections 2.2.4 and 2.3.3) the way in which the study of epidemics has illuminated important aspects of spatial diffusion theory and attracted contributions from leading statisticians throughout this century. N. T. J. Bailey's *The Mathematical Theory of Infectious Diseases* (1975) provides a comprehensive review of this work. Epidemic waves generally meet requirements (1) and (3) of section 3.2 in that they characteristically occur in the form of multiple waves (epidemics) which are recorded in public-health statistics in many countries. Not all epidemic diseases meet criterion (2): for example, influenza is typified by virus changes which may make one diffusion wave have a different attack rate (in terms of severity or the age group most markedly affected) from another wave. Many epidemics do not meet criterion (4): some infectious diseases have an epidemic pattern, with occasional epidemic peaks; others are endemic in large communities but re-invade smaller or more isolated communities in the form of discrete waves.

Critical examination of the several epidemic diseases available for study led the authors to select measles for special attention. In the remainder of this section we explain this choice.

3.3.1 Wave stability

Although written records of what appear to have been measles outbreaks go back to the Roman period, the causative agent was not identified until the middle of this century. In 1954, J. F. Enders and T. C. Peebles isolated the cause of measles as a virus; that is, a micro-organism which multiplies only within living susceptible cells. Since such viruses range in size from 20 μm to 250 μm in diameter, an understanding of their basic structure was dependent on the development of the electron microscope. The measles virus was found to be one of a group of viruses (the myxovirus group) which produces illnesses in man and other animals. In addition to measles, the group contains influenza, mumps, canine distemper and rinderpest. As far as present knowledge extends, the measles virus is not thought to undergo significant changes in structure and, unlike the influenza virus which has produced major mutations in a few decades, may be assumed to have stable diffusion parameters over the period studied here (see chapter 4). This assumption is strengthened by Ball, A. P. (1977, p. 238) who notes that, although laboratory research has produced measles viruses with attenuation – decreased virulence – no changes in basic type have yet been recorded. Measles epidemics may reasonably be treated as meeting constraint (2) in section 3.2.

3.3.2 Wave periodicity

Reports of measles cases indicate that outbreaks occur in distinct waves, often with a marked periodicity. Figure 3.1 shows the time series of reported cases between 1945 and 1970 for four countries, arranged in decreasing order of population size. Note that, in the United States, with a population of 210 million in 1970, epidemic peaks arrive every year, and in Britain (56 million), every two years. Denmark (5 million) has a more complex pattern, with a tendency to a three-year cycle in the latter half of the period. Iceland (0.2 million) stands in contrast to the other countries in that only eight waves occurred in the 25-year period, and several years are without cases.

Since countries frequently do not represent distinct epidemiological units, research has tended to concentrate upon more clearly defined examples of such units. Thus, Bartlett (1957) investigated the relationship between the periodicity of measles epidemics and population

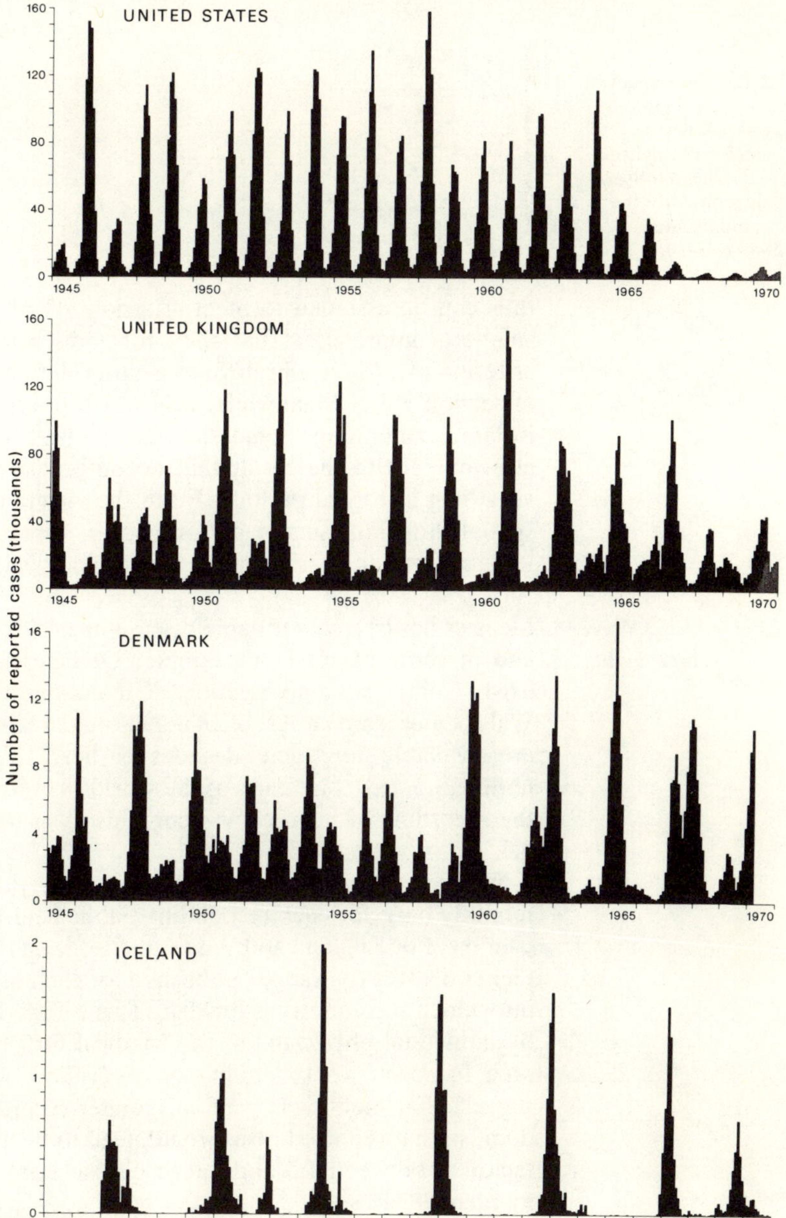

Fig. 3.1 Reported cases of measles per month, 1945 to 1970, for four countries arranged in descending order of population size. Note the characteristic cyclicity in all cases, the dramatic reduction in amplitude for the United States series after 1964 (because of vaccination programmes), and the fact that only Iceland has clear non-endemicity.

size for a series of urban centres. His findings for British cities are summarised in Figure 3.2. Note that the largest cities have an endemic pattern with periodic eruptions (Type I), while cities below a certain size threshold have an epidemic pattern with fade-outs. A distinction can be drawn between urban areas above about 10,000 people with a regular pattern of epidemics (Type II) and those where occasional epidemics may be missed, giving a more irregular pattern (Type III). Study of the two parts of Figure 3.2 suggests that, while measles epidemics display a periodicity in communities with a wide variety of population sizes and

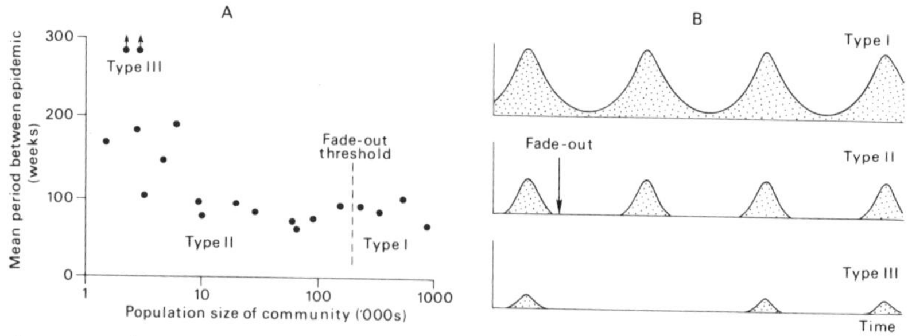

Fig. 3.2 (A) The impact of population size on the spacing of measles epidemics for 19 English towns. (B) Characteristic epidemic profiles for the three types indicated in (A). *Source:* Bartlett (1972).

thus can be assumed to meet criterion (1) of section 3.2, it is only in smaller communities that they form discrete waves and thus meet criterion (4). We shall return to a closer definition of this size threshold in section 3.4.1. Meanwhile, it is worth noting that, in very small and isolated communities, measles may not have been introduced from elsewhere, with the result that no outbreaks will have occurred over very long historical periods. From the viewpoint of building models of spatial diffusion, such cases are of less direct interest, although they remain fascinating from other epidemiological points of view.

3.3.3 Wave observability

Measles has been a notifiable disease in a few countries since the 1880s, and in some places (for example, Denmark) good historical records exist. Compulsory notification of infectious diseases in England and Wales dates from an Act of 1889, although records for a few urban areas are available for some decades earlier. Legislation requiring such notification exists in many of the world's countries, and those for which the recording of measles was compulsory in 1970 are shown in Figure 3.3.

Where collected, statistics are generally published on a weekly or monthly basis for each responding public health authority area within a country. For England and Wales, the relevant document is the Registrar General's *Weekly Return*, published for each of the local authority areas into which the country is divided. This is based on the records supplied by individual physicians to the Medical Officer of Health for a given area for each week (ending on a Friday). Detailed clinical studies suggest that measles is generally under-recorded in the United Kingdom, so that reported cases would need to be multiplied by a correction factor of between 1.5 and 2.0 to give a more realistic estimate of the number of cases.

Measles occurs throughout the world without any apparent relation to the ethnic or genetic background of the population infected, or to the environment in which they live. Building up a picture of the worldwide distribution of the disease is, however, made difficult because, as is evident from Figure 3.3, only a limited number of countries require compulsory notification of cases of the disease. There is an absence of records for much of Asia, while some countries with highly developed health services choose to note only deaths from measles (for example, West Germany, Australia and New Zealand). Between countries recording measles cases, the reporting rate varies dramatically (see Black, 1966).

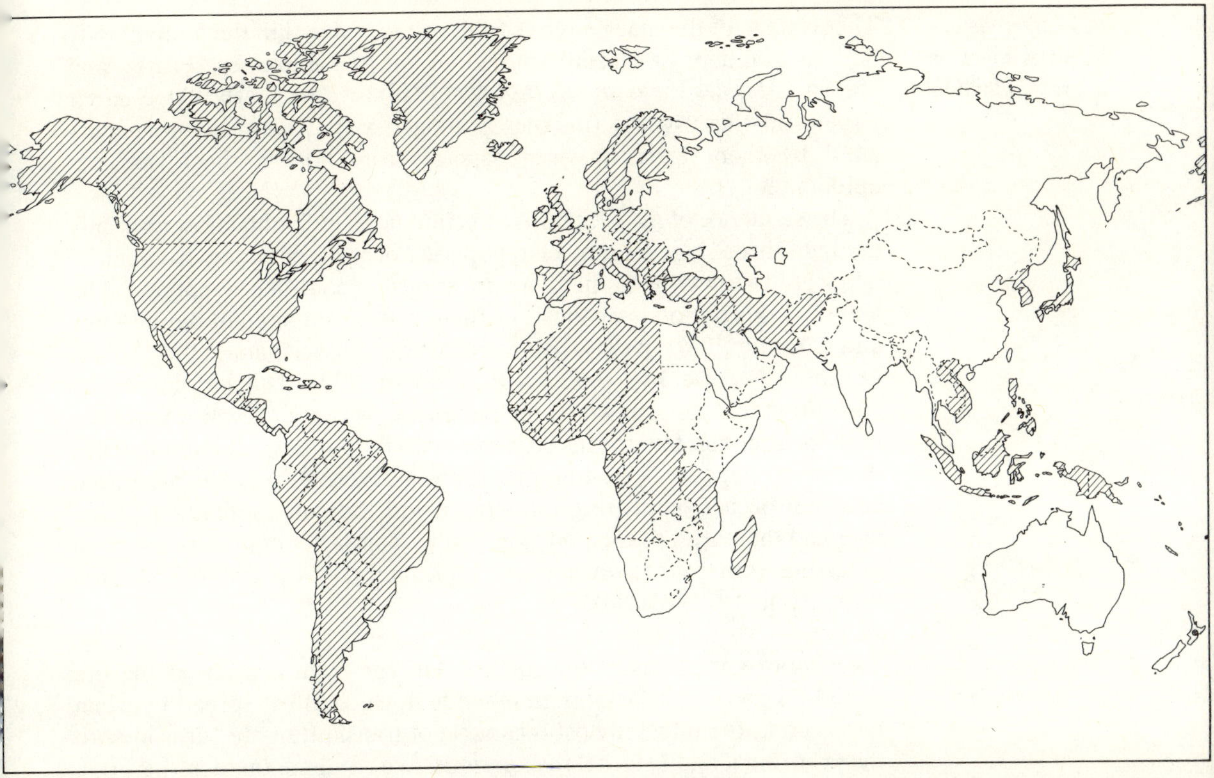

Fig. 3.3 Countries (hatched) reporting incidence of measles cases in 1970. *Source:* World Health Organisation (1970).

In contrast to most other human infectious diseases, measles has a high rate of incidence in exposed, unvaccinated populations. There are few reliable estimates in the literature of the proportion of a population that has had measles. In an early paper, Chapin (1925) cites figures for several cities – Aberdeen, Scotland, 90–95 per cent; Willesden, London, 93 per cent; and Providence, Rhode Island, 96 per cent – and concludes that '. . . it is probable that in England, Canada, and the United States [the countries he studied] over 90 per cent of urban populations contract measles at some time during their lives' (Chapin, 1925, p. 643). In contrast to the 1920s, Goodall's (1978) analysis of Icelandic populations suggests that the proportion of the population affected by their twentieth birthday can now be as low as 35 per cent. While the precise level will vary both historically and regionally, the very high incidence rates in comparison with other infectious diseases give some confidence in the reported data.

3.3.4 Wave propagation

An understanding of the way in which measles epidemics happen and are propagated as waves demands that we consider the virus itself. The explosive growth in the number of cases which characterises the upswing of a major epidemic implies that the virus is being passed from one host to many others. Here, we begin by examining (1) the life cycle of the measles virus within a single individual, and (2) its passage between individuals, before looking at (3) epidemic spread on a large scale.

(1) Life cycle of a measles attack on a single individual

The passage of the measles virus from cell to cell within the human body has been the most closely studied of the three phases. Fraser and Martin's *Measles Virus and its Biology* (1978) reviews nearly 500 research papers on this process (measles pathogenesis), while only 10 papers cited by them refer to virus passage from host to host (measles epidemiology).

The sequence of measles virus infection in an individual host normally involves three stages. First, a latent period occurs, extending from initial exposure to the virus to the first appearance of cold-like symptoms. The length of this period is variously estimated at 'seven or eight days' (Riley and O'Grady, 1961, p. 97), 'ten or eleven days' (McKhann, 1973, p. 25), to 'about two weeks' (Ball, A. P., 1977, p. 239). This is followed by a prodromal period, in which the patient shows upper respiratory catarrhal disorder and fever. This lasts from two to four days. It culminates in the third stage or external rash period. Here, a distinctive raised eruption occurs, appearing initially behind the ears, spreading to the face and thereafter to the body and limbs. This latter period is described as lasting from 'four to seven days' (McKhann, 1973, p. 25) to 'about ten days' (Ball, 1977, p. 240).

(2) Virus transmission between hosts

Two important pieces of information emerge from a study of the life cycle of a measles attack on an individual which affect spread between hosts. First, the infected host is capable of transmitting the virus in both the prodromal and external rash periods. We combine these in this book as an infectious period. Second, the prodromal period is the most critical in the rapid spread of the disease since a host (for example, a child) will display only cold symptoms, and will not generally be isolated from other potential hosts (such as other children). Given the variation cited above in the lengths of the various phases, we have adopted here the average values given in Chapin (1925, p. 651) of eight to twelve days for the latent period, and seven to nine days for the infectious period (see Figure 3.4). These estimates allow us to view the transmission process of the disease in terms of a chain structure. Figure 3.4 shows the shortest length of chain (8 days), the longest (21 days) and, thus, a typical chain of around 14 days. Empirical studies suggest that the mean length of the chain may, in fact, be slightly shorter than 14 days.

(3) Virus transmission under epidemic conditions

The chain mechanism described above accounts for the continued existence of the virus under endemic conditions. For an epidemic to occur, we must assume that an infected host (an infective) has access to a large number of potential hosts (susceptibles). Burnet and White (1972, pp. 15–16) describe measles as:

> a typical childhood disease in which a single attack is followed by lifelong immunity . . . [Of] all infections its ecology is the simplest to understand. A child becomes infected perhaps by someone from another city. From this child a number of five-, six-, or seven-year-olds are infected perhaps at school and a fairly rapid spread occurs to all exposed children not yet insusceptible by virtue of a previous attack. Almost every susceptible child exposed to contact . . . will contract the disease. The epidemic will spread progressively through a city,

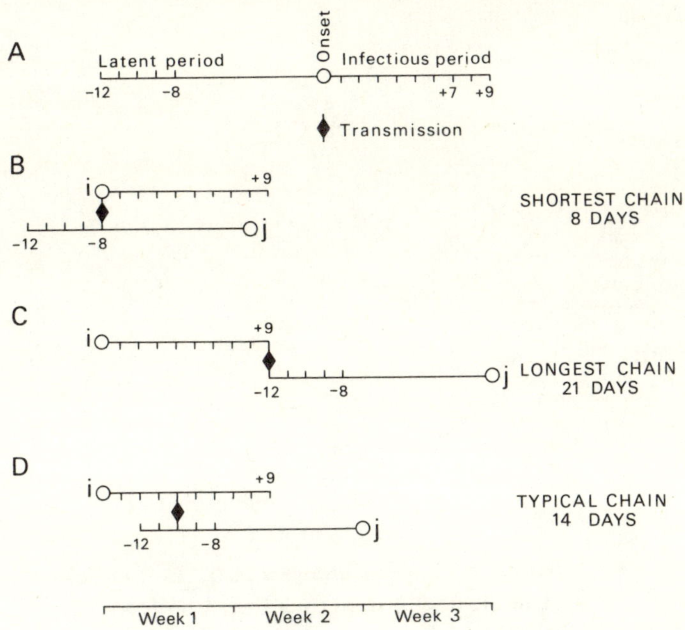

Fig. 3.4 The infection process as a chain structure. Schematic model for measles contacts between an infective (*i*) and a susceptible (*j*). Open circles denote onset of infection. In the shortest chain (B), infective *i* makes his contact on day 1 of his infectious period, and the susceptible *j* is 'latent' for as short a time as possible. The longest chain arises when *i* transmits on his last possible day of infection and *j* is latent for as long as possible (C). In the epidemiological literature, the average chain length (that is, the average time between the observation of symptoms in one case and the observation of symptoms in a second case directly infected from the first) is referred to as the *serial interval* of the disease.

twelve or fourteen days between successive crops of infectives. As each child passes through his infection he becomes immune and the virus finds greater difficulty in spreading. Eventually measles disappears from the community.

As we shall show later (chapter 4), another crop of susceptible children is born and, 'sooner or later, the measles virus re-enters the community and the cycle is repeated' (Burnet and White, 1972, p. 16).

The distinctive age incidence of measles attack is illustrated in Figure 3.5. This is based on Chapin's (1925) classic study of 14,376 measles cases in Providence, Rhode Island. It shows that the attack rate is at its highest in the sixth year (the first year of school life for most children) and declines thereafter. A quarter of the cases studied by Chapin had occurred by the end of the second year of life, a half by the end of the fourth year, and three-quarters by the end of the sixth year. Only one tenth of the cases occurred after the age of eight.

Such a youthful distribution of cases has important geographical implications, in that the population most at risk (i) has low spatial mobility compared with adults, and (ii) is commonly organised into an areal framework of local school districts which helps to guide the spread of the disease. Wells (1955) investigated every student infected in an American school, Swarthmore High, and was able to trace infective to susceptible contacts to within the school in 60 per cent of the cases. Further studies by Riley and O'Grady (1961, p. 113) confirm Wells' findings on the great importance of the school for virus spread, but emphasise that other conditions which bring children close together in enclosed atmospheres (school buses, Sunday school services, family gatherings) all play a part. Some light is shed on spread *within* the family

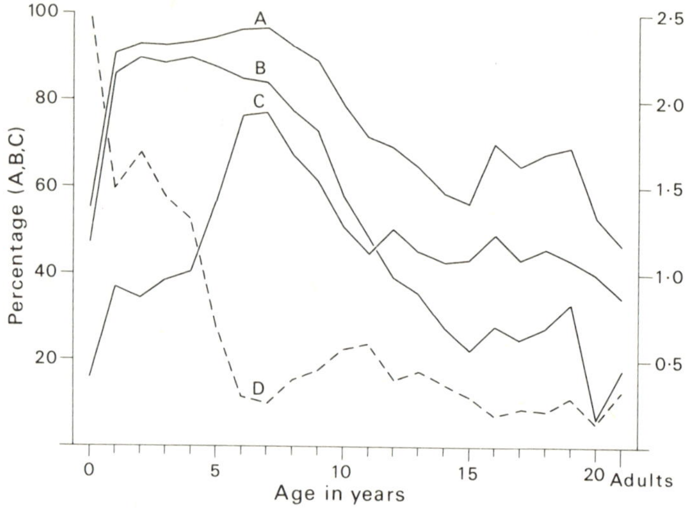

Fig. 3.5 Attack rates for measles by ages for 14,376 cases in Providence, Rhode Island, 1917–23. Institutional and non-resident cases have been excluded. Define α = total population at risk, β = all reported measles cases, γ = primary cases, δ = secondary cases. Then the overall attack rate is $100\beta/\alpha$(line A), secondary attack rate is $100[\delta/(\alpha-\beta)]$ (line B), primary attack rate is $100\gamma/\alpha$ (line C), and secondary cases per primary case is δ/γ (line D). *Source:* Chapin (1925, Table II, p. 639).

unit by Chapin's analysis of 6,345 measles cases in Providence, Rhode Island, over the period 1917 to 1923. Figure 3.6 is based on Chapin's data and shows the average interval between primary and secondary cases within families. Note that the secondary wave peaks between 11 and 15 days after the initial case. Less than 8 per cent of cases occur after the sixteenth day from the first infection in a family, a fact which has important implications in defining a quarantine or isolation period.

It is important to note that, although the strong age bias outlined here still persists, recent studies describe a more complex pattern. The average age of attack is higher where (i) there are long intervals between measles outbreaks, and (ii) a population is vaccinated (Griffiths, 1973). An extreme case of the first condition occurred in the Faroes, where the 1846 measles epidemic attacked people of all ages up to 65 years. Those who escaped infection were predominantly immunes who had survived the 1771 epidemic, the previous recorded date of a measles outbreak in the Faroes (Panum, 1940). The age distribution of measles cases in Iceland is shown later in Figure 8.1.

3.4 The choice of island communities

The decision to analyse spatial diffusion processes through the behaviour of epidemic waves (section 3.3) led to a consideration of scale and location. Given the choice of measles epidemics, it was clear at the outset that, as noted in section 3.3.3, the patchy nature of statistics from country to country would rule out a worldwide examination. Since any study would have to be restricted to a particular region, we required that the region selected met the observability criterion of section 3.2. In particular, we would expect the area to display distinct, non-overlapping epidemic waves, and to have records of exceptional quality in terms of reliability, historical length and spatial detail.

3.4.1 Discrete waves

We have already noted that continuous measles records are characteristic of large communities, while discrete waves are characteristic of smaller communities. In terms of Figure 3.2B, a region with Type II

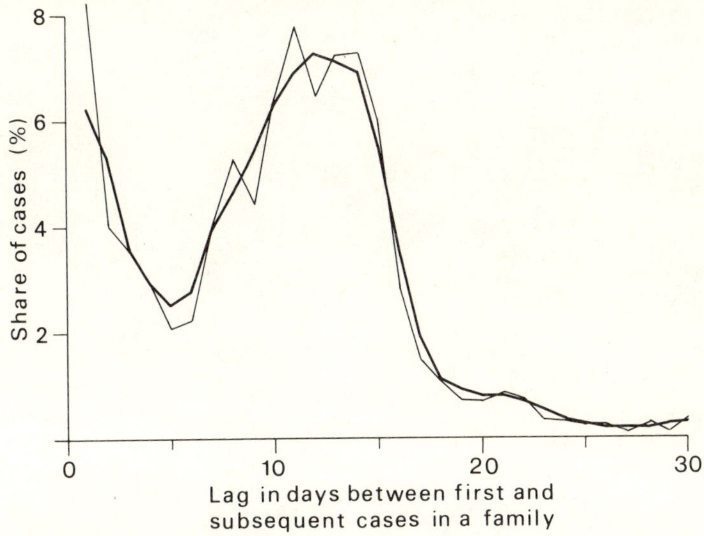

Fig. 3.6 Lag in days between first measles case in a family and first day of sickness for subsequent cases. Based on a study by Chapin (1925, p. 650) of 6,345 cases in Providence, Rhode Island. Light line is raw data, heavy line is three-day running mean.

measles – regular but discrete – would be strongly preferred for spatial diffusion study. Bartlett's (1957, 1960) analysis of British and American cities indicated that the number of cases needed to sustain endemicity (Type I waves) is 4,000 to 5,000 measles cases per annum. Given the reporting rates and incidence at the times Bartlett wrote, this number of cases would have been generated by a city of around 250,000. In some earlier work on measles epidemics (Haggett, 1972; Cliff *et al.*, 1975), we explored the possibility of studying the characteristics of Type II waves in small cities and rural areas below the Bartlett threshold. Unfortunately, the complexity of the 'swash and backwash' diffusion patterns discovered in these urban systems made the separation of the characteristics of one wave from another virtually impossible.

Insular communities have had a central place in biogeographical work since Charles Darwin (MacArthur and Wilson, 1967) and they have played some small part in attempts to understand the impact of measles epidemics (for example, Panum's (1940) account of the Faroes, and Gould, Hermann and Witte's (1971) work on the United States Pacific islands). Their isolation has meant that measles was introduced from time to time from continental areas where it was endemic, but the sporadic pattern of waves that ensued was more characteristic of Bartlett's Type III than Type II. Figure 3.7 gives Black's (1966) findings on the relationship between endemicity and population size for 18 island communities. Only those islands, notably Hawaii with a total population of 550,000, sustained continuous records of measles infection over the 16-year study period. The figure also indicates the estimated reporting rate obtained by comparing the number of cases reported with the birth-rate and with serological tests. Of the five islands with rates in excess of 40 per cent, only one (Iceland) displayed a Type II pattern (see Figure 3.2); all the remainder were much smaller in population size and had irregular Type III patterns.

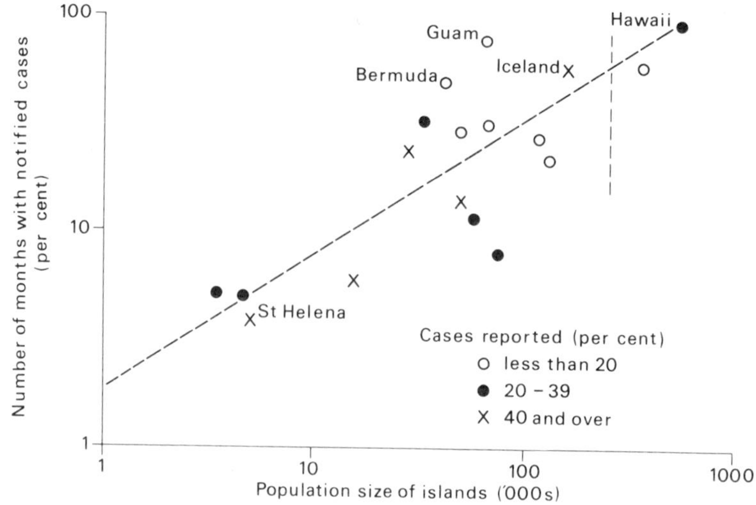

Fig. 3.7 Fade-out of measles epidemics in relation to population size for 18 island communities. Vertical pecked line denotes endemic/non-endemic size threshold. Regression line is also shown. *Source:* Black (1966).

3.4.2 Iceland as a laboratory area

The selection of Iceland from those islands reporting measles proved, in retrospect, to be an even more fortunate choice than we had initially expected. We comment later in the book on the quality and range of that country's public-health and epidemiological records (chapter 4); it is sufficient to note here that they are exceptionally high in comparison, not only with other islands, but also with the United States and the United Kingdom.

Two aspects of the Icelandic population as a laboratory for spatial diffusion studies are examined here. General discussions of Iceland's demography appear in Baldursson (1975) and Preusser (1976).

(1) Overall population trends

Figures 3.8 and 3.9 show the demographic history of Iceland since 1751. From Figure 3.8, it is evident that the population was stable at around 40–60,000 for the period 1751–1900, when a remarkable growth set in; the population approximately quadrupled between 1900 and 1970 to about 200,000. Up to 1950, this growth was concentrated mainly in the capital, Reykjavík. Since then, Reykjavík and the rest of Iceland have grown in population at about the same rate. The excess of immigrants over emigrants during this century has accounted for part of this remarkable growth but, as we see from Figure 3.9, the decline in infant mortality since 1850 and the higher birth-rates of the twentieth century (especially since 1940) are the main reasons.

The increasing youthfulness of the Icelandic population stands in sharp contrast to the ageing population of other western nations. Since measles is mainly a children's disease, we might expect the size of measles epidemics to increase in proportion to the increase in number of children, all other things being equal. It is evident from Figure 3.9C that this has not happened, and we touch on reasons for this in section 5.5.1. The increasing youthfulness of the population during the period, 1945–70, a time period we use in the modelling work of chapters 6 and 7,

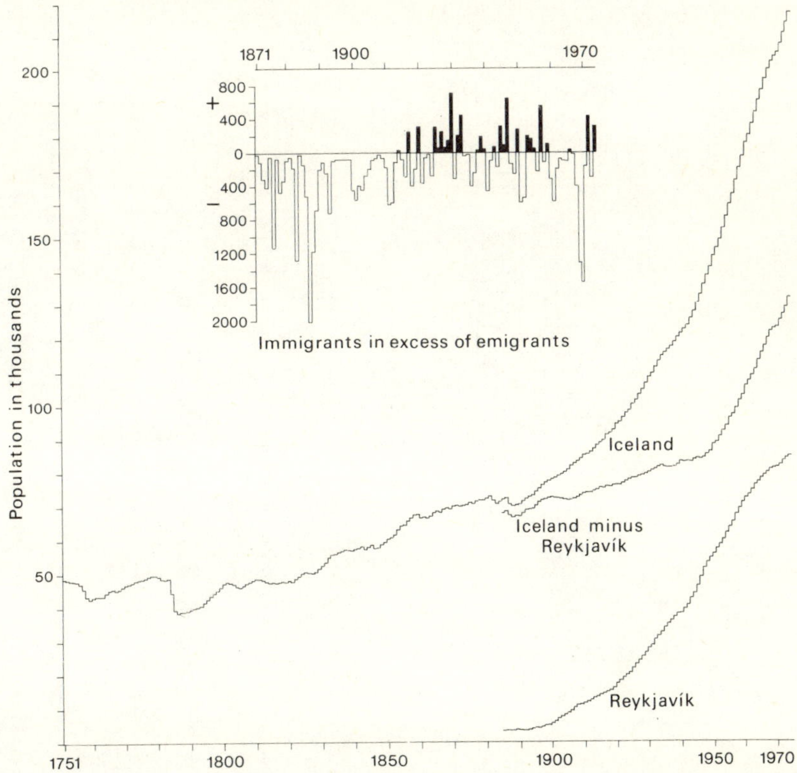

Fig. 3.8 Population totals and migration history of Iceland, 1751–1974. *Source:* Statistical Abstract of Iceland (1974).

is made clear in Figure 3.10. In this diagram, change is defined for each medical district in Iceland as:

(a) $\dfrac{\text{1970 population under 20}}{\text{1945 population under 20}}$ on the vertical axis,

and

(b) $\dfrac{\text{1970 total population}}{\text{1945 total population}}$ on the horizontal axis.

Log scales are used to give equal weight to change ratios less than and greater than one. The index numbers identify the medical districts named in Figure 4.2 and mapped on Figure 4.1. The bottom part of the diagram is an enlargement of the area contained within the pecked lines on the upper part. The 45° line passing through the origin of the graphs represents the case where the population under the age of 20 years for a place has remained a constant proportion of the total population for 1945–70. Places below the line have ageing populations; places above the line have more youthful populations. Figure 3.10 shows that only five of the 50 medical districts in Iceland had ageing populations in the period 1945–70. The identity numbers of the areas are 17, 30, 38, 40 and 42 which, from Figure 4.1, are all located on either the extreme north-west or north coasts of Iceland.

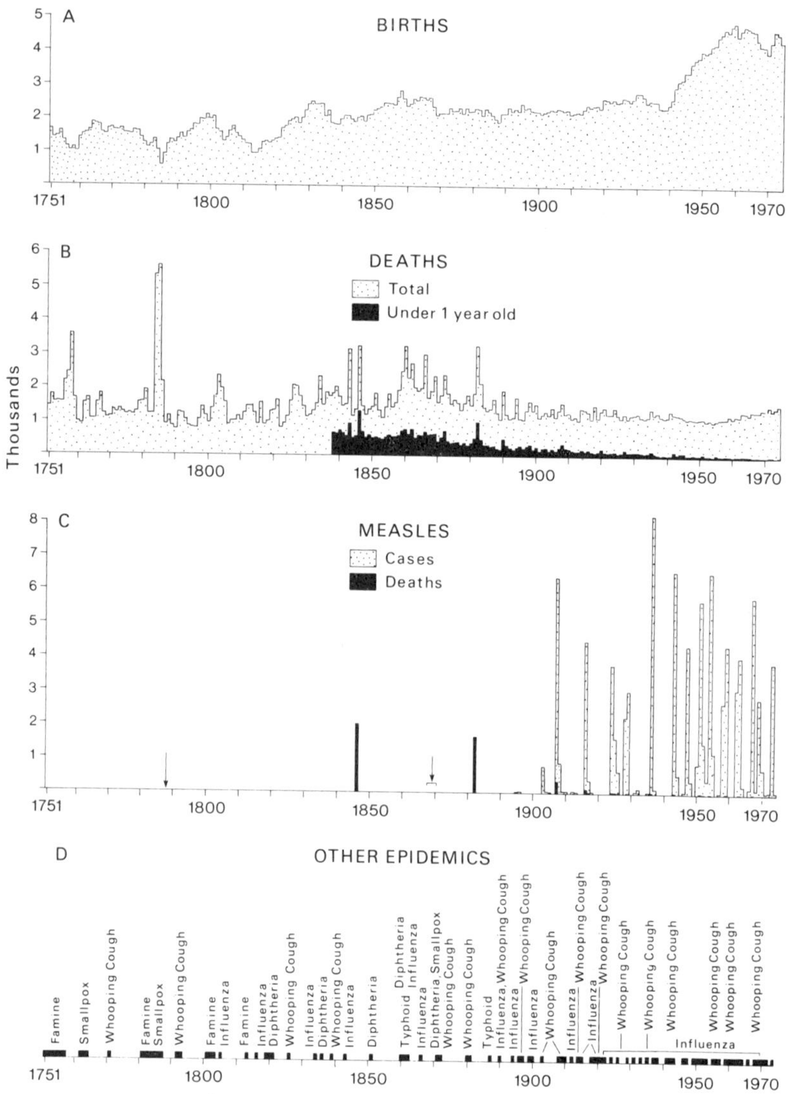

Fig. 3.9 Births, deaths and epidemic history of Iceland, 1751–1974. *Sources: Tölfræðihandbók* (1974, pp. 8–11); *Heilbrigðisskýrslur* (1911–20, p. 10).

(2) Low density and isolation

Iceland has the lowest population density of any country in Europe. The entire 1970 population could have been present at the first Wembley Cup Final in 1923 (the White Horse Final), although the stadium would have occupied an area equivalent to all of England and Wales south of a line running east to west through Coventry! Figure 3.11 shows the location of individual habitations (as dots) and built-up areas (black) in Iceland, 1970; most are single isolated farmsteads. The coastal concentration of communities is marked. Inland penetration of settlement is confined to the bottoms and lower slopes of valleys extending back from the fjord inlets. The overall impression is of population distributed around the coast much like the beads on a necklace. In terms of the spread of measles epidemics, an important question we ask in section 5.3.3 concerns the extent to which the diffusion process is tied to this unusual necklace distribution. The degree of isolation of settlements

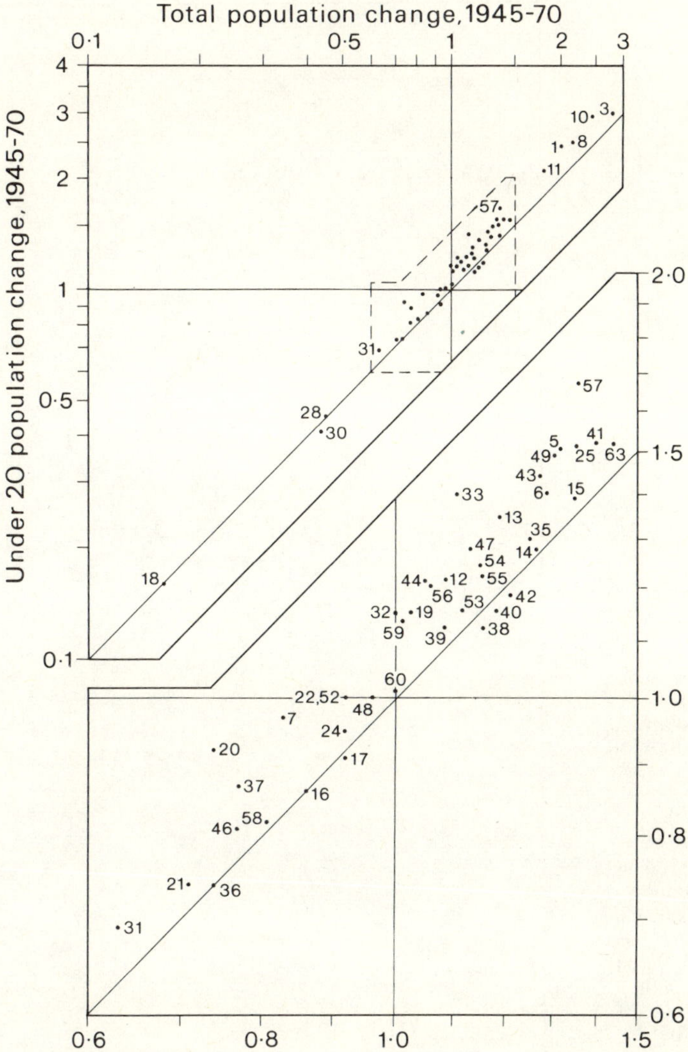

Fig. 3.10 Temporal change in the age structure of the Icelandic population. Change is defined by 1970/1945 population characteristics (see text). Numbers index the medical districts as listed in Figure 4.2. *Source: Heilbrigðisskýrslur* (1945, 1970, Tables III and IV).

around the coast means that it is often possible to treat such communities as separate epidemiological cells from a modelling point of view, giving a spatial equivalent to the discrete epidemic waves in time discussed in section 3.2.

Regional changes in population distribution in Iceland are striking. Figure 3.12 covers the period 1945–70. Settled areas are stippled. The proportional circles give the population of each of the medical districts in 1970, and the figures give the percentage change between 1945 and 1970. The rapid population increase in Reykjavíkur may be contrasted with the heavy depopulation of districts in the north-west, north and east; yet despite this, we noted in connection with Figure 3.10 that, with five exceptions, the medical districts involved here have become 'younger' over the period 1945–70. Population changes on a micro-scale

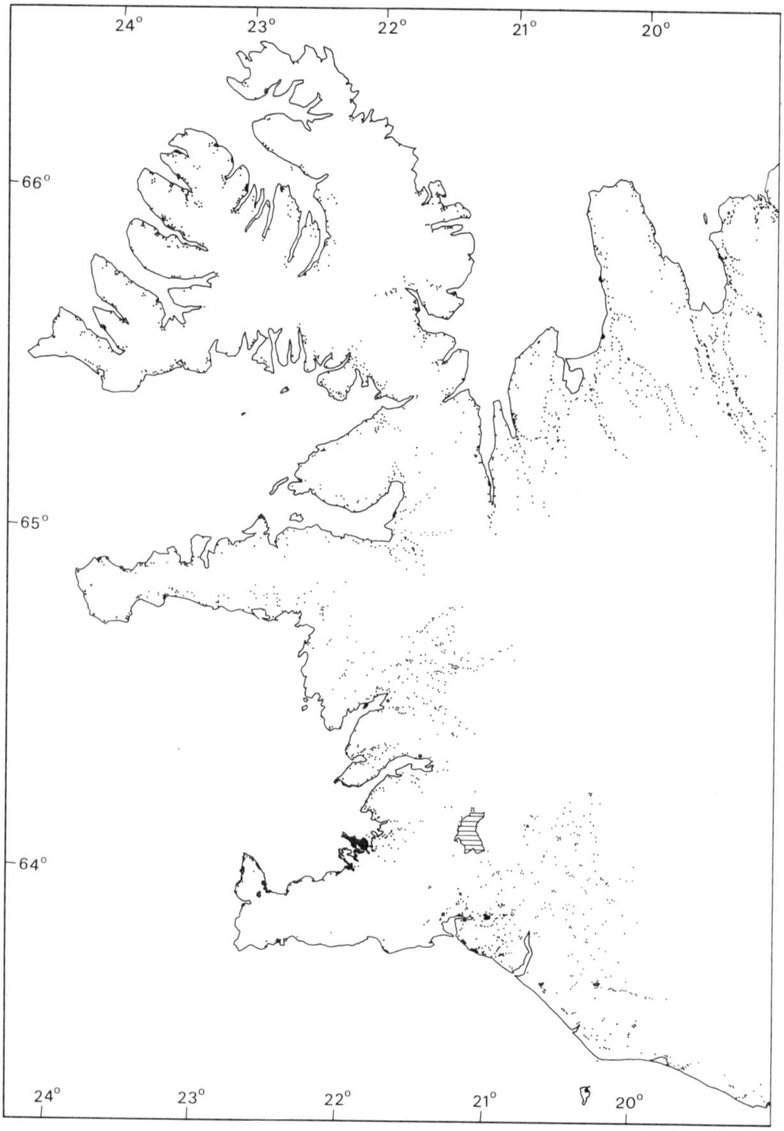

Fig. 3.11 Settlements in Iceland. Location of individual habitations (dots) and built-up areas (black). Most settlements shown are single farmsteads. Note the general coastal concentration of settlement with inland penetration along the valleys extending from the fjord inlets. Lakes are cross-hatched. Based upon the 9 sheets of the 1 : 250,000 map series of Iceland prepared by Landmælingar Íslands and the Geodetic Institute, Copenhagen *c.* 1970.

(Figure 3.13) reveal the detailed pattern of rural depopulation in two areas of Iceland. In the north-west region (Figure 3.13A), the pattern has been one of total abandonment of settlement except in two of the broader, more southerly, lowland embayments. In the north-east region (Figure 3.13B) the pattern has been one of retreat of settlement down-valley with time, particularly in the direction of the coastal settlement of Vopnafjörður.

Iceland illustrates the isolation of population in a striking manner at several scales. For a measles attack to occur on an Icelandic farmstead, the virus has to cross several hundred miles of sea, travel from a seaport or airport to the rural community, and eventually to the farm itself.

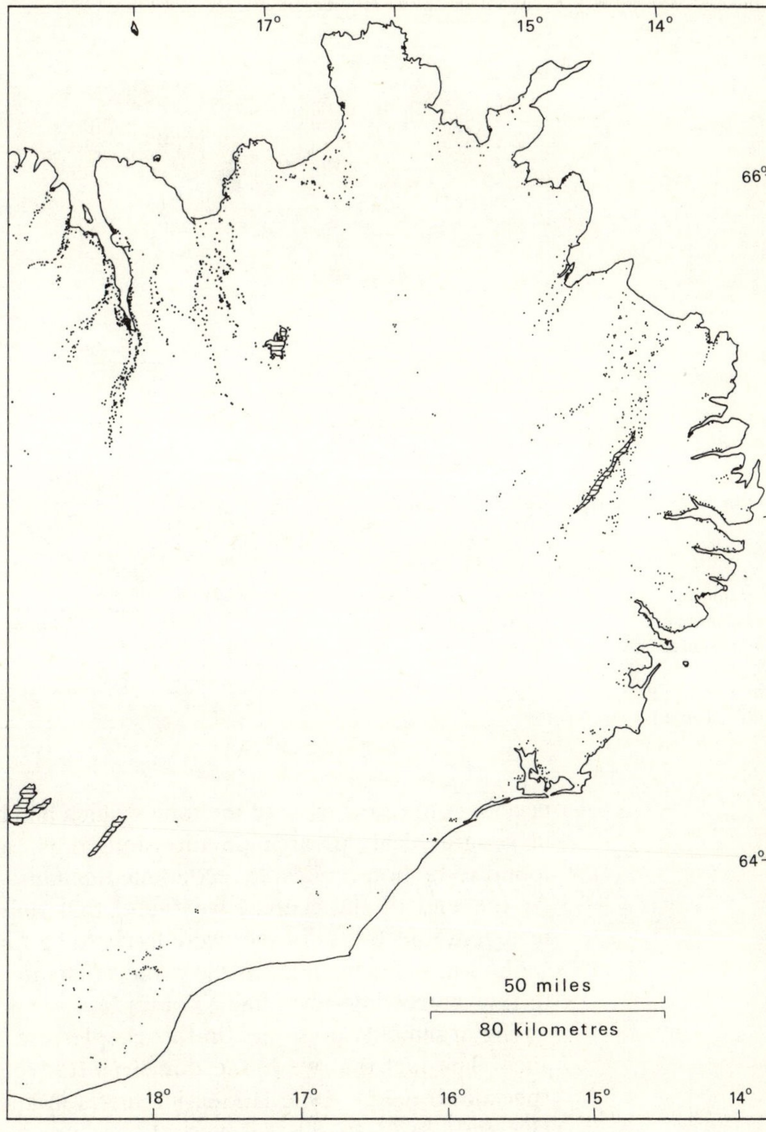

Fig. 3.11 (contd)

Figure 3.14 sketches the kind of movements necessary to overcome these barriers; in the next two chapters we use historical records to establish whether spatial diffusion of the disease did occur in this manner.

3.5 Conclusion

In this chapter, we have set out the reasons which led us to pursue our study of spatial diffusion in the directions that we report in the next two chapters. We began by arguing that any productive empirical study of spatial diffusion would need to meet four conditions – replicability, stability, observability and isolability – and we set out to find data which stood up to these requirements. One by one, we found it

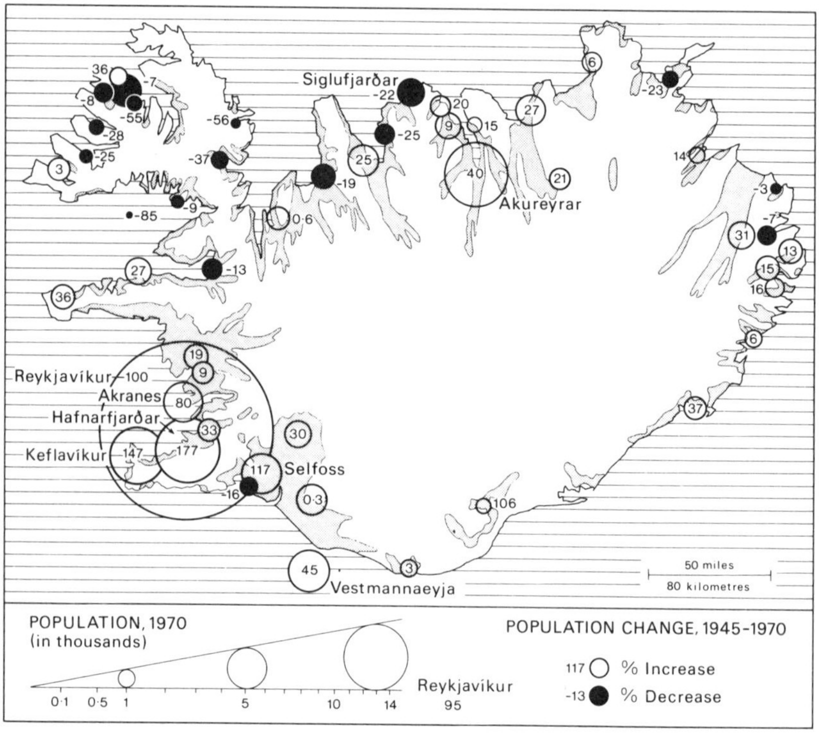

Fig. 3.12 Regional population change in Iceland. Settled areas are stippled. *Source: Heilbrigðisskýrslur* (1945, Table I; 1970, Table I).

necessary to reject most of the topics which had been studied previously in geographical research on diffusion; thus, social innovations were found to be non-replicable, economic fluctuations unstable, and so on. At the end of the search, we found that only the waves set up by recurrent infectious diseases were likely to be suitable for the modelling we had in mind for later in the project (chapters 6 and 7). Even here, further narrowing-down had to occur.

The arguments presented in this chapter are, we believe, of importance. The fact that we found ourselves studying a very restricted and specialised field – Type II measles waves in a single island community (Iceland) over an 80-year period – is not a matter of accident or intuition. It has, rather, been forced upon us by the contribution we wanted to make to spatial diffusion studies. It is, despite its intrinsic interest, essentially a means to this end.

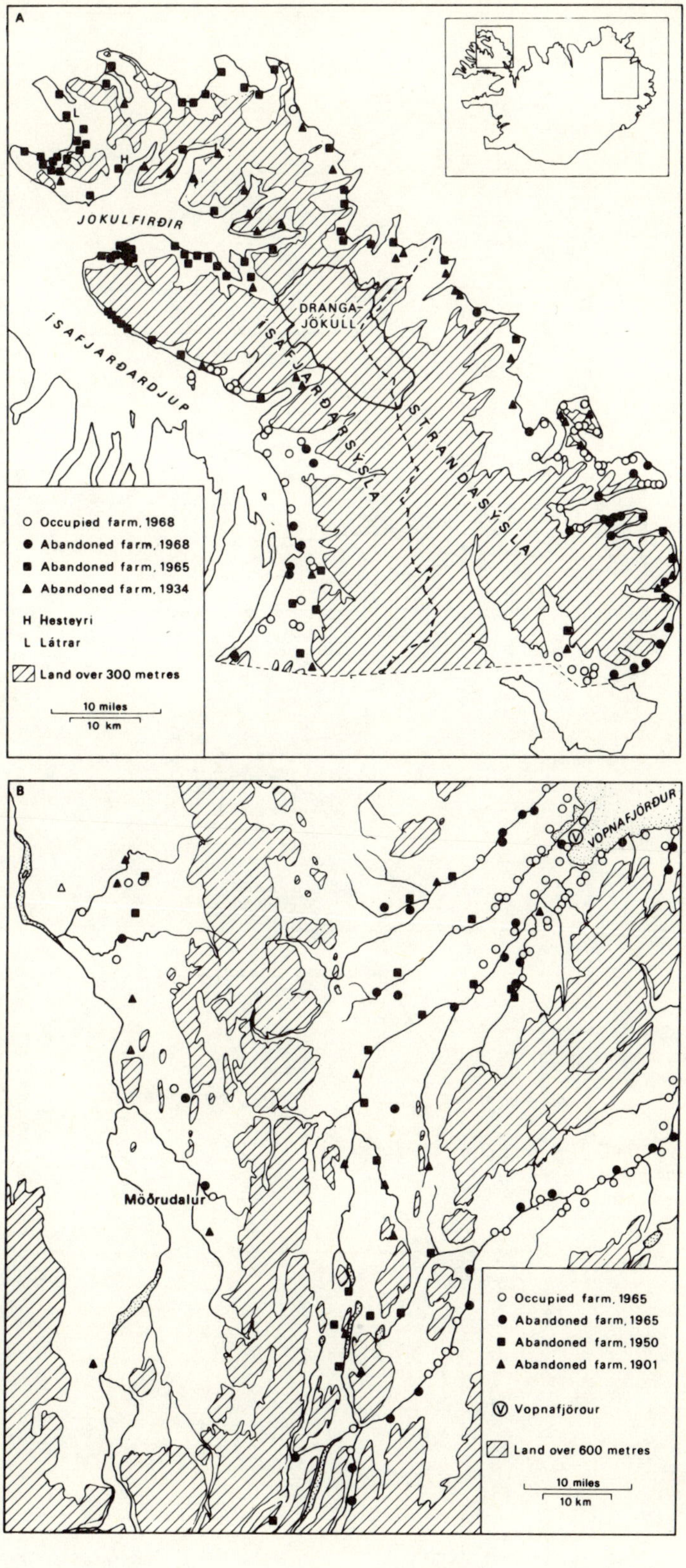

Fig. 3.13 Patterns of rural depopulation in two regions of Iceland. *Sources:* Thorarinsson (1961, p. 529); Preusser (1976, pp. 174, 209).

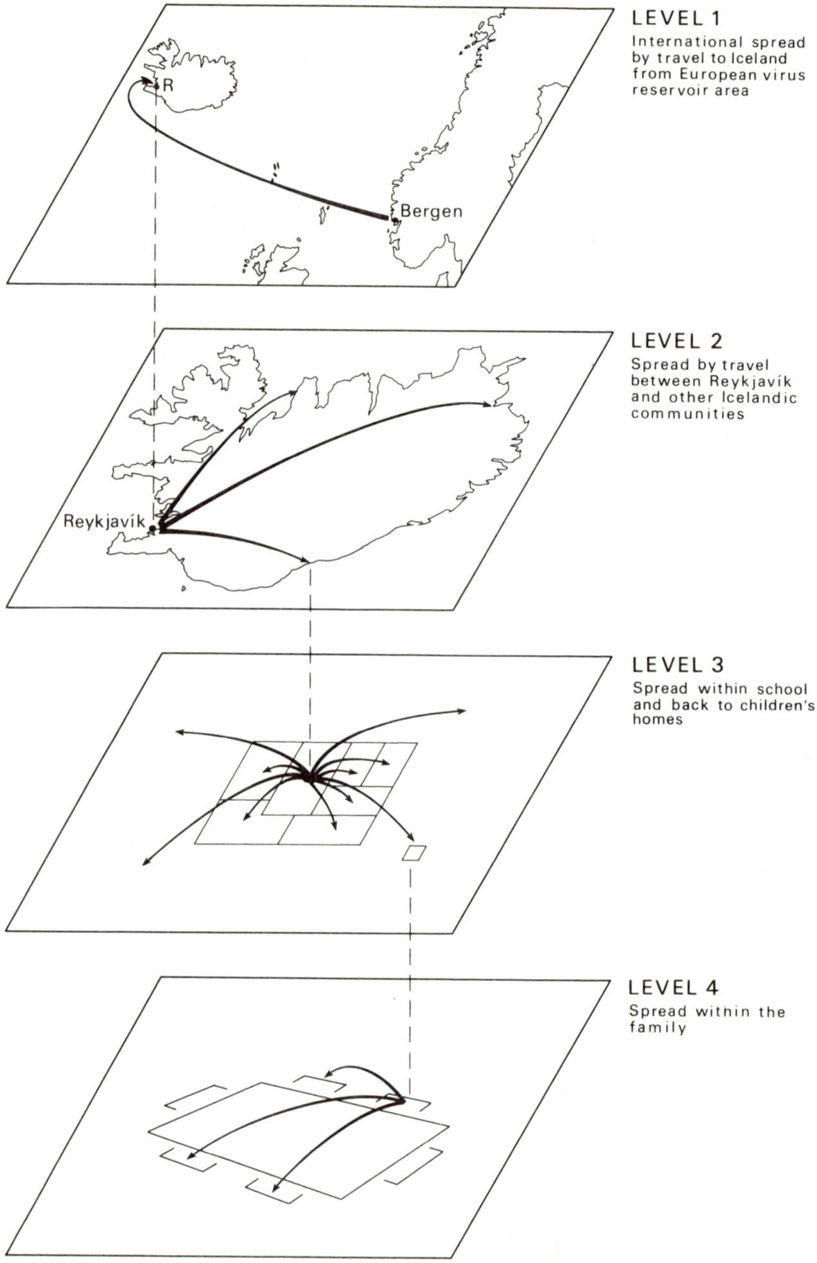

Fig. 3.14 Hypothetical sketch of the spread of measles virus into a farm family in rural Iceland. The arrows indicate the probable number of contacts in a 10-day period. At levels 1 and 2, the movements are likely to be those of young adults; at 3 and 4, children.

4 Measles epidemic cycles in Iceland

4.1 Introduction

In this chapter, we examine the data as recorded in our basic source, *Heilbrigðisskýrslur* (Public Health in Iceland). *Heilbrigðisskýrslur* was first published in 1896, and between then and 1975, which we have taken as the finishing date for our main study, 16 distinct measles epidemic waves passed through Iceland (see Figure 3.9). The information presented in *Heilbrigðisskýrslur* is in two forms, namely:

(1) Details of the number of cases of measles reported in each medical district in each month for all the epidemic waves except those of 1904 and 1907. For these first two waves in our data series, figures are given only monthly for Iceland as a whole, and annually by district, rather than being both spatially and temporally disaggregated.

(2) Written summaries of the course of each epidemic. These summaries are prepared from the annual reports filed in Reykjavík by the doctors in charge of public health in each medical district. The reports contain details of the size and severity of the various epidemics in each medical district. In addition, and crucially from a geographical point of view, many of the reports relate in some detail the spatial course of the epidemic in the medical districts. For such districts, information is given about the date of introduction of the disease into the district, where it came from and which farms and other communities were subsequently infected. This level of detail makes the data uniquely valuable for the study of a diffusion process. In many cases, we have, for the first time, been able to reconstruct the history of a spread process almost completely independently of any modelling or inferential methods. The reports vary in the amount of information given and seem to be readily divisible into two periods: (a) pre-1945, when size, severity and spatial spread information is provided, and (b) post-1945, when the spatial information is often lacking.

Because of the unique quality of the data for the study of diffusion processes, we give in this chapter and in the Appendix to the book full details of the information available. The Appendix contains the actual month-by-month records of measles cases reported for the various spatial units in each epidemic wave. In this chapter, we map from the data and the written reports the number of cases reported in each medical district for the various epidemic waves, and the diffusion links between medical districts as detailed in the written reports. The chapter is concluded with an examination of the spatial and temporal regularities displayed in the diffusion process from one epidemic to the next.

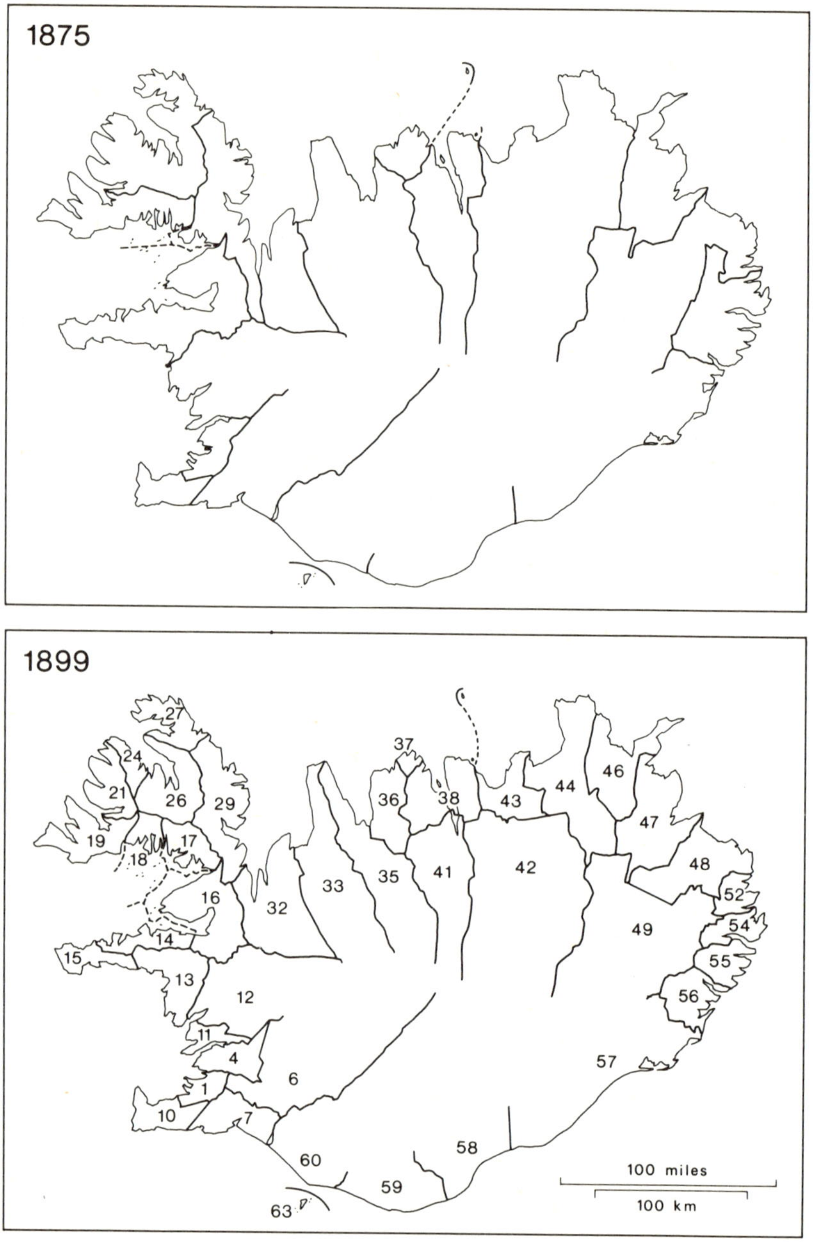

Fig. 4.1 Medical districts in Iceland as defined by the legislation of 1875, 1899, 1907, 1932 and 1955. The 1945 map defines a consistent set of medical districts used for all the formal modelling for the period 1945–70 (see chapters 6 and 7). Stipple indicates areas affected by boundary changes. The identity numbers of the medical districts correspond with Fig. 4.2.

4.2 The medical districts

The basic reporting unit for disease data in Iceland is the medical district. As one might expect for a study period of 80 years, there have been many changes in boundary locations and numbers of medical districts, and our first task is to tie the data reported in the Appendix to the appropriate geographical locations. Unfortunately, detailed maps of medical districts are not available, and we have worked from source material in the following way.

The Icelandic unit roughly equivalent to the English parish or the American township is the *hreppur* (commune). Medical districts are

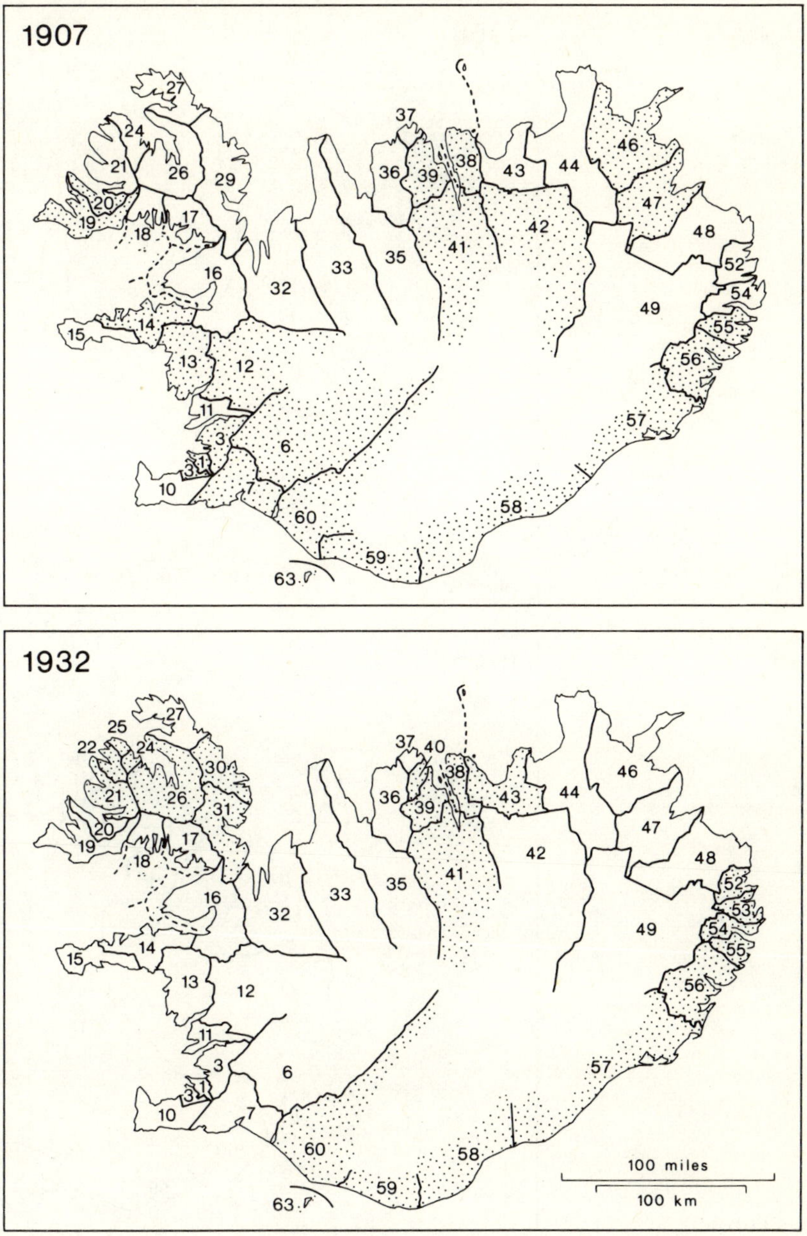

Fig. 4.1 (contd)

composed of *hreppar*. Sometimes a particular *hreppur* will be split between medical districts, but this tends to be the exception rather than the rule. Major revisions of the boundaries of medical districts were undertaken in the following years 1875, 1899, 1907, 1932 and 1955. With the exception of 1875, at these revisions, legal documents were prepared detailing which *hreppar* comprised which medical districts. Using these legal documents and base maps of the *hreppar* we have prepared the series of maps of the medical districts shown in Figure 4.1. The 1875 map shown in Figure 4.1 is less reliable. The legal document for this

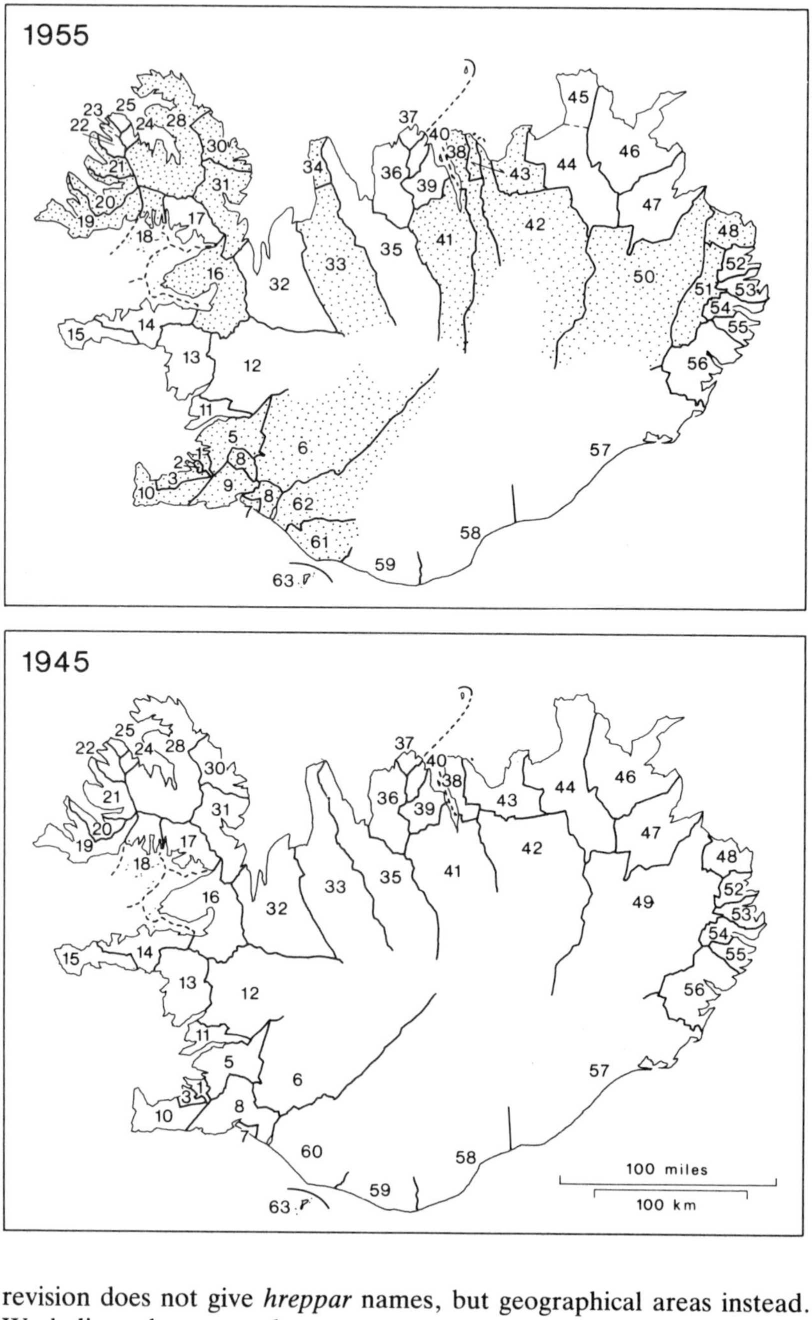

Fig. 4.1 (contd)

revision does not give *hreppar* names, but geographical areas instead. We believe, however, that any errors are minor. On the maps, those medical districts whose boundaries were changed at a given revision from their location at the revision immediately preceding are stippled.

The identity numbers of the medical districts given on Figure 4.1 correspond with Figure 4.2. At each major boundary revision, names of medical districts were often changed, and new districts were created by dividing or amalgamating old districts in response to population changes. The branching diagram indicates all the known district changes of this sort and their date of occurrence. Thus, from Figure 4.2, we see that medical district (1), Reykjavíkur, existed throughout the study period, but that district (3), Hafnarfjarðar, was first created in 1907 by an amalgamation of Kjósar (4) with part of Reykjavíkur (1). Minor boundary changes were sometimes made between the major revisions. Details of these changes are recorded in either *Heilbrigðisskýrslur* or *Mannfjöldaskýrslur*, and the changes are incorporated in Figure 4.2.

The inferential and modelling work on the diffusion waves contained in chapters 5–7 is based on the period 1945–75. This choice was made because, as noted, the description of the spread process contained in *Heilbrigðisskýrslur* is considerably weaker for the post-war, as opposed to pre-war period. We thought it was important to see how successfully models can use or detect the kind of spatial regularities we know to exist from the historical record in the pre-war period. The year 1945 lies mid-way between two major boundary revisions of the medical districts, those of 1932 and 1955. In 1945, the names of many medical districts were changed compared with 1932, but boundary changes were minimal. Changes in boundaries since 1945 are documented, and we have had no difficulty in defining the consistent set of medical districts shown on the 1945 map of Figure 4.1. We have employed these districts for all the analytical work covering the period 1945–70 and in the Appendix for the data tables of that period. The data tables in the Appendix for other dates are given for the medical districts existing at the boundary revision then in force.

4.3 The epidemic waves (1896–1975)

The diagrams, Figures 4.3–4.18, have been produced in a standard form. The last diagram of each set is the simplest; it uses proportional circles to record the total number of cases reported in each medical district during the course of the epidemic. The histograms show (a) the time series of reported cases for each month of the wave for Iceland as a whole, with the sample Pearson measures of skewness ($\sqrt{b_1}$) and kurtosis (b_2) of the histogram, and (b) the time series of reported cases by month for Reykjavíkur. To define $\sqrt{b_1}$ and b_2, let x_t denote the number of measles cases reported in month t for Iceland. The mean lag time in months from the start of an epidemic until all attacked areas are reached is given by (coding the starting month as $t = 1$)

$$\bar{t} = \sum_{t=1}^{T} t x_t / n, \qquad (4.1)$$

where T is the number of months in the epidemic and

$$n = \sum_{t} x_t .$$

The rth central moment about $\bar{t}$ may be written as

$$m_r = \sum_{t=1}^{T} [(t - \bar{t})^r x_t] / n , \qquad (4.2)$$

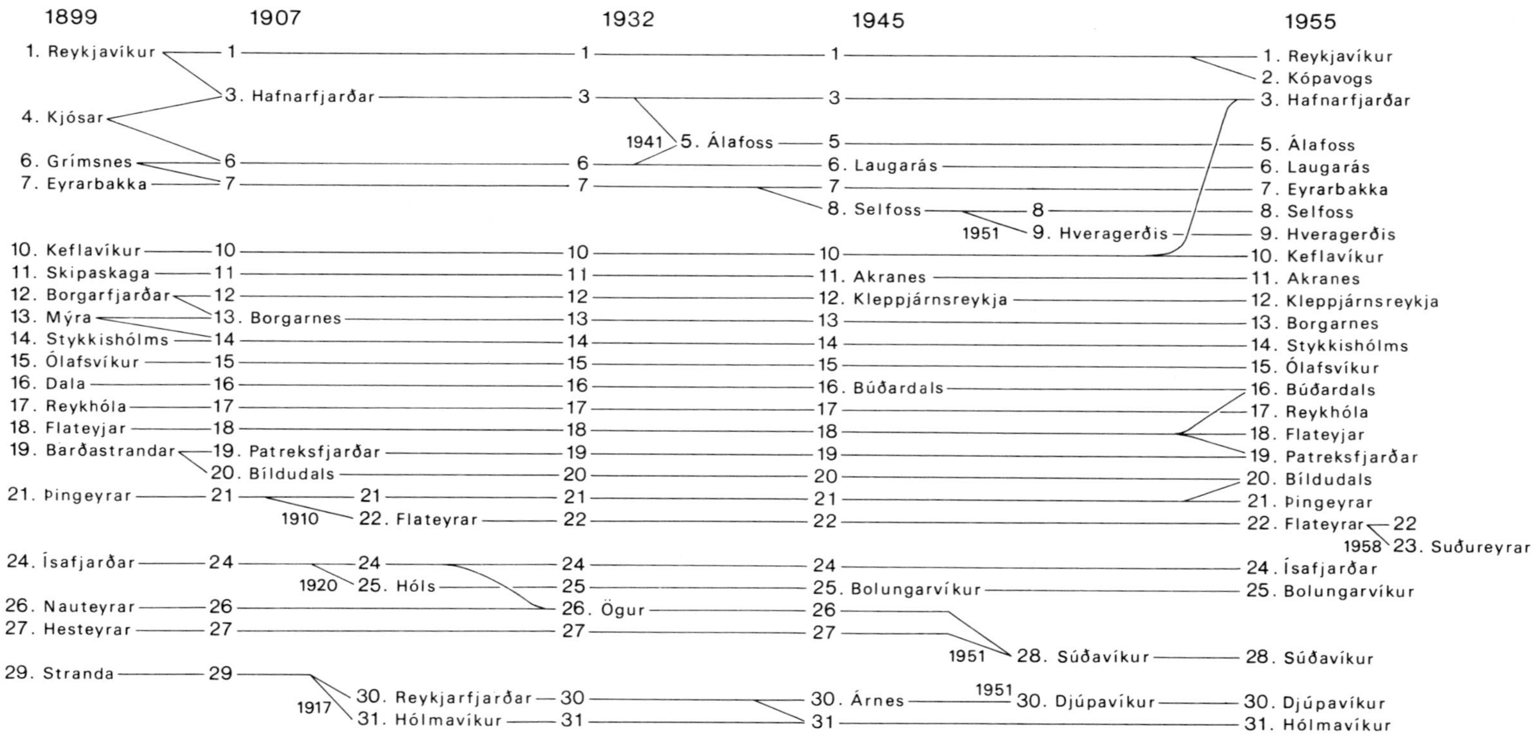
1899
1907
1932
1945
1955
1. Reykjavíkur
3. Hafnarfjarðar
4. Kjósar
6. Grímsnes
7. Eyrarbakka
10. Keflavíkur
11. Skipaskaga
12. Borgarfjarðar
13. Mýra
14. Stykkishólms
15. Ólafsvíkur
16. Dala
17. Reykhóla
18. Flateyjar
19. Barðastrandar
21. Þingeyrar
24. Ísafjarðar
26. Nauteyrar
27. Hesteyrar
29. Stranda
13. Borgarnes
19. Patreksfjarðar
20. Bíldudals
1910
22. Flateyrar
1920
25. Hóls
1917
30. Reykjarfjarðar
31. Hólmavíkur
1941
5. Álafoss
26. Ögur
6. Laugarás
8. Selfoss
11. Akranes
12. Kleppjárnsreykja
16. Búðardals
25. Bolungarvíkur
30. Árnes
1951
9. Hveragerðis
1951
28. Súðavíkur
1951
30. Djúpavíkur
1. Reykjavíkur
2. Kópavogs
3. Hafnarfjarðar
5. Álafoss
6. Laugarás
7. Eyrarbakka
8. Selfoss
9. Hveragerðis
10. Keflavíkur
11. Akranes
12. Kleppjárnsreykja
13. Borgarnes
14. Stykkishólms
15. Ólafsvíkur
16. Búðardals
17. Reykhóla
18. Flateyjar
19. Patreksfjarðar
20. Bíldudals
21. Þingeyrar
22. Flateyrar
1958
23. Suðureyrar
24. Ísafjarðar
25. Bolungarvíkur
28. Súðavíkur
30. Djúpavíkur
31. Hólmavíkur

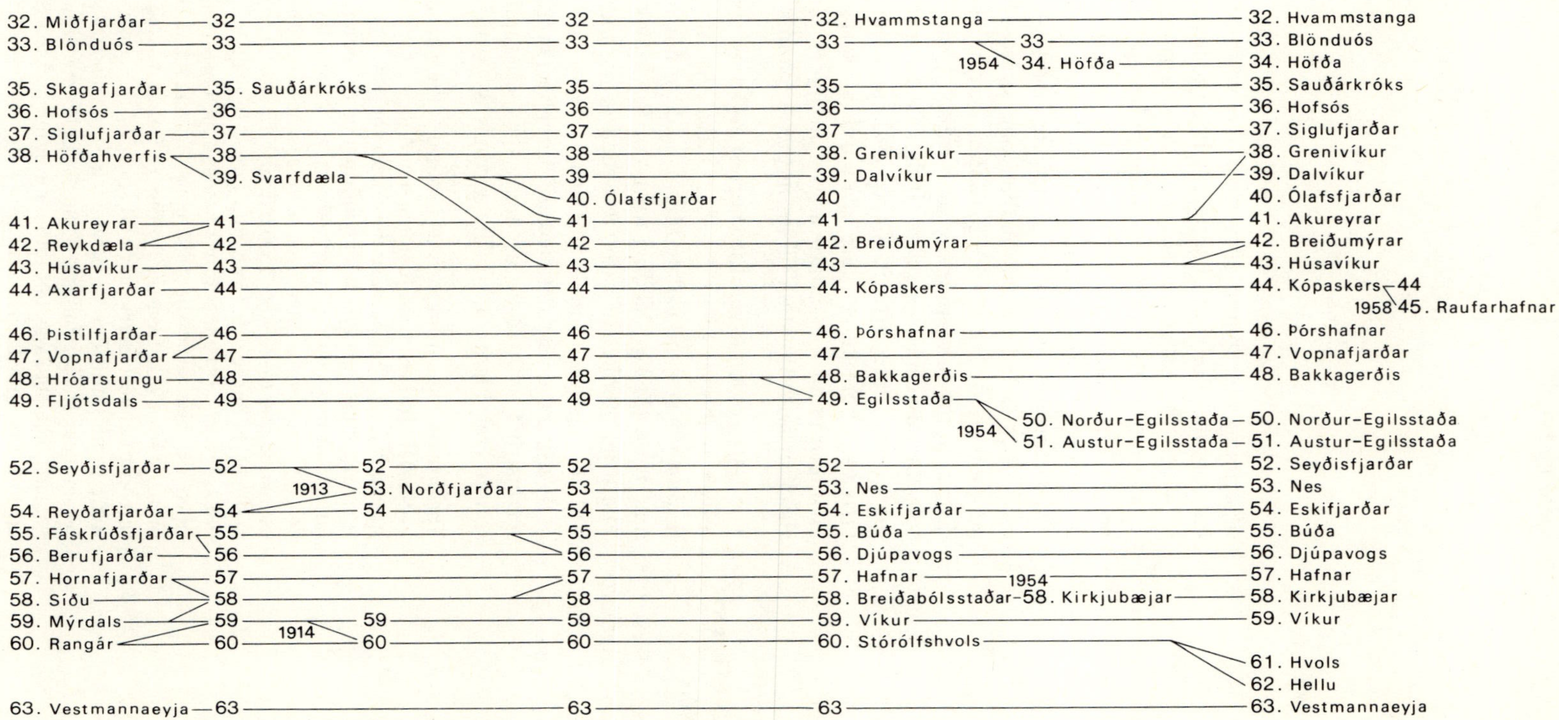

Fig. 4.2 Changes in medical district names from 1899 to 1958 shown as a branching diagram. Numbers correspond with the areas shown in Figure 4.1.

yielding finally

$$\sqrt{b_1} = \frac{m_3}{m_2^{3/2}}, \tag{4.3}$$

and

$$b_2 = \frac{m_4}{m_2^2}. \tag{4.4}$$

The bond diagrams have been constructed from the written reports describing the spatial spread of the various epidemics. The arrows indicate the direction of spread, while the numbers indicate the months in which the disease was reported as arriving in the medical district concerned. Although the coastline of Iceland has been omitted from the bond maps, they are drawn at the scale both of the accompanying proportional circles map and of Figure 4.1. They may, thus, be superimposed on the appropriate medical district base. Several epidemics lasted for more than one year. The convention has been adopted on the bond maps that links showing the arrivals of measles in a district in the first epidemic year are solid, and links showing arrivals in subsequent years are pecked. If the disease spread to a given place more than once, each arrival is recorded, and the month numbers of the arrivals, where known, are given in their serial order. Any ambiguities in interpreting the month arrival numbers can be resolved by cross-checking with the data tables in the Appendix of the book.

4.3.1 The early epidemic waves

Wave I: April to November 1904 (Figure 4.3)

The 1904 epidemic was the shortest and most spatially confined of the 16 waves analysed. In its seven months' duration, it spread only to the fishing villages and isolated farmsteads of north-west Iceland, and at no time were the two leading towns of Reykjavík and Akureyri affected. The total number of cases recorded in the public health report is 822, with an unknown number of deaths.

By using the very detailed account given in this report, it is possible to reconstruct with some accuracy the geographical pattern of measles spread (see Figure 4.3). The account is worth reproducing verbatim:

> The disease came from Norway in April to the whaling stations in Hesteyrar and Ísafjarðar. In Hesteyrar it stopped and there were no further infections, but it spread in Ísafjarðar because the doctor there was not informed at an early date. It spread most rapidly after a confirmation ceremony at Eyri in Seyðisfjörður [a farmstead and church in Ísafjarðar] on 22nd May. The disease caught hold despite preventive measures and reached Ísafjörður in June. The doctor estimated that there were 1500 patients, but he knew of only 23 deaths. It spread to Þingeyrar but reached only four farms. In Dala, it affected only one farm. The disease reached Nauteyrar in June, and the doctor said most people who did not catch the disease in the 1882 epidemic caught it then. In July, measles was brought by a boy from Ísafjörður to Látrar í Aðalvík in Hesteyrar, where it spread to almost every home in some of the communes, but not in others. It went from Ísafjörður to Stranda in June and reached most homes in four communes. Then a Faroese fishing vessel came with sick men to Siglufjörður in August. The ship was put into quarantine and the disease did not spread. The doctors say the disease was generally mild and deaths few. The doctor in

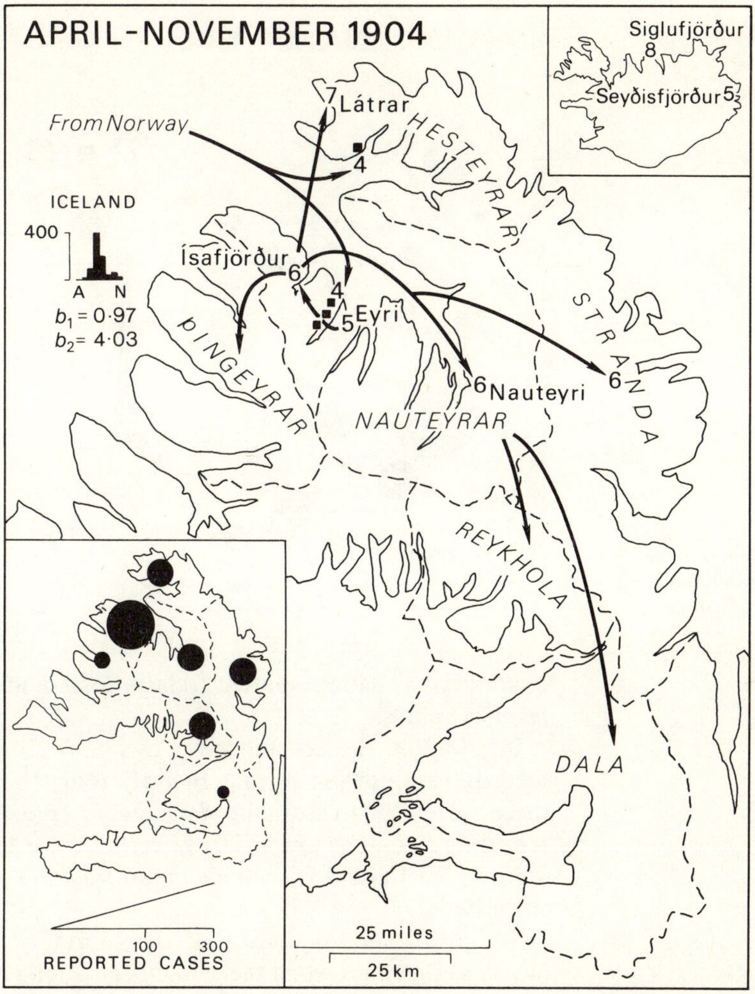

Fig. 4.3 Spread of the epidemic of 1904. Squares indicate whaling stations. In this and each of the following figures (Figures 4.3–4.18 inclusive) the circle areas are proportional to the total number of measles cases reported in each medical district affected by the epidemic. The histograms give the number of reported cases by month for Iceland as a whole, with the sample Pearson measures of skewness ($\sqrt{b_1}$) and kurtosis (b_2). Note that, on the diagrams, we have omitted the radical sign from $\sqrt{b_1}$ for clarity. A separate histogram for Reykjavíkur is drawn where data are available. Where arrows are shown, these indicate the *known* direction of spread as reported by medical officers of health for each district in their annual reports. The numbers (1 through 12) against medical districts and place names indicate the month of the year in which cases were first recorded. See text for further details. All maps are based on data and reports in the annual volumes of *Heilbrigðisskýrslur*. Medical districts not affected by an epidemic are stippled.

Ísafjarðar said the disease got worse as it went on. The most common complications were ear infections, diarrhoea and pneumonia, which caused most of the deaths. In May [of the following year], a Norwegian seaman came to Seyðisfjörður in Seyðisfjarðar, but he was isolated in hospital and the disease did not spread.

(*Skýrslur um heilsufar og heilbrigðismálefni á Íslandi,* 1904, p. 87)

The account underlines three factors of prime importance in understanding both the maps and the descriptions of the epidemic waves which follow. First, it highlights the role of a single infected individual (the index case) whose spatial mobility plays a crucial part in starting an outbreak in a given community. Fishermen (or the crew of whalers in the 1904 outbreak) are of special interest in the Icelandic case. Second, it indicates the importance of communal activities which bring susceptibles together at a critical period; the confirmation ceremony at Eyri on 22 May 1904 illustrates this point. Third, it describes the countermeasures taken to control the spread of disease by placing ships in

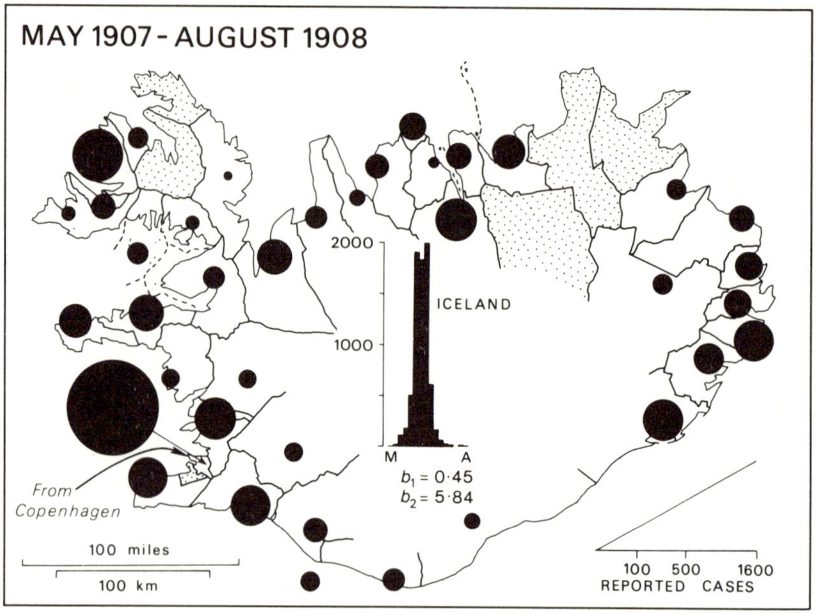

Fig. 4.4 Spread of the epidemic of 1907–8. See caption for Figure 4.3.

quarantine, isolating an infected farmstead, and by putting patients into fever hospitals.

In addition, the account gives us one of our few indications in the records of reporting errors. In Ísafjörður, the doctor estimated that there were 1,500 cases; the data record (see Appendix) gives 310, a reporting rate of as low as 20 per cent if the estimate is to believed (cf. sections 3.5.1 and 6.4.3, where a reporting rate of 40 per cent or more is suggested).

We also gain some idea of the mortality that could accompany measles epidemics when there had been a long gap since the last major epidemic (in 1882). In this context, the following quotation from *Heilbrigðisskýrslur* (1911–20, p. xxvi) is relevant.

> Although the figures are not completely reliable as regards the earlier epidemics, and allowing for the fact that the disease [measles] varies greatly in severity, it is obvious that after 1882, a major change occurred in the death rate. The disease is no longer accompanied by high mortality as it was before. . . . Measles will be a fatal illness in most places when it recurs very infrequently.

Indeed, as Figure 3.9 shows, the 1882 epidemic was a major killer (of the order of 1,700 deaths; the 1846 epidemic produced 2,026 deaths).

Wave II: May 1907 to August 1908 (Figure 4.4)

A 2½-year gap followed the end of the 1904 epidemic. When the next wave came, it was much larger. Unlike its predecessor, it affected all parts of the island, and was not confined to any particular region. First cases were reported in the early summer of 1907. The epidemic reached its peak that winter and persisted until the late summer of the following year. The total number of cases reported was 7,398; 354 deaths were believed to have occurred (cf. quotation below). The attack rate was 89.2 cases per 1,000 population, compared with 10.4 for wave I.

Measles were first introduced into Reykjavík from Copenhagen, and the disease spread rapidly to all districts. As with the 1904 outbreak, the start of the epidemic can be traced in detail from the official public health reports, viz.:

> Measles came in the early summer of 1907; first to Reyjavík by ship from Copenhagen. Persons sick on ship were taken to the isolation hospital and those who had not had measles previously were isolated. Healthy ones were let out if they promised they had had measles before. Among these was a young man who went to Stykkishólmur. Shortly after, came news of measles in Stykkishólmur. It was spread by the young man. . . . Stykkishólmur was isolated and visitors to the town were confined in homes where there was no-one of measles age. They were let out of the town in two weeks' time. Among them was a young girl from Reykjavík. She went home with an isolation certificate from the doctor in Stykkishólmur. Now Reykjavík was being visited by the King [of Denmark] and the town was full of people. It appears that the girl had a mild case of measles and went into the streets before this was appreciated. . . . The disease spread speedily in Reykjavík and could not be contained. From there, the infection spread rapidly over the whole country, especially from October 1907–February 1908. It then died away slowly, terminating in August 1908. Deaths from the disease and complications are not known, but most doctors say it was rather severe and a number of children died.
>
> (*Heilbrigðisskýrslur*, 1907–8, pp. 4–5)

The report goes on to show that the girl who went out into the crowded streets to see the King, and so triggered off the Reykjavík epidemic, had been no less infectious in Stykkishólmur. While in quarantine there, she was visited by an old woman who, because of her age, was assumed to have already had the disease. This turned out to be untrue; the virus infected the old woman and soon spread widely around that community. Since no news was sent to Reykjavík immediately, the link between the two cases was unsuspected.

Only small areas in the north-west fjords (including areas heavily affected in the preceding wave) and the north-east of Iceland escaped wave II. Detailed statistical returns are not available for this epidemic and, thus, the contact pattern cannot be established with accuracy.

Wave III: April 1916 to May 1917 (Figure 4.5)

An interval of nearly eight years separated the second and third waves. A scatter of cases had been reported in the intervening years (56 notifications in all), but no major epidemics had occurred. The long gap may be attributable in part to the decreased shipping contacts with Iceland once World War I had broken out in Europe, but a more important factor were the stringent isolation measures adopted once a measles case had been diagnosed. These preventive measures were taken on the initiative of the local doctor in each community:

> In the year 1912, measles were carried from Höfn to Mýrdals and infected three farmsteads. Stefán Gíslason set about taking precautions and stamped them out. In the year 1913, they were carried to Reykjavík from Denmark, and had appeared in three households before preventive measures were taken. Jón Hj. Sigurðsson isolated the sufferers in hospital and stamped out the disease.
>
> (*Heilbrigðisskýrslur,* 1911–20, p. xxiii)

Prevention also depended on a measure of self-help by the threatened

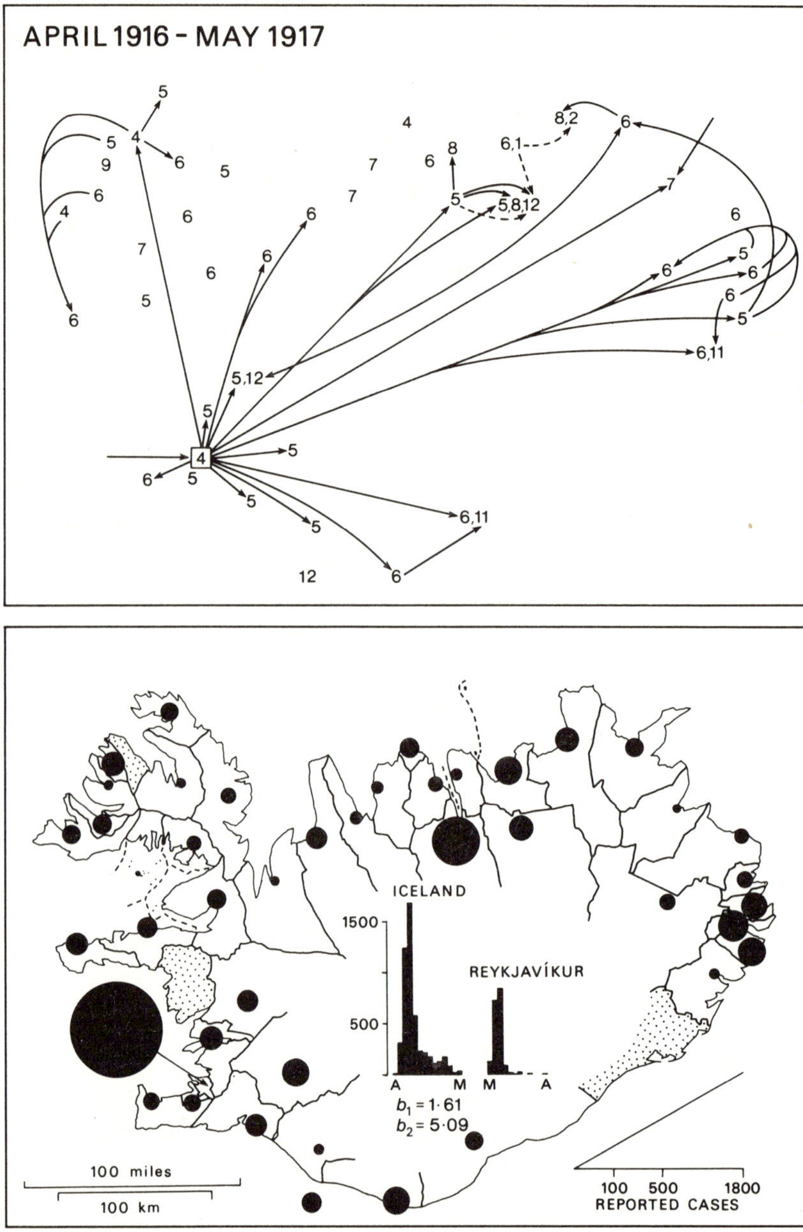

Fig. 4.5 Spread of the epidemic of 1916–17. See caption for Figure 4.3.

population. The report for Fljótsdals argues that '. . . it is easy in the countryside to avoid the disease'. Certainly this appears to have been true where those in isolated farmsteads were aware of the danger and were able to cut down contact with known centres of infection. Nevertheless, in some districts infection continued to penetrate. In Axarfjarðar, farmsteads which had isolated themselves effectively from the 1882 and 1907 epidemics were struck and people in their eighties caught the disease. One predisposing factor appears to be the high degree of contagion. For example, the report for Blönduós draws attention to the ease with which the infection can be spread: 'it is not necessary to have direct contact between an affected and unaffected person . . . a single schoolboy talked with farm people out in the open, but infected the whole household nonetheless' (*Heilbrigðisskýrslur*, 1911–20, p. 70*). Other reports speak of known contacts occurring when two people met on a country track.

The third wave was of somewhat lower intensity than its predecessor, with 4,944 reported cases (an attack rate of 55.0 per 1,000 population). Fewer deaths (118) resulted, a rate of 23.9 per 1,000 cases of measles. The epidemic reached its peak in July 1916, only four months after onset, and declined steadily over the succeeding year. The strongly marked skewness and speed of spread may well reflect the exceptionally long gap between the waves. This would allow a considerable build-up of susceptibles. The geographical pattern of spread is an intricate one. The virus was introduced into Reykjavík by a sailor from Norway in April 1916. The disease spread within the next two months both to other centres within the south-west and to major regional centres in the rest of Iceland. The bond maps show how these secondary centres acted as repeater stations from which further diffusion of the disease occurred. Thus, cases in Ísafjarðar spread measles into other districts in the north-west (for example, Nauteyrar and Olafsvíkur in June 1916), while cases in Akureyrar spread the disease into other northern districts (Reykdæla and Höfðahverfis in August 1916). Reykjavík continued to be the main centre of spread for the remainder of the year. Although cases continued to be reported until May 1917, it is important to note that all districts except one affected by the epidemic began to record cases by August 1916 (only four months after the start of the epidemic). The exception was Vestmannæyja which reported its first case in December.

Wave IV: June 1924 to August 1926 (Figure 4.6)

The gap of seven years which separated the third and fourth waves was similar to that between waves II and III. For the reasons given under wave III, this long gap made it likely that the epidemic, when it came, would be widespread. This fourth wave yielded 6,130 reported cases, giving an attack rate of 61.2 cases per 1,000 population. Thirty-four deaths were attributed to measles, a mortality rate of 5.6 per 1,000 reported cases.

The most distinctive temporal feature of the fourth wave is its bimodal shape. The outbreak began in June 1924 and peaked in October. This was followed by a small secondary wave, starting in the summer of 1925 and peaking in November. A high proportion of the cases in the main wave occurred in Reykjavíkur; the smaller secondary wave comprised lesser, but locally severe, outbreaks in the north and east. The main wave again started in Reykjavík with an infected case from Bergen in Norway. As in the third wave, other regional centres were affected within the next couple of months, but the pattern of subsequent spread is more complex. Secondary reinfection of communities, after the first attack had been contained, is a feature of 1925. These reinfections are due mainly to contacts within Iceland, but in one

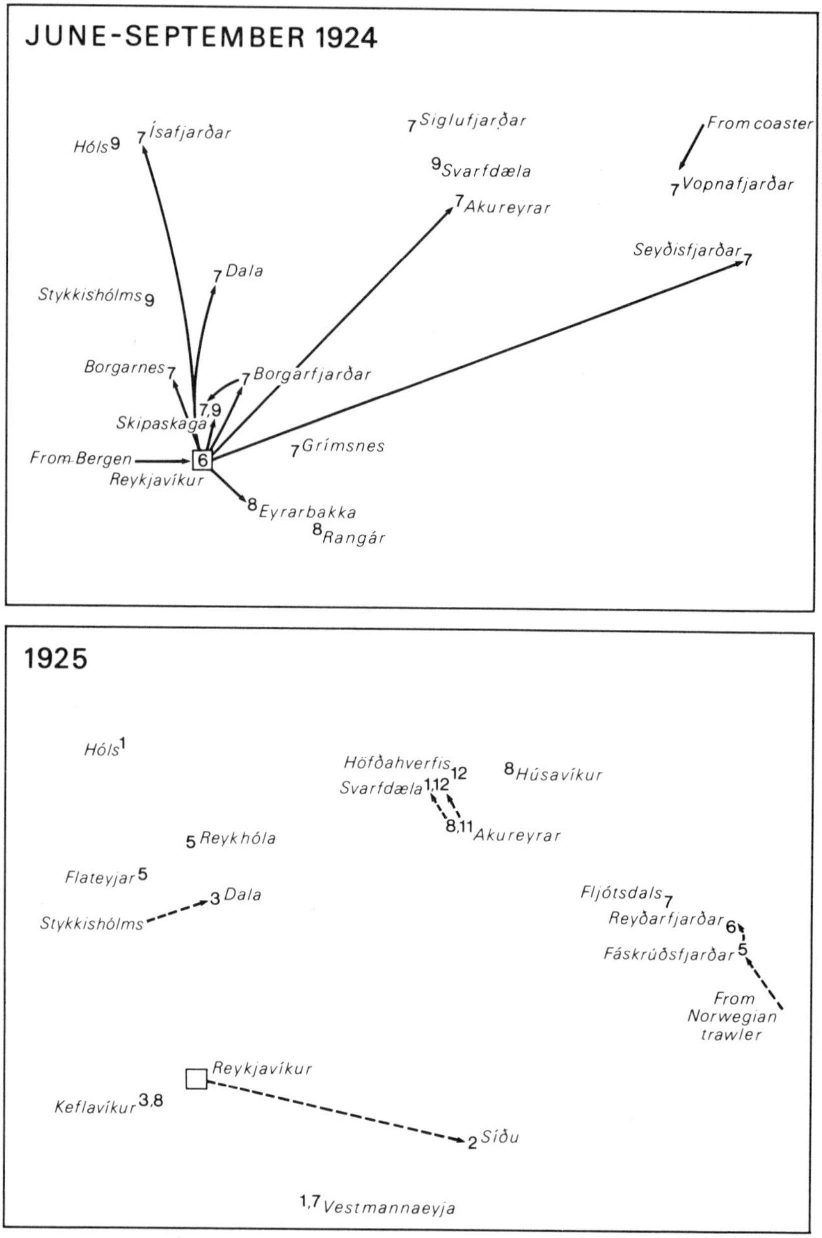

Fig. 4.6 Spread of the epidemic of 1924–6. See caption for Figure 4.3.

eastern district (Fáskrúðsfjarðar), cases were reported from May 1925 as a result of contact with an infected crew member from a Norwegian trawler.

By the 1920s, the falling death-rate from measles was allowing a more measured attitude to be taken to the appearance of the disease. The doctor's report from Svarfdæla reflects this:

> It is doubtful whether anti-measles precautions are worthwhile. In my opinion it would be desirable for measles to occur every year . . . They are more severe if long periods elapse between outbreaks.
>
> (*Heilbrigðisskýrslur*, 1921–5, p. 109*)

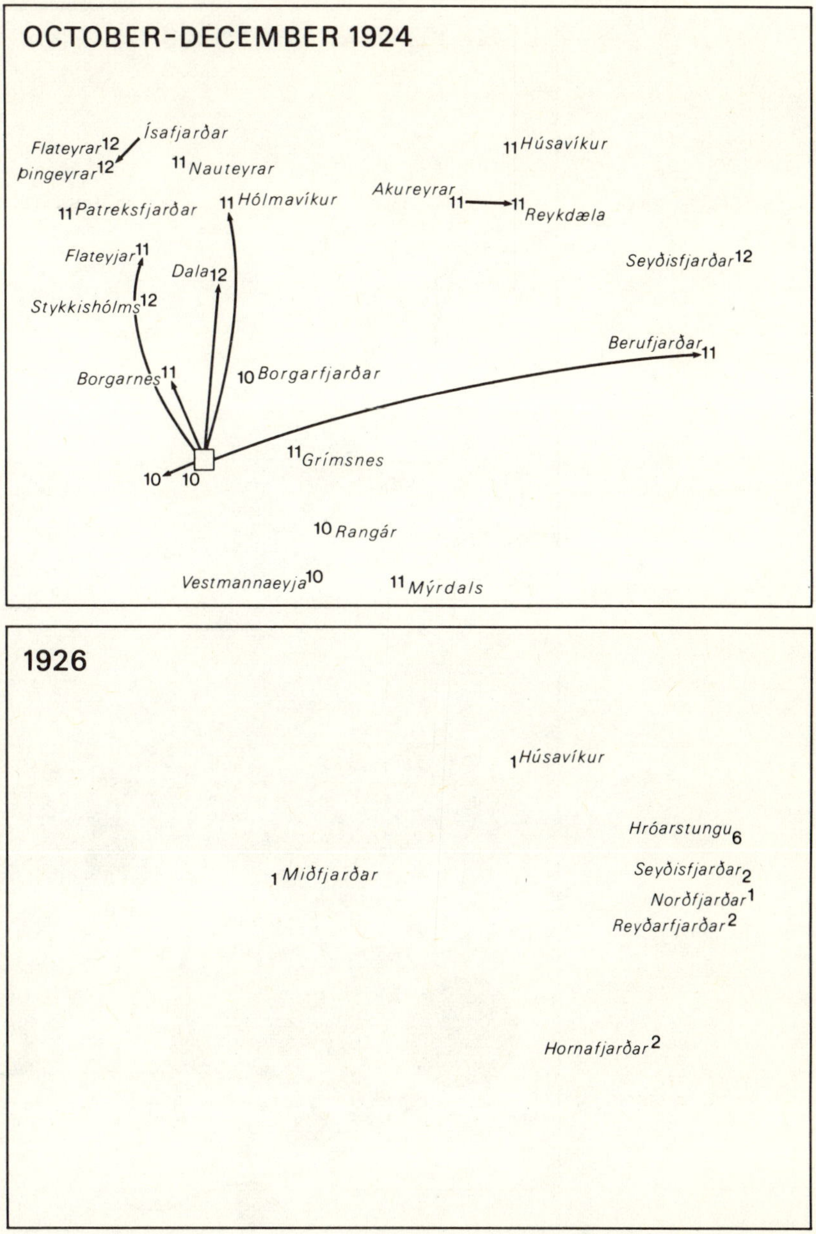

Fig. 4.6 (contd)

This change in control policy – away from containment and isolation, and towards exposure – reflected the realisation that adults are more severely affected than children, and that the economic loss attributable to the illness is thus a higher one. In districts which had not been affected since 1907, the number of immune people (i.e., those who had already contracted the disease) was small, so that an exceptional burden of transport fell on them during epidemic years when they alone brought in essential goods from other trading centres. The problem is summarised by Sigurjón Jónsson:

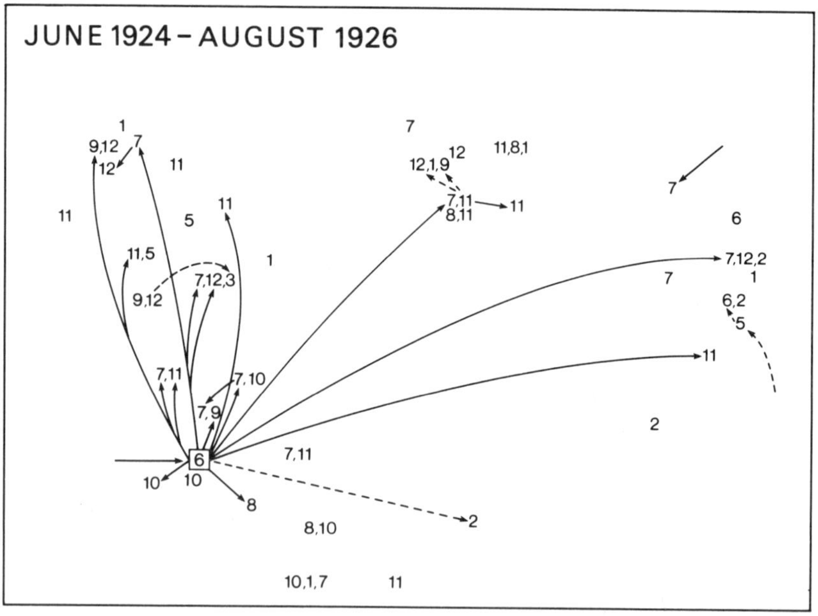

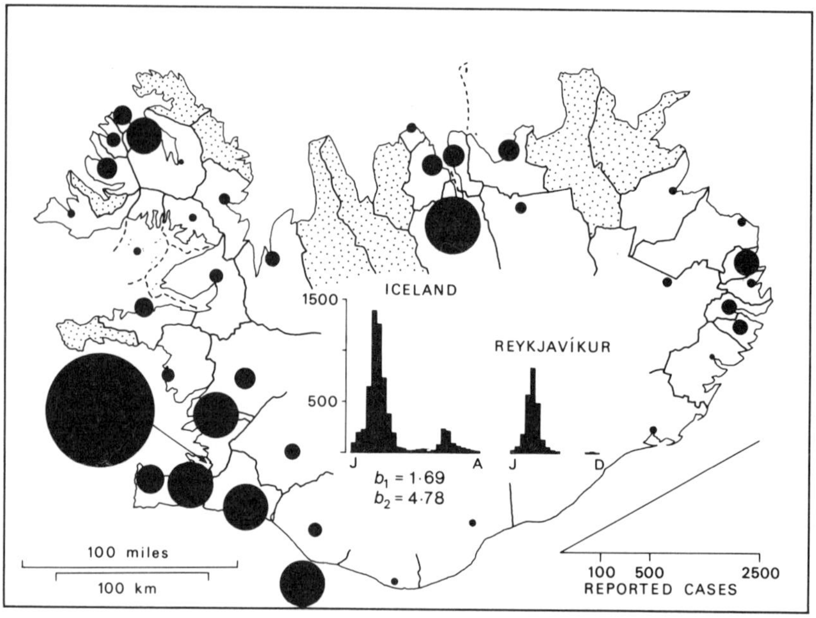

Fig. 4.6 (contd)

It seems very likely that the final result of widespread avoidance of the disease by preventive action will be a critically severe nationwide epidemic, as happened before, where all the inhabitants of a homestead are struck down together, and no-one can shield himself or assist in the nursing of others. The experience of past years shows that epidemics are less harmful in their effects if only short periods elapse between them . . .

(*Heilbrigðisskýrslur*, 1921–5, p. xiii)

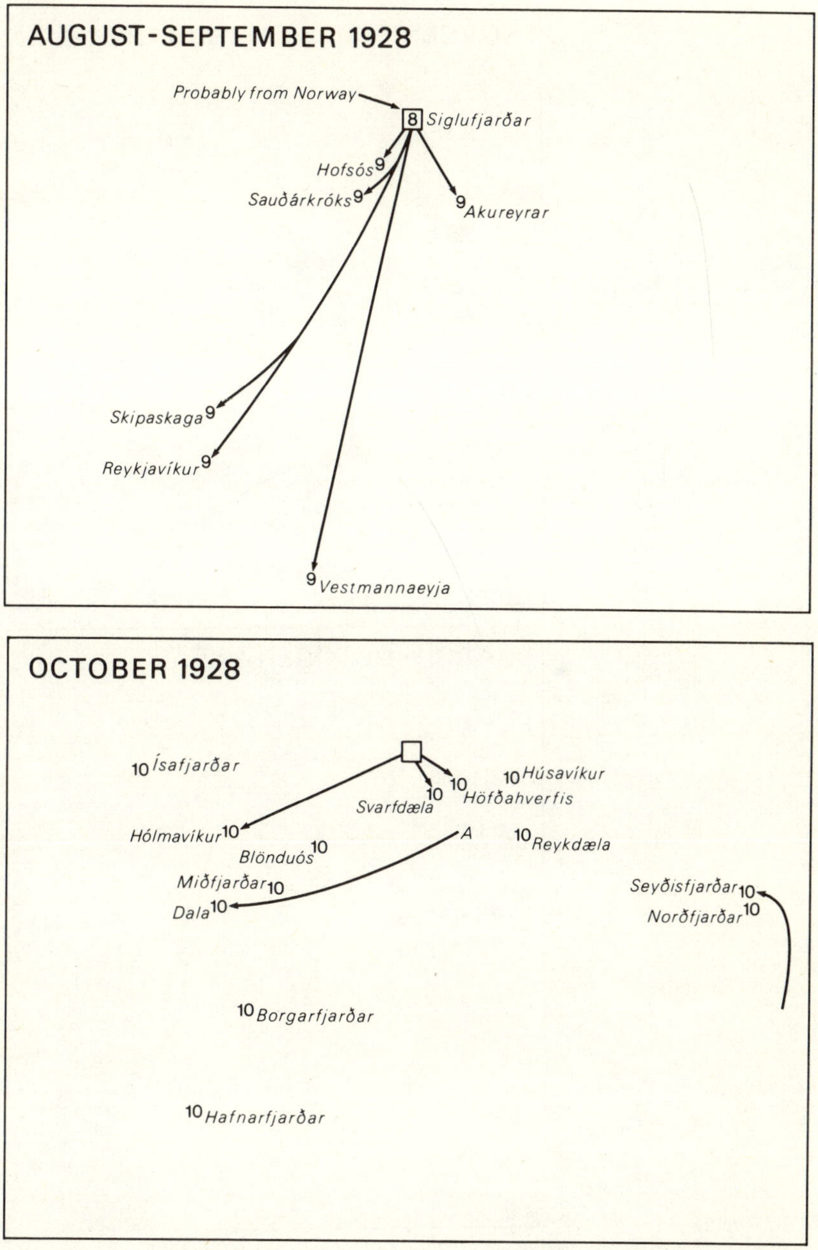

Fig. 4.7 Spread of the epidemic of 1928–9. See caption for Figure 4.3.

Wave V: August 1928 to December 1929 (Figure 4.7)

The fifth wave came hard on the heels of the fourth, separated from it by a gap of only two years. It is not surprising to find, therefore, that this wave was both less intense and less prolonged than its predecessor. The total number of reported cases was 5,317, an attack rate of 50.8 per 1,000 population. The number of deaths attributed to measles was 16, a death-rate of 3.0 per 1,000 cases. The wave had a single peak in January 1929.

The pattern of diffusion through the Icelandic community was a distinctive one. The starting point in this wave was Siglufjarðar on the

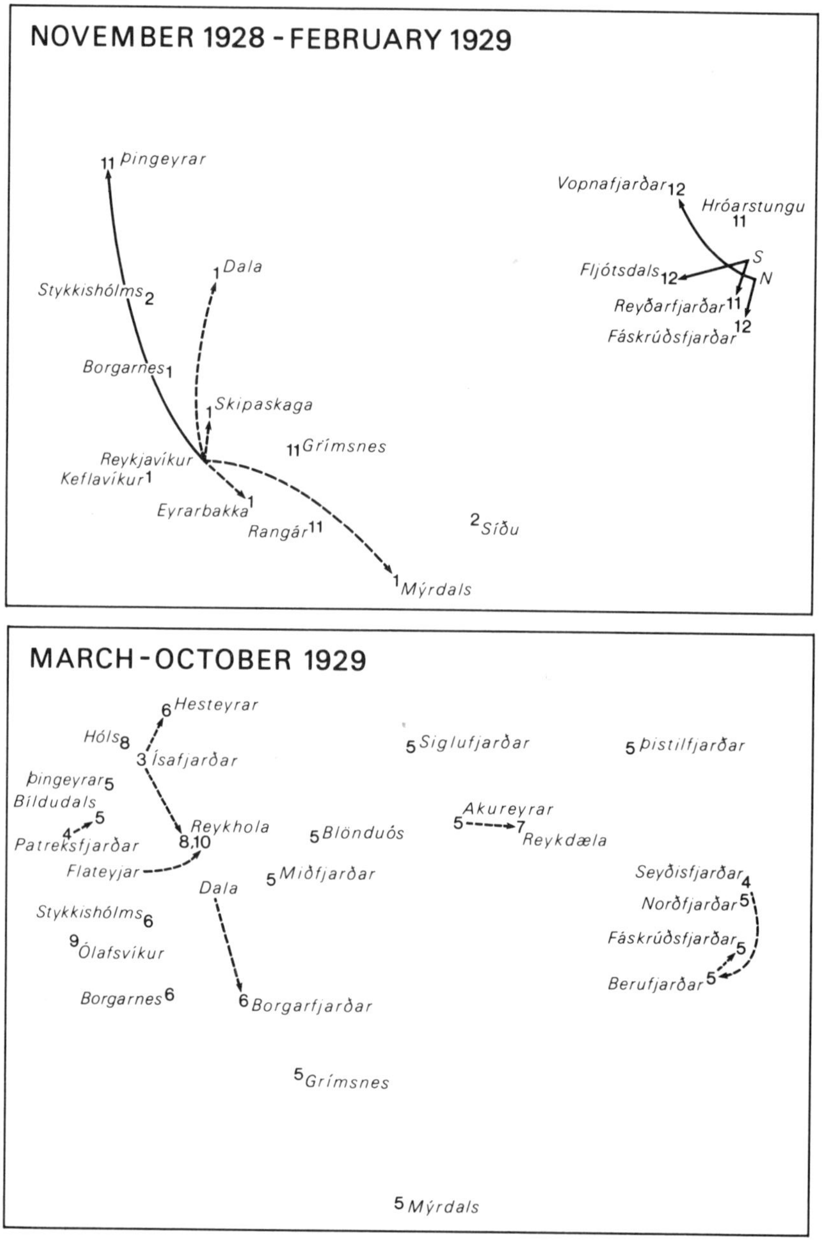

Fig. 4.7 (contd)

north coast, with an introduction from Norway into the fishing port of Siglufjörður. Within the next month, cases were being reported both from other districts in the same part of the north coast, and from Reykjavíkur and Vestmannaeyja in the south-west. Three separate subsystems can be identified thereafter: (a) continued spread from the original northern centre in the autumn of 1928 through the remaining northern districts; (b) secondary spread from Reykjavíkur in the winter months of 1928–9 to other western and south-western districts; and (c) spread between the eastern coastal districts, also in the winter months of 1928–9. The provenance of the third subsystem is not clear, but both

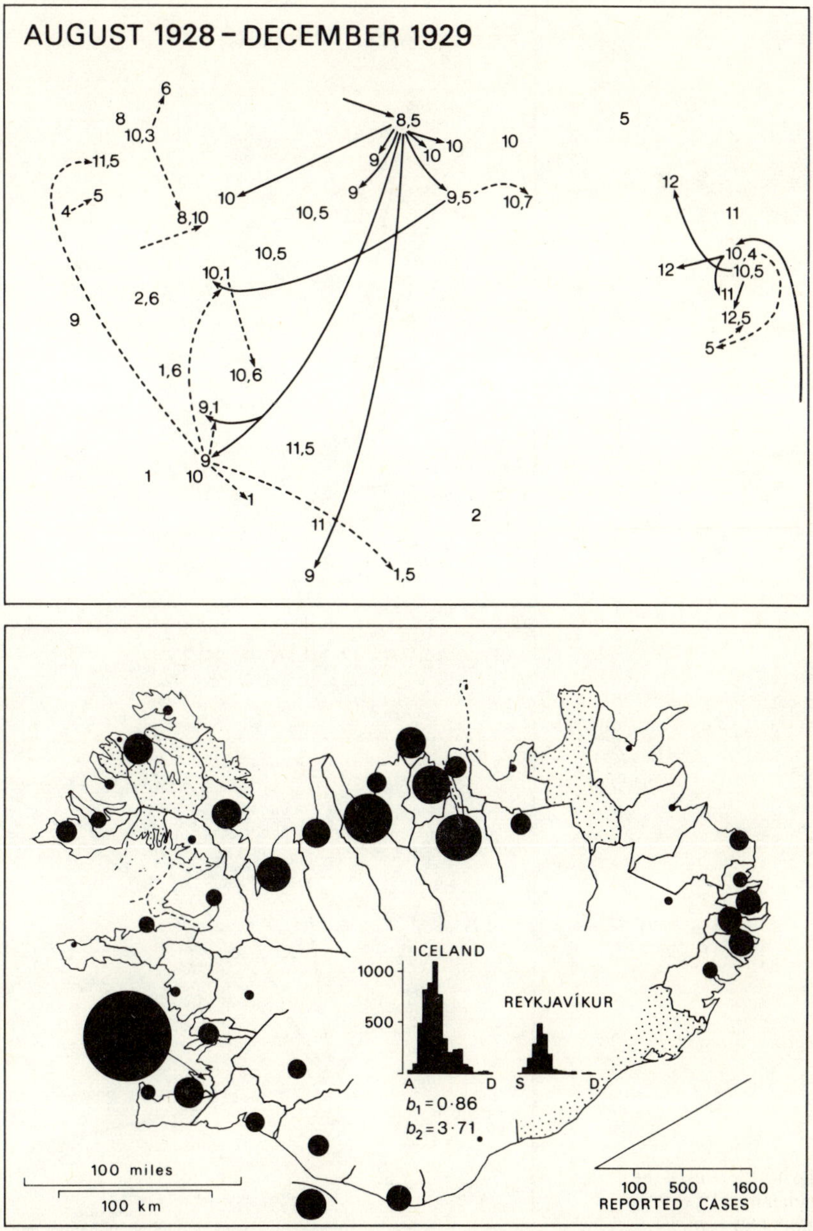

Fig. 4.7 (contd)

Seyðisfjarðar and Norðfjarðar were reporting cases in October 1928, presumably stemming from the original Siglufjarðar introduction.

The comments by country doctors on this epidemic point to the relative mildness of the disease and its progress by 'fits and starts' (Eyrarbakka) or 'travelling sluggishly' (Hólmavíkur) across the landscape. The ability of the measles virus to be transferred easily continued to attract comments. For example, the Hólmavíkur report describes the progress of a man who, claiming to have already had measles, walked around half the district. 'At one farmstead he only [briefly] met the couple who lived there . . . the children did not see the guest but . . . all

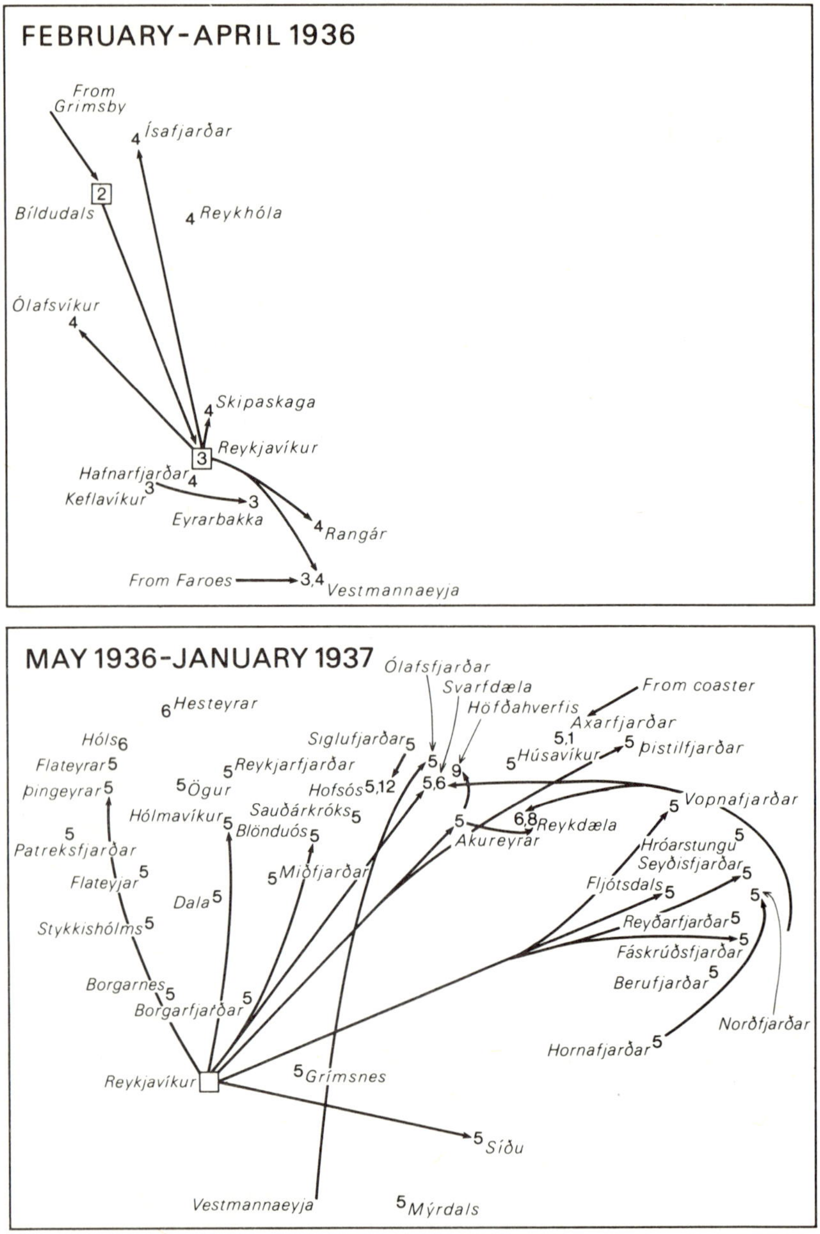

Fig. 4.8 Spread of the epidemic of 1936–7. See caption for Figure 4.3.

in the household caught measles at the same time (*Heilbrigðisskýrslur*, 1928, p. 9).

The mildness of the disease in some areas may well have affected the accuracy of the reported cases. The Reyðarfjarðar report (*Heilbrigðisskýrslur*, 1929, p. 25) suggests the 65 reported cases 'were demonstrably much too low, the mild cases being hardly noticed'. Again in Fáskrúðsfjarðar, the attacks were so mild that the doctor was not called, and the report acknowledges that 'I obtained the number of sufferers from an intelligent man who lives there' (*Heilbrigðisskýrslur*, 1929, p. 25).

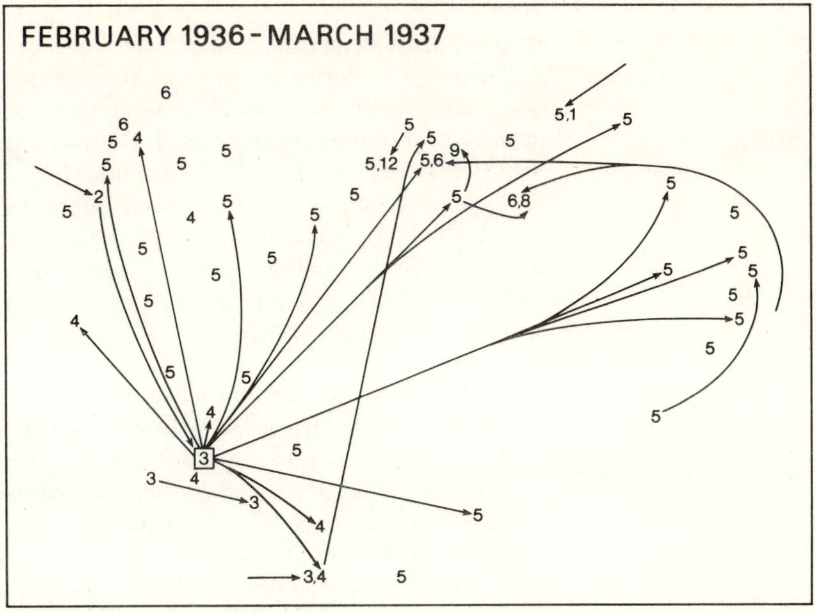

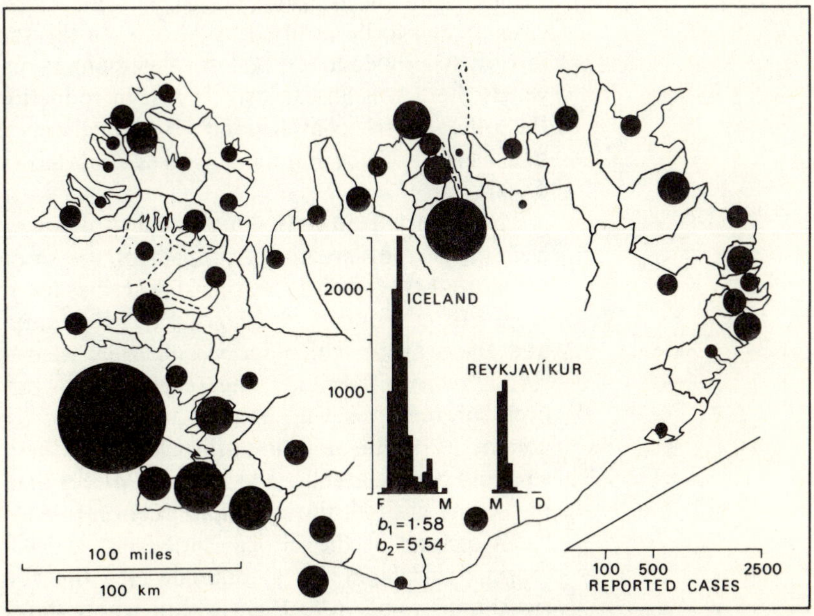

Fig. 4.8 (contd)

The assiduousness with which cases were reported also varied. The Höfðahverfis report declares that '. . . all sufferers have been accounted for, whether or not I was consulted' and that the names of victims were recorded '. . . so as to see later who had been suffering from measles' (*Heilbrigðisskýrslur*, 1928, p. 10). Where, however, the doctor was absent, the accuracy of the records was bound to suffer. In Seyðisfjörður, only four cases were recorded between April and June 1929 while the local doctor was on leave, although '. . . nearly all the households in the trading hamlet had been visited by measles' (*Heilbrigðisskýrslur*, 1929, p. 24). We thus know that under-reporting does occur, but the degree of error is very variable between both medical districts and epidemics.

The doctors' reports lay stress on the role of boat crews in passing the disease between the coastal settlements. Even after the wave had passed, quarantine arrangements for ships remained in force. Thus, the Siglufjarðar report for 1932 relates how boats were loaded under the supervision of the police to prevent infected crew members bringing measles ashore. Similarly, the Seyðisfjarðar report describes the work of the local 'committee for the prevention of disease' (*Heilbrigðisskýrslur*, 1932, p. 26) in placing quarantine orders on ships with crews suspected of having the disease.

Wave VI: February 1936 to March 1937 (Figure 4.8)

The only measles wave to hit Iceland in the 1930s was both intense and short-lived in comparison with the two waves that had preceded it. A total of 8,408 cases was reported within a 14-month period, an attack rate of 71.9 per 1,000 population. The number of deaths reported as due to measles rose compared with wave V to 60 (a death rate of 7.1 per 1,000 reported cases).

The speed of spread of wave VI is shown dramatically in Figure 4.8. From Bíldudals, the infection was transferred to Reykjavíkur, where cases began to be notified by March. In the same month, measles was introduced independently into Vestmannaeyja. From April 1936 onwards there was an explosively fast introduction of the disease into all the other districts of Iceland. By May, only four districts remained unaffected and the number of cases reported in the month rose above 2,000.

The reports from individual medical districts give a particularly rich account of the spread and impact of the disease. That for Bíldudals (*Heilbrigðisskýrslur*, 1936, p. 26) describes the return of the fishing boat *Geysir* from Grimsby, England, on 11 February after a four-day voyage and the way in which individual crew members spread the disease through the settlement. The return home was marked by an intense cycle of reunions with family and friends; as the report laconically comments of one man (identified as G.O.) 'he had been in contact with so many people and been to so many places that it was impossible to get in contact with all those he had been in touch with'. We also obtain a clear picture of the critical index case (E. J.) from Bíldudals who 'popped his head for a moment into the room adjacent to G.O.'s sickroom', went on to Reykjavíkur where 'he subsequently fell ill with measles and the disease spread out from there'.

A second characteristic of the reports for 1936 is that they make the first mention of index cases being carried by long-distance bus. The arrival of measles at Þistilfjarðar in May and at Axarfjarðar in August is traced to a bus driver and a bus passenger respectively. With long journeys, the virus could be spread to all passengers and the Síðu report suggests that, although 'one infected person joined the bus at Reykjavík, he had infected everyone else on board the bus before it was realised he was ill' (*Heilbrigðisskýrslur*, 1936, p. 31; cf. section 5.5.4). Education was also becoming an increasingly important medium for the transmission process. For example, measles was brought back to Fljótsdals by two girls who went to study in Reykjavík and returned home with the disease at the end of the summer term.

By the 1930s, a number of Icelandic physicians were again trying to cure those suffering from the disease or to give patients immunity to the disease by injecting convalescent serum. (This strategy had been first tried in the 1924–6 epidemic but was largely abandoned in 1928–9). After the epidemic, doctors in six of the country districts report that they had tried such injections, generally with encouraging results. The Borgarnes medical officer complained, however, that '... though it seemed to be a sure preventive, it was so expensive that very few were able to avail themselves of it' (*Heilbrigðisskýrslur*, 1936, p. 26). Despite four decades of worldwide research, the efficacy of convalescent serum alone remains sufficiently unclear to provoke a recent *Lancet* editorial (28 October 1978) arguing for further clinical trials. In the Iceland 1936–7 epidemic, the number of cases treated was such a small fraction of the infected population that it must be doubtful if the sporadic experiments with convalescent serum had any major impact on the sequence of disease diffusion.

Wave VII: February 1943 to July 1944 (Figure 4.9)

The seventh measles wave arrived during World War II when Iceland was occupied by British and American forces. The external provenance of the disease is unknown but, given the severing of links with Denmark and Norway (both then German-occupied), we may speculate that the most likely source was allied servicemen stationed at the Keflavík air-base or at the Hvalfjörður naval base, both located in south-west Iceland. The precise epidemiological role of these non-Icelandic population enclaves is impossible to measure, but it is worth noting that, from wave VII onwards, one of them (Keflavík) remained a potential source for virus introduction (cf. section 5.5.2).

Like its predecessor, the seventh wave was relatively intense and lasted a little over a year. It came six years after the end of the 1936–7 epidemic and generated 7,155 cases, an attack rate of 56.8 cases per 1,000 population. The improvements in medical care (notably the sulpha drugs) over the decades are shown by the fact that only 18 deaths are ascribed to complications of measles such as pneumonia in this wave, a rate of only 2.5 per 1,000 recorded cases (one third of that in wave VI).

The outbreak appears to have originated in Reykjavík. It reached other parts of Iceland within three months of the starting date, making it the second fastest wave of those studied in terms of its spatial spread. As Figure 4.9 indicates, the recorded bonds form a clear pattern of direct links from the capital city to all parts of Iceland, with the exception of some of the eastern fjords. These were also reached by July 1943. Secondary connections between the northern and eastern districts persisted well into 1944. Contact patterns are generally fully reported, and 19 vectors can be plotted.

It is evident from the individual medical district reports that, by the 1943 epidemic, even social conventions had their place in the spread of

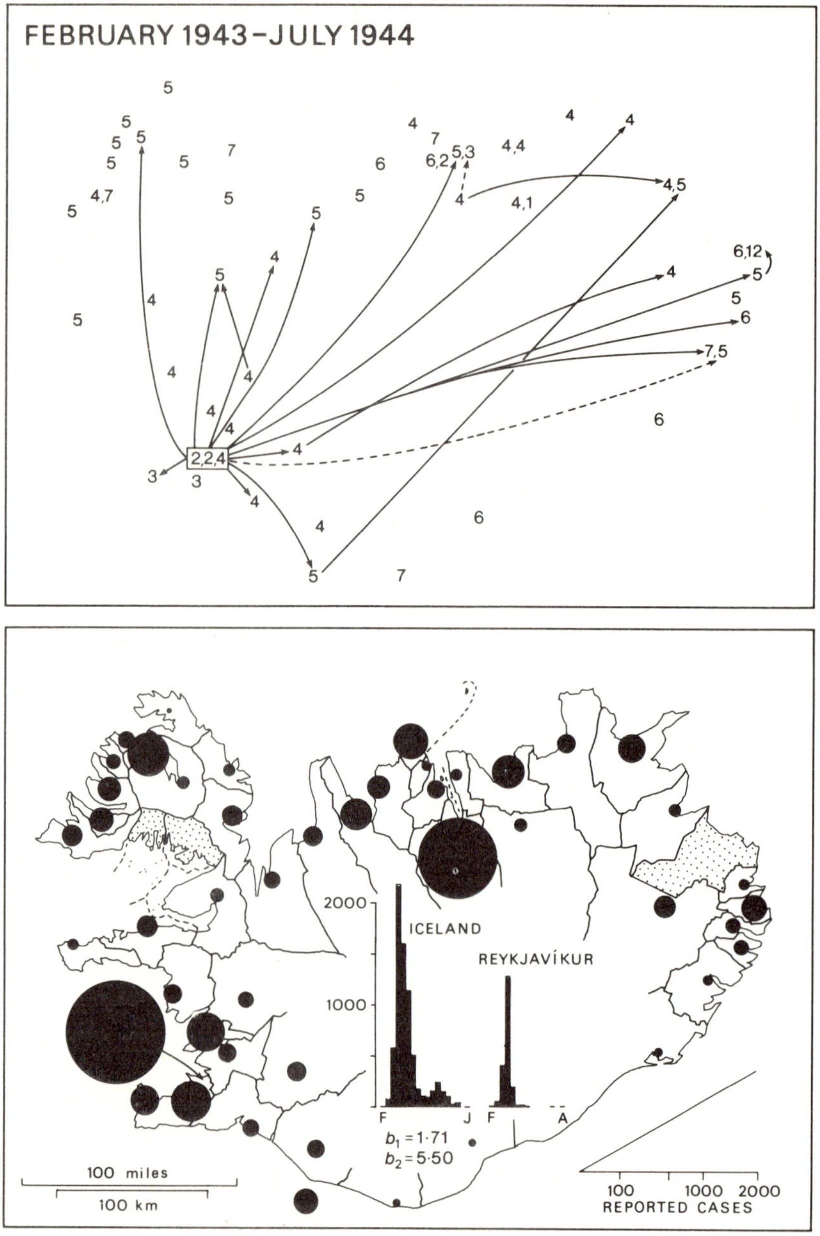

Fig. 4.9 Spread of the epidemic of 1943–4. See caption for Figure 4.3.

the disease. The submission by the medical officer for Vopnafjarðar vividly describes the plight of the young man from Foss who caught the infection while attending a local dance. He was unlucky enough to invite a girl already infected with measles to be his partner. In the words of the report, 'while he was standing in front of her, she was seized with a violent fit of coughing, so that there was a little delay before the invitation could be accepted' (*Heilbrigðisskýrslur*, 1943, p. 31). In such embarrassing moments are the links of a spatial diffusion process forged!

The seasonal patterns of the 1943 epidemic attracted comment from a number of district physicians. Thus, at Þingeyrar, measles are described as 'beginning their career' in the spring. The first index case coming into Fljótsdals likewise arrived in April (a schoolboy returning from boarding school) but the spread was confined to only two farmsteads. However, '. . . when people started to move about more and to come in from other districts (i.e., when the snow thawed and travel across the island became possible) then the disease appeared once again and spread considerably as summer came on' (*Heilbrigðisskýrslur*, 1943, p. 32).

4.3.2 The post-war epidemic waves

With the end of World War II, the epidemiology of the Icelandic population entered a new phase. The decades of relative isolation, in which the only external links were seaborne, were characterised by large measles epidemics (often with a distinct regional character as described in section 4.3.2), separated by generally long, quiet periods when the island was free of the virus. From 1945 onwards, any epidemiological isolation was increasingly broken down. Seaborne links with continental Europe were re-established, while air services brought an ever larger flow of both Iceland-bound and trans-Atlantic passengers into Keflavík. The epidemiological response in terms of measles waves is summarised in Table 4.1. The post-war waves were smaller than all the pre-war ones (except 1904–5) in terms of cases per 1,000 population, and were more frequent with usually a less pronounced regional character. The long, quiet periods between epidemics were shortened (in Table 4.1, gap length is the number of months between the end of one wave and the beginning of the next) and the number of sporadic cases (outbreaks) in these gaps increased. To an ever-increasing extent, the behaviour of Icelandic measles waves moved towards the regular patterns of Western Europe and eastern North America (see Figure 3.1). Given also, as noted in section 4.1, that information about the spatial transmission process is largely absent from the accounts in *Heilbrigðisskýrslur* for the post-war waves, our treatment of them here is much briefer. Apart from the statistical character of each wave given in Table 4.1, we can satisfactorily comment only upon the speed and extent of spread of each epidemic. Certain exceptions do exist, like wave IX, which is well documented.

Wave VIII: November 1946 to August 1948 (Figure 4.10)

The epidemic was spread over a 22-month period, and was the first of several post-war waves which moved rather slowly through the Icelandic population (*see* $\bar{t}$ in Table 4.1). Cases were first reported in Reykjavíkur. Although we do not know the contact pattern, it is interesting to note that the regional centres of Akureyrar (north coast) and Egilsstaða (eastern fjords) reported in the second month, followed by Ísafjarðar (north-west fjords) in month three.

Wave IX: January 1950 to March 1952 (Figure 4.11)

The epidemic lasted for 26 months. Its average lag time to reach all areas, $\bar{t}$ in equation (4.1), was 15.45 months, making it the slowest moving of all the 16 waves (see Table 4.1). The epidemic established itself in Reykjavík in February, although an isolated case had been

Table 4.1. *Characteristics of the 16 Icelandic measles waves, 1896–1975*

Wave and years	Total cases	Cases per thousand population	Deaths	Deaths per thousand cases measles	Time gap (months)	T	$\bar{t}$	s	$\sqrt{b_1}$	b_2
I 1904–5	822	10.4	23*	?		8	4.53	1.23	0.97	4.03
					29					
II 1907–8	7,398	89.2	354	47.9		16	7.05	1.52	0.45	5.84
					91					
III 1916–17	4,944	55.0	118	23.9		14	4.80	2.46	1.61	5.09
					84					
IV 1924–6	6,130	61.2	34	5.6		26	7.61	5.22	1.69	4.77
					23					
V 1928–9	5,317	50.8	16	3.0		17	6.15	2.45	0.86	3.71
					73					
VI 1936–7	8,408	71.9	60	7.1		14	5.41	2.14	1.58	5.54
					70					
VII 1943–4	7,155	56.8	18	2.5		16	5.74	2.67	1.71	5.50
					29					
VIII 1946–8	4,791	35.3	6	1.3		22	8.42	3.74	0.77	3.04
					16					
IX 1950–2	6,645	45.2	11	1.7		27	15.45	3.52	−0.28	4.86
					3					
X 1952–3	1,872	12.5	1	0.5		10	5.22	1.77	0.14	3.52
					10					
XI 1954–5	7,787	49.9	4	0.5		21	9.05	2.92	1.24	5.98
					27					
XII 1958–9	7,102	42.1	3	0.4		22	11.29	2.03	0.59	5.58
					27					
XIII 1962–4	7,405	40.4	6	0.8		26	10.54	3.54	1.86	7.58
					29					
XIV 1966–8	6,152	30.4	4	0.7		22	5.85	2.40	2.17	11.76
					1					
XV 1968–70	3,625	17.8	0	0.0		27	13.32	3.96	0.14	3.97
					21					
XVI 1972–4	3,953	18.2	0	0.0		16	6.46	2.33	1.42	5.19

* Ísafjörður only.

T, $\bar{t}$, $\sqrt{b_1}$ and b_2 are defined in equations (4.1), (4.3) and (4.4); $s = \sqrt{m_2}$ in equation (4.2).

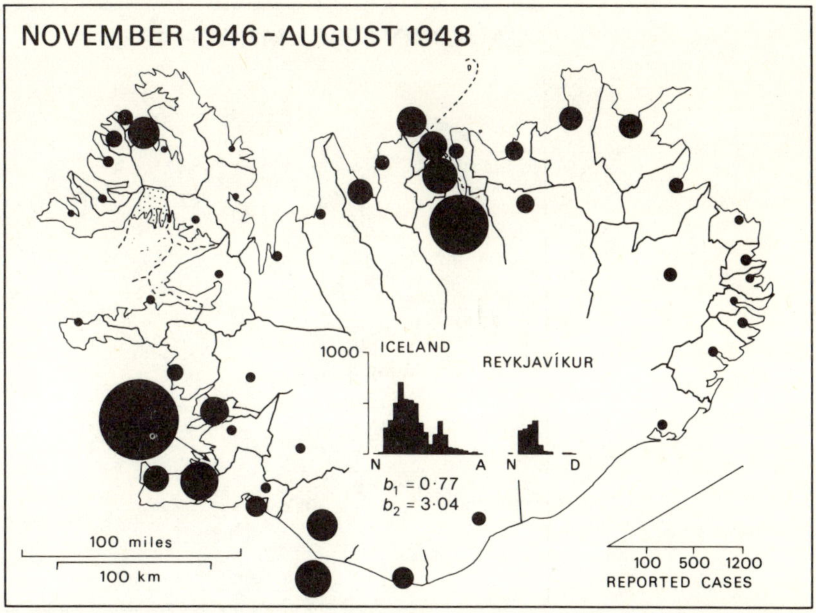

Fig. 4.10 Spread of the epidemic of 1946–8. See caption for Figure 4.3.

recorded in the north-west fjords in the preceding month. For the first 12 months of the wave, spread was confined largely to districts north of Reykjavíkur in the western half of the island. The disease spread from Reykjavíkur to the eastern fjords in the second quarter of 1951, but the epidemic was regionally concentrated in west Iceland throughout. The quality of evidence about the diffusion process for this wave is high. As Figure 4.11 shows, 21 bonds can be plotted and all but six of these radiate from Reykjavíkur.

Wave X: July 1952 to April 1953 (Figure 4.12)

The tenth epidemic was the smallest and regionally most distinct of the waves since that of 1904. Thus, 1,872 cases were reported, and these were spatially concentrated in two areas – the Akureyri region in the north, and the eastern fjords. Only isolated cases were reported from districts in the western and southern parts of the island. More than 30 cases were registered from four eastern fjord districts in July. Their number and multiple provenances cause us to suspect either (a) a single, unrecorded introduction into the area in a preceding month, or (b) unreported cases carrying over from the ninth wave. The unusual regional concentration arises from the fact that this epidemic infected largely those pockets of susceptibles 'missed' by the previous wave, which had finished only three months previously. Comparison of Figures 4.11 and 4.12 shows that the areas in which this wave flared up were the ones in which cases were reported late in the previous epidemic.

Wave XI: March 1954 to November 1955 (Figure 4.13)

This was the largest of the post-war waves. The epidemic lasted 21 months and moved relatively slowly ($\bar{t}$ = 9.05 in Table 4.1). It was, however, widely distributed throughout the island; only three of the medical districts failed to report infection. The first registered cases

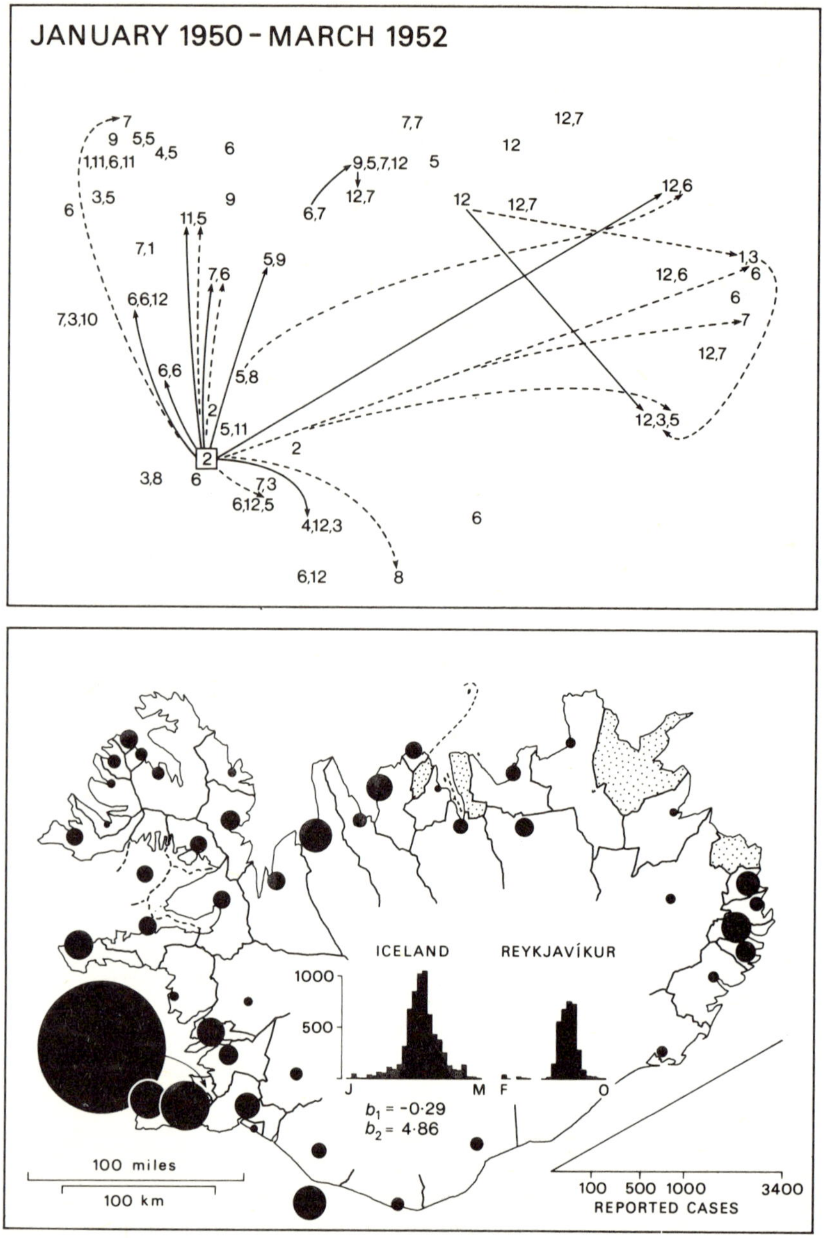

Fig. 4.11 Spread of the epidemic of 1950–2. See caption for Figure 4.3.

were located in Akranes in March, but it was not until Reykjavíkur was infected two months later that generalised diffusion occurred. The pattern of spread from Reykjavíkur shown in Figure 4.13 indicates that 9 of the 12 index cases traced originated in the capital. The three remaining vectors describe local movements between north-coast districts.

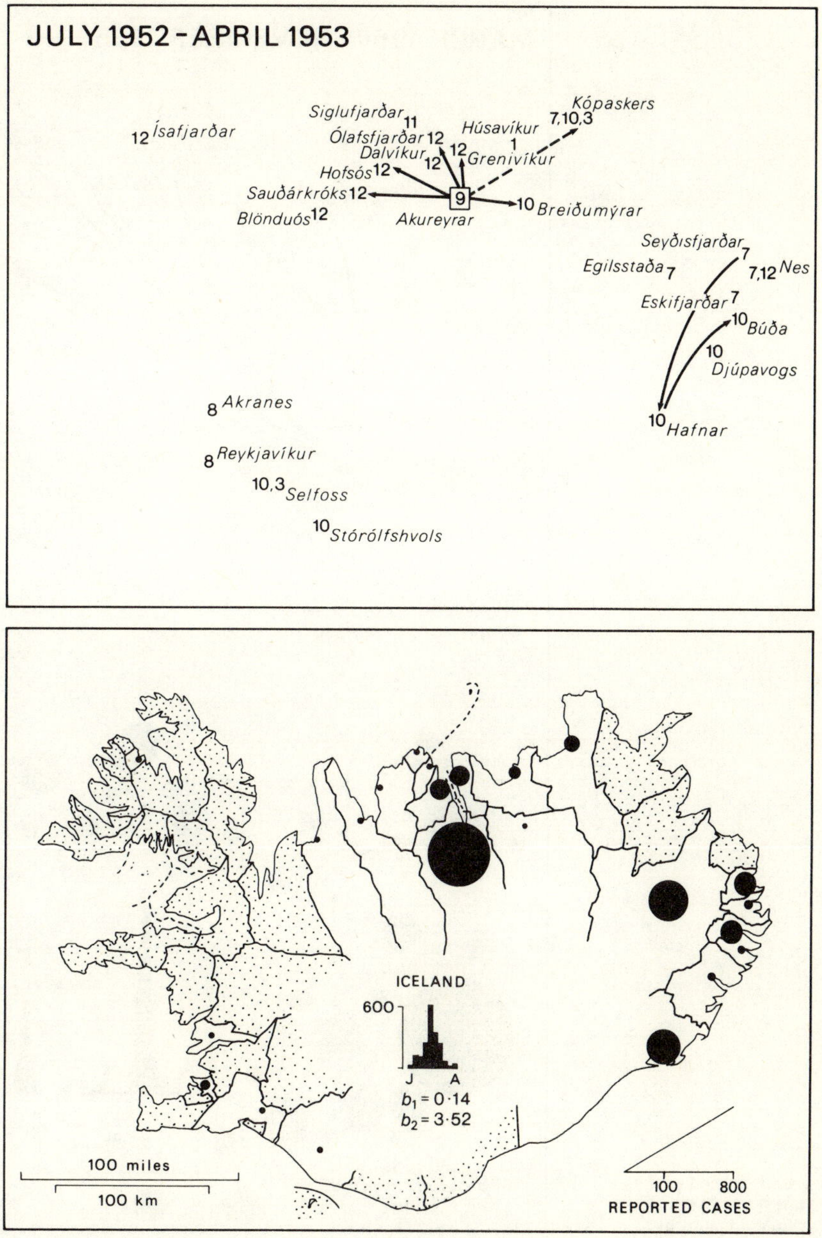

Fig. 4.12 Spread of the epidemic of 1952–3. See caption for Figure 4.3.

Wave XII: March 1958 to December 1959 (Figure 4.14)

This epidemic, like wave XI preceding it, was slow-moving ($\bar{t} = 11.29$) and was of similar size and intensity to wave XI except in north-east Iceland.

Wave XIII: April 1962 to May 1964 (Figure 4.15)

In contrast to its two predecessors, this wave erupted rapidly throughout the island but died away only slowly. The histograms in Figure 4.15 show that the disease built up to epidemic proportions in Reykjavíkur more slowly than in Iceland as a whole, but that the capital peaked at

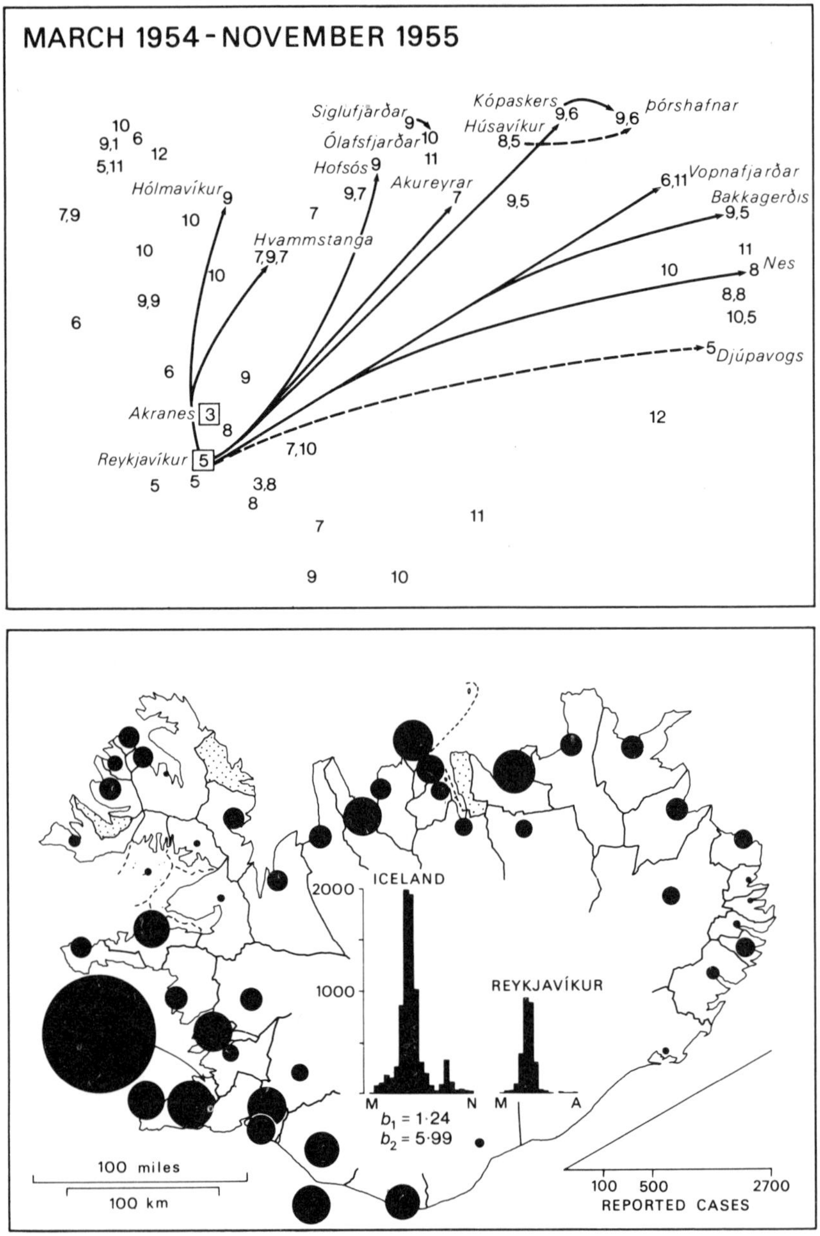

Fig. 4.13 Spread of the epidemic of 1954–5. See caption for Figure 4.3.

about the same time. A common pattern in previous epidemics was for Reykjavíkur to lead the rest of Iceland by several months.

Wave XIV: November 1966 to August 1968 (Figure 4.16)

Only six measles cases were reported in the 29-month gap after the close of wave XIII. The simultaneous reporting of measles from three medical districts in November 1966 marked the onset of one of the fastest-moving epidemics of the post-war period ($\bar{t} = 5.85$). Within three months of the arrival of the wave, half the districts were reporting cases,

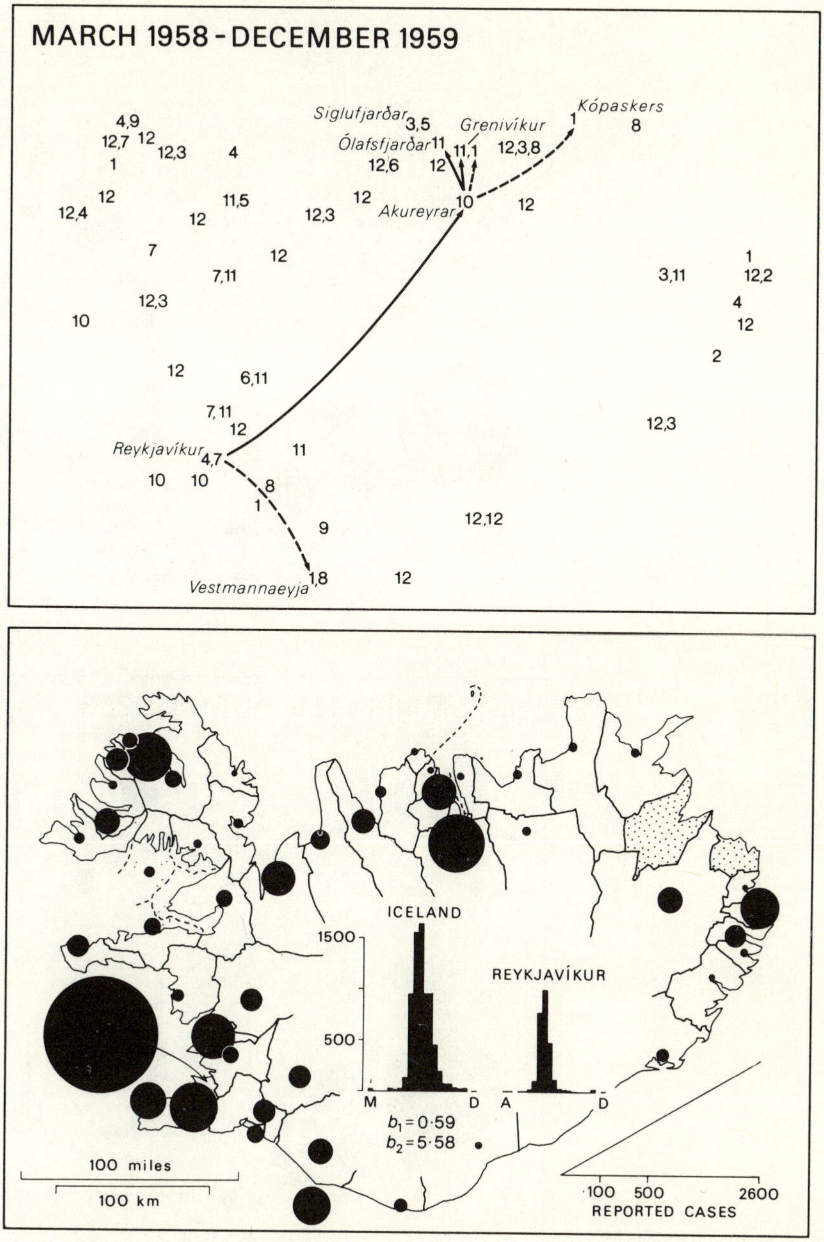

Fig. 4.14. Spread of the epidemic of 1958–9. See caption for Figure 4.3.

and within six months, half the cases in the epidemic had occurred. This early peaking is shown clearly in the histograms for Iceland and Reykjavíkur in Figure 4.16.

Wave XV: October 1968 to December 1970 (Figure 4.17)

The penultimate wave examined was the second smallest in the post-war period. Unlike its predecessor, it was very slow-moving ($\bar{t} = 13.32$). This slow build-up is shown particularly well in the histogram for Reykjavíkur in Figure 4.17; note the very different form of that histogram from

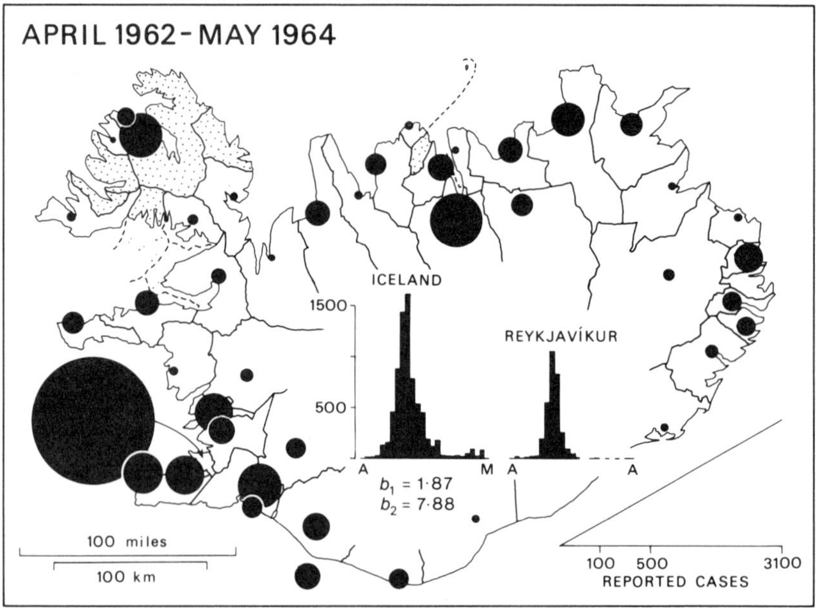

Fig. 4.15 Spread of the epidemic of 1962–4. See caption for Figure 4.3.

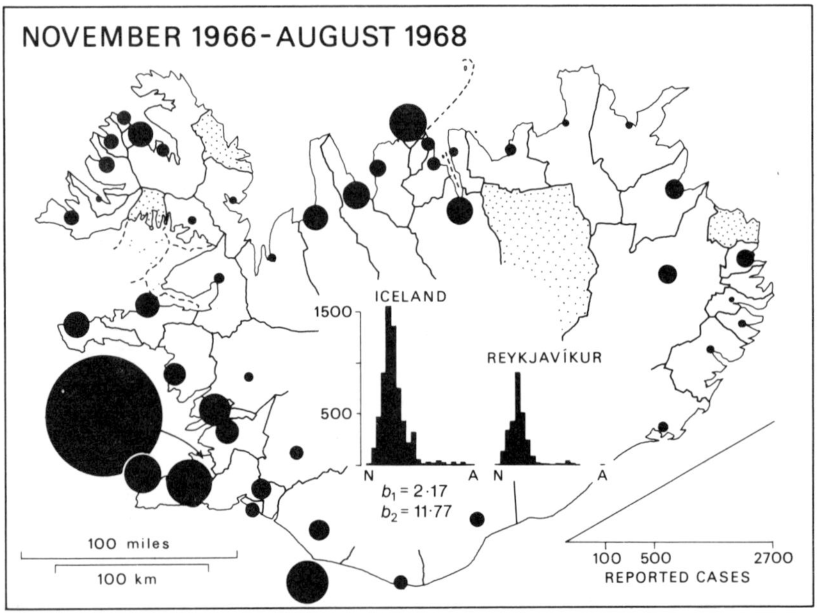

Figure. 4.16 Spread of the epidemic of 1966–8. See caption for Figure 4.3.

those in previous diagrams. A major outbreak began in Selfoss in January 1969, but the monthly totals for Iceland did not exceed 100 cases until July 1970, when the typical epidemic pattern began to emerge. Only one month separates the beginning of this wave from the end of the previous one, and it is highly likely that, in reality, the two formed a continuous epidemic with two peaks separated by an endemic trough.

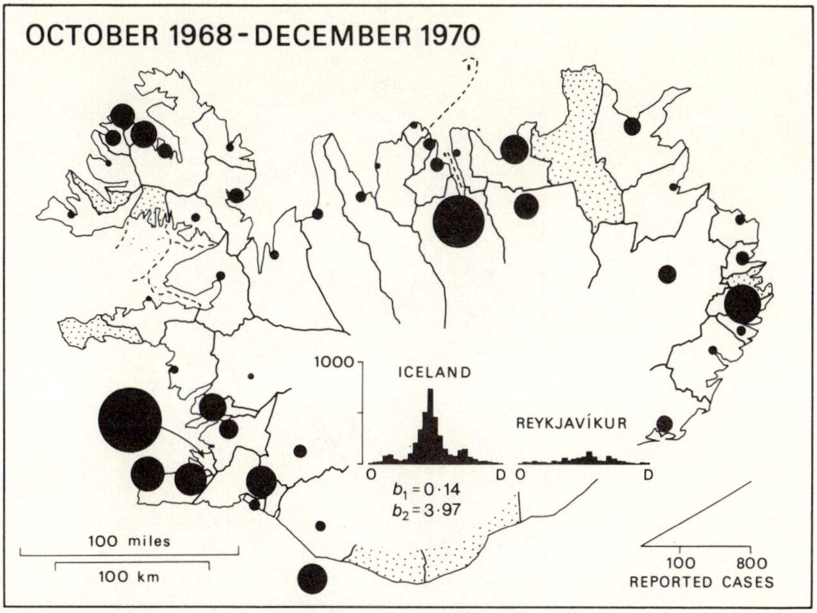

Fig. 4.17 Spread of the epidemic of 1968–70. See caption for Figure 4.3.

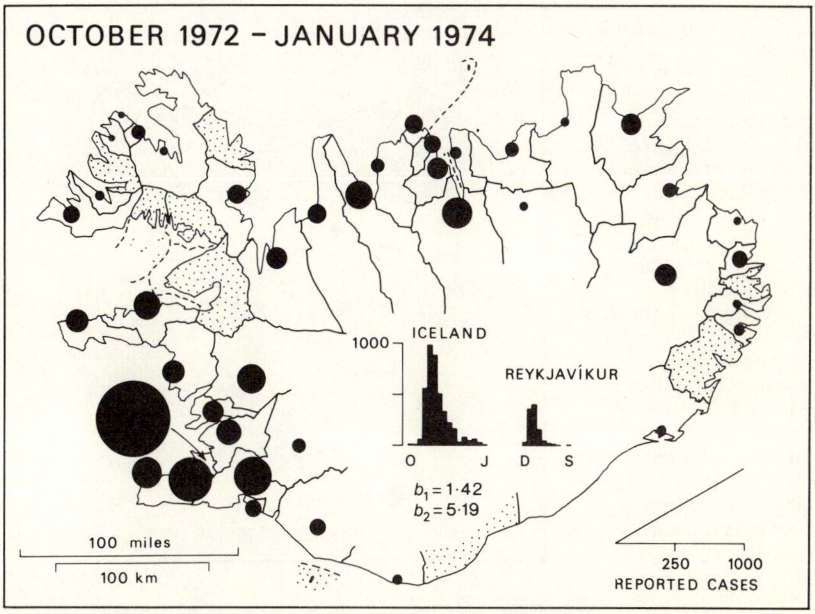

Fig. 4.18 Spread of the epidemic of 1972–4. See caption for Figure 4.3.

Wave XVI: October 1972 to January 1974 (Figure 4.18)

A gap of nearly two years separated this, the last wave studied, from its predecessor. Like wave XV, it was small in size, but it differed from it in that the conventional epidemic profile shown in the histograms re-established itself – that is, positively skewed distributions indicative of a more rapid build-up than fade-out phase to the epidemic (see Figure 4.18). Along with wave XIII, this epidemic was atypical of most analysed in that the disease took off more rapidly in the rest of Iceland

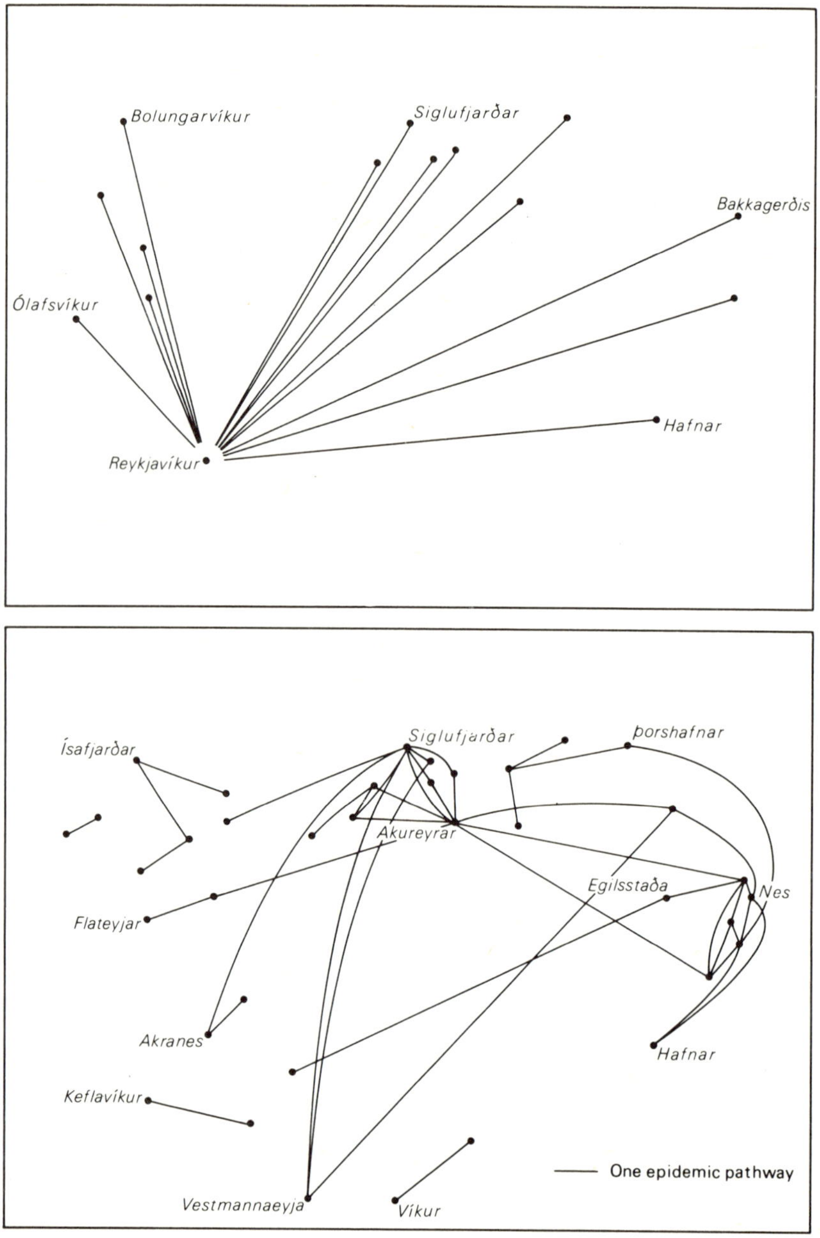

Fig. 4.19 Internal epidemic pathways. Bond persistence diagrams showing known direction of spread between medical districts in the epidemics from 1904 to 1974. Links involving Reykjavíkur (upper) and *not* involving Reykjavíkur (lower) are shown separately at three levels of intensity. Note that, as in Figures 4.3–4.18, all bonds are conventionally drawn as smooth lines connecting pairs of areas; they do not attempt to describe the actual routes followed, which were often peripheral movements by sea between the coastal settlements.

than in Reykjavíkur, although both peaked at the same time. The wave displayed some regional distinctiveness; the areas around Reykjavíkur and Akureyrar were relatively badly hit, whereas the north-west and eastern fjords escaped fairly lightly.

4.4 General regularities in the waves

A basic question which can be asked about the bond diagrams included in Figures 4.3–4.18 is 'do *epidemic pathways* exist, along which measles regularly seem to move from one place to another when an epidemic is in progress?' That is, we are interested in the extent to which the bonds

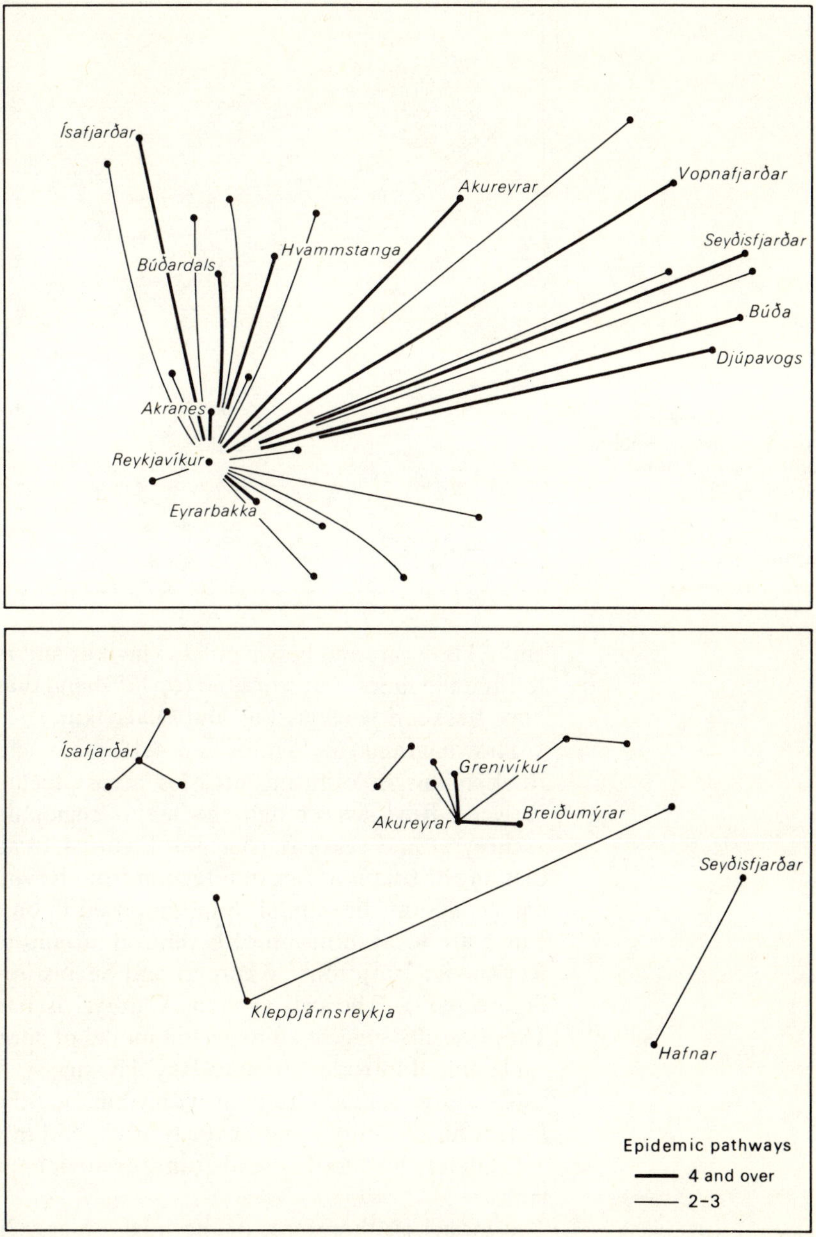

Fig. 4.19 (contd)

shown persist from epidemic to epidemic. Figure 4.19 is a *bond persistence diagram*, constructed from the individual link maps in Figures 4.3–4.18. The diagram gives the number of times measles are known to have spread from place to place along the links shown in all epidemics between 1904 and 1974. The upper illustrations indicate the known epidemic pathways between Reykjavíkur and other areas, while the remaining pair shows the epidemic pathways between districts excluding Reykjavíkur. For example, it can be seen from the top right-hand diagram in Figure 4.19 that measles spread between Reykjavíkur

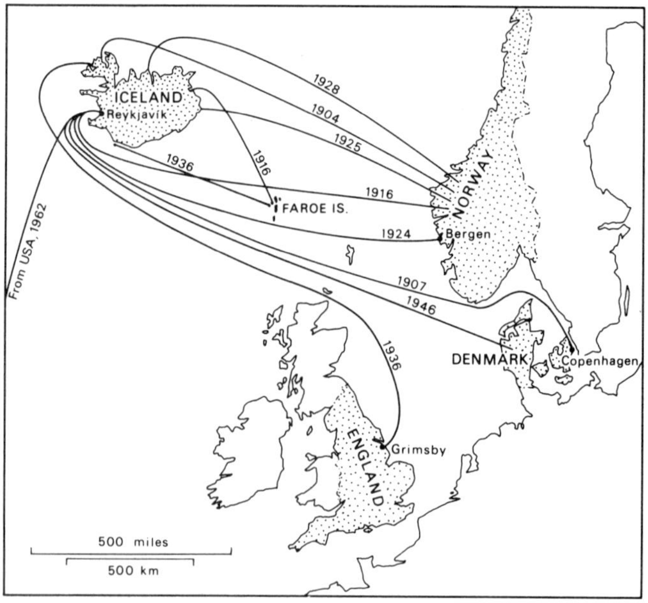

Fig. 4.20 External epidemic pathways. Known countries of origin for the Icelandic epidemic waves. Up to 1943, all introductions are known; after World War II, the record is incomplete.

and Akureyrar, and between Reykjavíkur and Isafjarðar, in at least 4 of the 16 epidemics, but from the top left-hand diagram that it moved only once between Reykjavíkur and Ólafsvíkur.

The diagrams in Figures 4.3–4.18 make clear the central role of Reykjavíkur in diffusing measles across Iceland. Strong bonds exist between Reykjavíkur and the major regional districts of Ísafjarðar, Akureyrar and Seyðisfjarðar; but Figure 4.19 also makes clear the fact that any district is at risk of infection from Reykjavíkur once the disease has arrived in the capital. Superimposed upon this primate city dominance are local diffusion cells centred around the main urban areas of Reykjavík, Ísafjörður, Akureyri and Seyðisfjörður (lower illustration, Figure 4.19). The cell around Akureyri is particularly well defined. These results suggest an expected model of spread in any epidemic as:

(1) initial introduction into Reykjavíkur;

(2) early spread from Reykjavíkur to the regional centres of Ísafjörður, Akureyri and Seyðisfjörður, and in the Reykjavík area;

(3) later, localised spread from the regional centres to their hinterlands.

The model is, therefore, of the mixed hierarchical/contagious type as discussed in connection with Figures 2.4 and 2.16.

The written reports in *Heilbrigðisskýrslur* not only permit some reconstruction of the internal spread process, but they also indicate the country of origin of many of the epidemic waves which reached Iceland. These international epidemic pathways are mapped in Figure 4.20. The Scandinavian connection is most marked. Perhaps a little surprising, in view of the role of Keflavík airforce base as a troop staging post and as a transit passenger point for flights between Europe and the United States, is the fact that only the 1962 epidemic is known to have originated in the United States.

4.5 Conclusion

In this chapter, we have used the historical record to try to identify the main components of a spatial diffusion process for recurrent measles waves. As described in section 4.4, a three-component model seems to be present in most epidemics, namely:

(1) initial introduction from the rest of the world, or at a very early stage from elsewhere in Iceland, to the capital, Reykjavík;

(2) spread from the capital to regional centres in the north-west (Ísafjörður), north (Akureyri) and east (Seyðisfjörður) of the island (that is, down the urban-size hierarchy), and contagious diffusion around Reykjavík in south-west Iceland;

(3) localised spread out from the regional centres to their hinterlands.

In addition, the reports on the 16 waves by the various medical officers have been used to discover socio-economic and geographical factors which affect the rate of operation of the diffusion process. These factors seem to be:

(1) the role of communal activities such as haymaking, school terms and social events in turning isolated cases into major epidemics;

(2) the effect of the decreasing world isolation of Iceland upon the waves – the gap between epidemics and attack rate per 1,000 population has declined steadily throughout the century. The pre-war waves were noticeably wider apart, more severe and, as a result of fewer recurrences, produced higher mortality levels than did the post-war waves;

(3) the role of ship movements in spreading the disease around the coast from port to port, and of bus traffic and journey-to-school trips in across-island diffusion;

(4) the use of quarantine and serum vaccinations to contain the spread process;

(5) the tendency of the pre-war epidemics to mushroom in the late spring after the thaw improved communications and thus permitted increased spatial mobility;

(6) the fact that under-reporting of cases does happen, but that there is great variety from district to district in the extent to which this occurs.

In the next chapter, some elementary statistical methods of analysis are applied to the data described in this chapter, especially for the period 1945–74. We shall find that many of the empirical regularities identified there can be reasonably interpreted only in terms of the factors isolated above in the documentary accounts.

5 Identifying diffusion processes – the historical record

5.1 Introduction

In the descriptions of the last 16 measles epidemics to affect Iceland (section 4.3), we concentrated on the characteristics unique to each wave. In this chapter, we move from questions of particularity to those of generality, and try to identify those features in the spread process which are common to all waves. By asking questions at a general level, we hope to be able to identify some of those diffusion processes of key significance in the transfer of an infectious disease from one community to another.

The approach followed in this chapter is to move upwards through various geographical scales of analysis. Thus, we begin at the finest scale with the individual records of the medical officer in each district. We follow this by statistical analysis at the district level itself. Finally, we move up to the higher spatial level at which the districts are organised into regions. The results from each of the three levels are then reviewed in the light of the changing geography of Iceland over the period under study.

5.2 Diffusion at the micro-scale: contemporary accounts by Icelandic doctors

The picture of the diffusion of measles epidemics presented in the preceding chapter rests on the records of a handful of qualified men. In 1970, there were 308 medical doctors resident in Iceland; in 1900, there was only one fifth of that number. Health work at the local level is supervised by a district physician who reports directly to the Director of Health. In the more populous town districts, where there are other practising doctors, the district physician is concerned largely with preventive medicine and public-health work. But, in the remoter rural districts where he is the only doctor, the care of the sick occupies the greater part of his time (Sigurjónsson, 1975, p. 296).

Jónsson (1940, p. 162) has provided a vivid account of the work of the rural doctor in such districts, where the distance from the doctor's residence to an outlying farm might be as much as 70 miles:

> Over this the doctor must make his way, often across mountains and uninhabited areas, or over desert sands and unbridged rivers. At the best such journeys are made on horseback, but in winter when even this method of travelling is impossible the doctor has often to go on foot, or on skis; in other places the journeys are made by motor boat across fjords and bays and even round promontories which project right out into the open oceans. At such times it may take the doctor the whole of a long day or even days to reach his patient and cost him and those who have come to fetch him unbelievable difficulty. But all this may now be said to be of rare occurrence and most of the inhabitants are now within reach of the telegraph and almost without exception within a telephone call of all the inhabited parts of their respective districts.

In addition to the qualified doctors are the paramedical staff, notably the qualified midwives. Again, there are major differences between the towns and the sparsely-settled districts. In the latter, confinements may be so rare that midwives are part-time, often farmers' wives.

When working with the data used in this book (see Appendix), we thus need to bear in mind the extent to which medical services would have been stretched in major epidemics – especially in the early part of the study period. In particular, despite the known high quality of the data compared with other countries, reports like that quoted above go a long way towards explaining why the reporting rate may be only about 40 per cent of the number of cases which actually occurred (see below and sections 3.5.1 and 6.4.3).

5.2.1 Reported number of cases

The incidence of infectious diseases in each medical district in a given month is reported by the district physician to Reykjavík; these figures form the raw material for the tables given in *Heilbrigðisskýrslur* and the Appendix. We have not been able to estimate with certainty the accuracy of the figures given from internal evidence. Clearly, reported cases represent a lower bound for actual cases in a readily diagnosed disease such as measles. The incidence of sub-clinical cases, or untreated cases in remote areas, would augment the recorded figures. For examples of the variation in levels of reporting from district to district, see the discussion of wave V in section 4.3.1. Notwithstanding these doubts, as noted in section 3.5.1, Iceland would appear to be a country with relatively high accuracy of disease reporting. In terms of much of the modelling used later in this book, the absolute numbers of cases are not critical to a great deal of the analysis; the relative size of outbreaks and their absence (or presence) in particular locations are of more direct relevance. One factor which would disturb the findings at a local scale would be strong variations from place to place between reporting levels. We have no direct evidence on this point, although it is noticeable that, in the 1880s, not all medical districts had a doctor present in all years. Thus, in the 1882 measles outbreak, the six areas failing to report measles are those in which a medical practitioner was not present. By the date of the first of the waves studied in detail (1904) the number of doctors was sufficiently large to minimise this risk.

5.2.2 Provenance of infections

In addition to providing monthly figures of numbers of cases, each district medical officer wrote an annual report to the Chief Medical Officer in Reykjavík. These annual reports are filed in the National Archives in Reykjavík. Sections from each report are published in the annual *Heilbrigðisskýrslur*, sometimes in full but mainly in abridged form, and arranged under individual diseases. Descriptions for measles outbreaks typically begin with a general comment for Iceland as a whole on the severity and age distribution of the outbreak. This is followed by the accounts for reporting districts, working in a clockwise direction from Reykjavík in a ring around the country.

As the maps in section 4.3 show, one of the crucial pieces of information contained in these accounts is identification of the index case for an outbreak, together with his (or her) provenance. Thus, Figure 4.3 for wave I shows both the external origin of the measles virus (Norway), and the subsequent movement of infected cases within north-west Iceland. Inspection of the sequence of maps given in chapter 4 for the 16 waves studied shows that the number of bonds recorded decreases over time. Given the transport conditions, the smaller population and the lower level of movements at the beginning of the century, it is not surprising that movements of index cases were easier to determine then than they were later in our study period.

5.2.3 Other information

As well as containing provenance data, the annual reports of district medical officers comment on other factors relating to the diffusion process. Central to this are accounts of the different methods used to reduce the spread of the disease. Among many reports, we may note that Flateyrar reported the isolation of a trawler which came from Reykjavík (*Heilbrigðisskýrslur*, 1921–5, p. 81*) while in Borgarfjarðar 'a ban was put on all assemblies' (*Heilbrigðisskýrslur*, 1921–5, p. 80*). Not all assemblies could, however, be avoided, and the annual gathering of farmers in September to co-operate in bringing down sheep from the hills had the inevitable consequence of sharply increasing the spread of the disease. In other cases, common sense over quarantine prevailed and 'people conscientiously avoided the farmsteads where the disease was' (*Heilbrigðisskýrslur*, 1911–20, p. 71*).

In addition to quarantine, early attempts at vaccination were also made. Thus, the medical officer for Borgarfjarðar in the 1924 wave comments: 'I tried to protect a few babies [very young children] against the disease with blood injections from one or other of the parents, beneath the skin. I consider it certain that this is the best protection' (*Heilbrigðisskýrslur*, 1921–5, p. 80*). Some make comical reading with the wisdom of hindsight. The report for Hofðhverfis for 1943 contains the following immortal lines: 'A man came to me in mid-July who had been given measles serum five weeks previously and was very lethargic. I gave him a good dose of serum. Two days after I saw him, the man was entirely covered with measles' (*Heilbrigðisskýrslur*, 1943, p. 31).

Through all accounts runs an indication of the economic importance of measles and its relation to the farming and fishing calendars. For example, measles was carried to Mýrdals from Reykjavík in June 1916 and 'although precautions were not officially taken, many homesteads did their best to protect themselves and tried not to contract the disease at haymaking' (*Heilbrigðisskýrslur*, 1911–20, p. 71*). At Stokkseyri, stress is again laid on avoiding loss of manpower at haymaking. Where a community felt the onset of the disease was inevitable, an attempt might be made to bring the infection forward to a more convenient time. Thus, the Borgarfjarðar report for 1916 records that, in May, 'measles attacked 33 to 34 farms; some of them wanted to get it over, and what is more even sought it' (*Heilbrigðisskýrslur*, 1911–20, p. 69*).

The reports go on to comment on the severity of each epidemic and the several complications to which it gave rise. Although the diagnosis of measles did not prove difficult, the attribution of deaths to measles

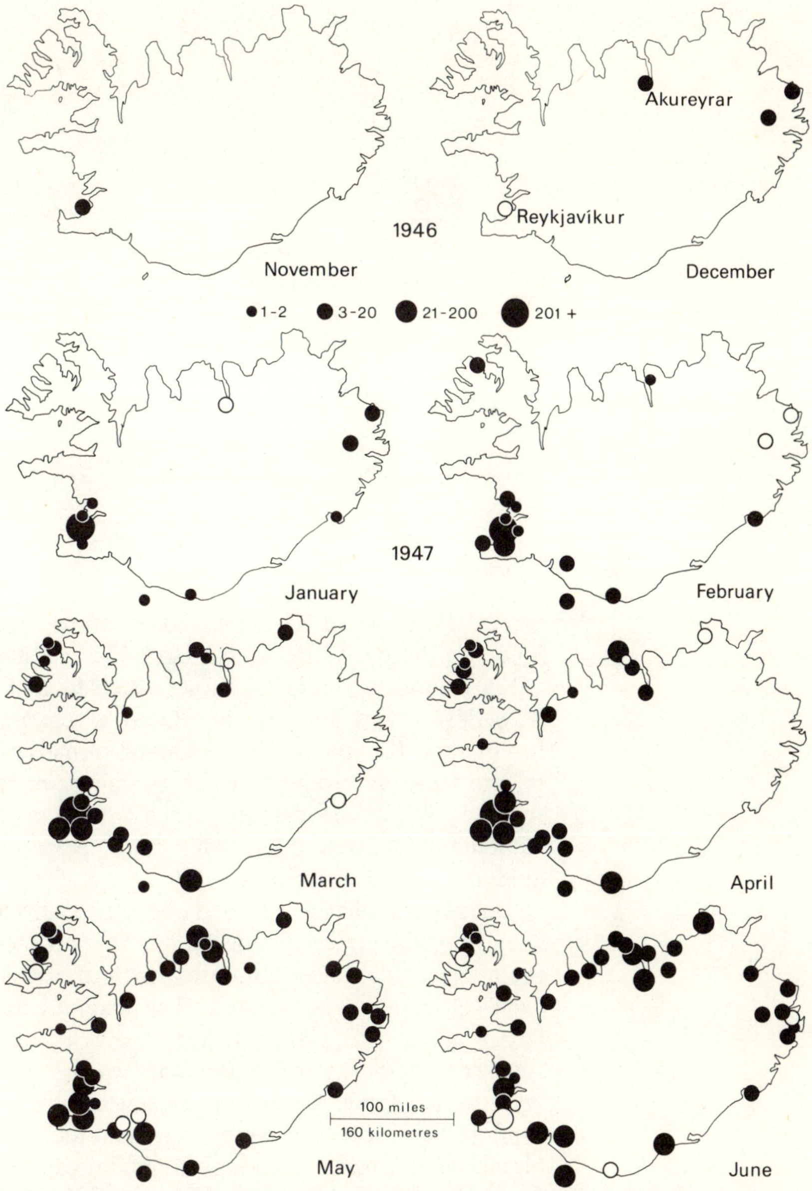

Fig. 5.1 Spread of measles on a monthly basis, Iceland, wave VIII. Circles indicate number of cases reported. Places reporting cases in month t but not in $(t + 1)$ are denoted by open circles. *Source: Heilbrigðisskýrslur* (1946 Table IV; 1947 Table IV).

certainly did. The report for Akureyrar notes that measles affected the elderly severely and, although six are counted as dying from this cause, 'the number would have been greater if subsequent illnesses are added in' (*Heilbrigðisskýrslur*, 1911–20, p. 70*).

5.3 Diffusion at the meso-scale: statistical reconstruction at the district level

5.3.1 Epidemic maps

Using the monthly data, a map was constructed to show the number of cases reported by each district at each time period. Since, as we have noted earlier (see section 4.2), the boundaries of the medical districts changed over time, it was necessary to edit the records by combining areas to ensure spatial comparability. An atlas of standardised distribution maps was produced for the eight waves in the Icelandic sequence,

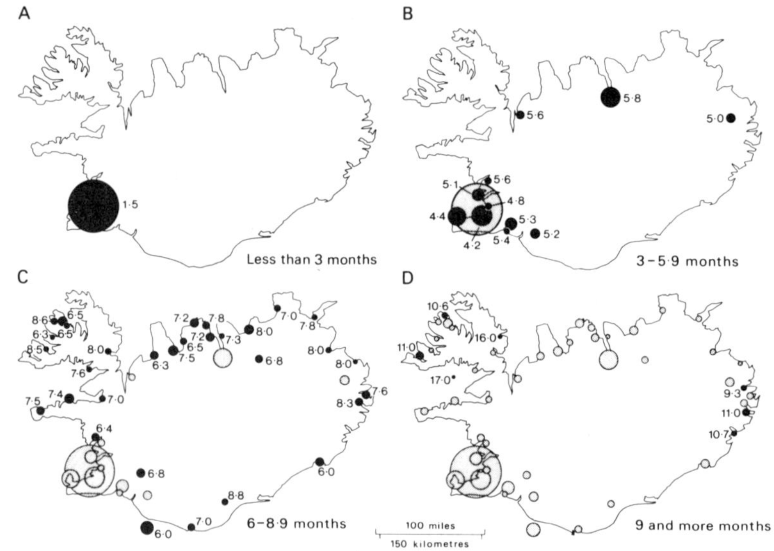

Fig. 5.2 Mean lag time in months from the start of all epidemics occurring between 1945 and 1970 (waves VIII to XV) before medical districts were reached. Stipple indicates districts shown as reached on earlier maps. Area of circles proportional to population size of districts in 1970.

wave VIII to wave XV, 1945–70, to allow some generalisations to be made on the basis of both cartographic and statistical methods.

For example, Figure 5.1 shows a sequence of eight monthly maps for wave VIII. Note the way in which the epidemic starts in the largest urban area, Reykjavík. The epidemic spreads rapidly to, and intensifies in, the Reykjavík region and in the towns of the south-west corner of Iceland. Wholesale spread to the north, north-west, and east-coast settlements follows later. This same pattern is repeated for other epidemic waves in Iceland.

The general picture outlined above is confirmed by Figure 5.2, which shows, for the eight epidemic waves that hit Iceland from 1945 to 1970, the average lag time (in months) from the start of an epidemic before each settlement was reached. The diagram demonstrates clearly that larger places and places nearer to Reykjavík are generally hit first; smaller settlements and settlements which are isolated from Reykjavík are reached later. While this evidence may, on the surface, seem to support the idea of a simple spread model for epidemics *down* the hierarchy of urban size and the contagious spread of epidemic waves *out* from the initial centres of introduction (cf. section 4.4), the interpretation is complicated by the high inverse correlation between population size of settlements and distance from Reykjavík. The smaller settlements are generally distant from the source areas, and so it is difficult, even with partial correlation analysis, to disentangle the size and distance effects. We encounter again the problem besetting the cholera data set analysed in section 2.3.3.

5.3.2 Centroid movements

Where a spatial distribution is changing rapidly from month to month, it may not always be possible to recognise the general trends in the direction of spread. One summary measure is to define a *centroid* for each map to show its mean 'centre of reported incidence'. Suppose that data are recorded for areas. The location of the jth areal unit whose disease incidence is to be measured may be given a horizontal cartesian co-ordinate u_j and a vertical map co-ordinate v_j (say for its geographical centre). Let the reported number of cases for the jth unit be I_j. The mean centre of the reported number of cases in the set of $j = 1, 2, \ldots, n$ regions is located at $\bar{U}$, $\bar{V}$ where

$$\bar{U} = \sum_{j=1}^{n} I_j u_j \Big/ \sum_{j=1}^{n} I_j \tag{5.1}$$

and

$$\bar{V} = \sum_{j=1}^{n} I_j v_j \Big/ \sum_{j=1}^{n} I_j . \tag{5.2}$$

The mean is one of the simplest of a series of measure of central location, each with particular advantages and drawbacks, developed by geographers. See the literature reviewed by Haggett, Cliff and Frey (1977, pp. 312–3). One especially useful measure is the Kuhn–Kuenne centroid. This is computed by choosing an initial location for the centroid at a map co-ordinate position $\hat{U}$, $\hat{V}$. This may be the spatial mean given in equations (5.1) and (5.2) or be based on observations of the map pattern. The true centroid of the distribution is now located by an iterative search procedure based upon repeated solution of the equations

$$\hat{U}_{(k+1)} = \frac{\sum_{j=1}^{n} I_j u_j d_{j(k)}}{\sum_{j=1}^{n} I_j d_{j(k)}} \tag{5.3}$$

and

$$\hat{V}_{(k+1)} = \frac{\sum_{j=1}^{n} I_j v_j d_{j(k)}}{\sum_{j=1}^{n} I_j d_{j(k)}} \tag{5.4}$$

until $\hat{U}_{(k+1)} - \hat{U}_{(k)} < \varepsilon$ and $\hat{V}_{(k+1)} - \hat{V}_{(k)} < \varepsilon$, where ε is an error level set by the researcher. In these equations, d_j is the distance between the latest centroid and the jth area, in addition to previously defined notation. The new centroid is denoted by the subscript $(k + 1)$. Although tedious to compute by hand, the procedure is readily programmed for a desk calculator, and yields an estimate for the centroid which is independent of the orientation of the map co-ordinate system.

By plotting centroids for successive periods and linking them in sequence, the general direction of movement can sometimes be captured. Figure 5.3 plots the successive locations of the Kuhn–Kuenne

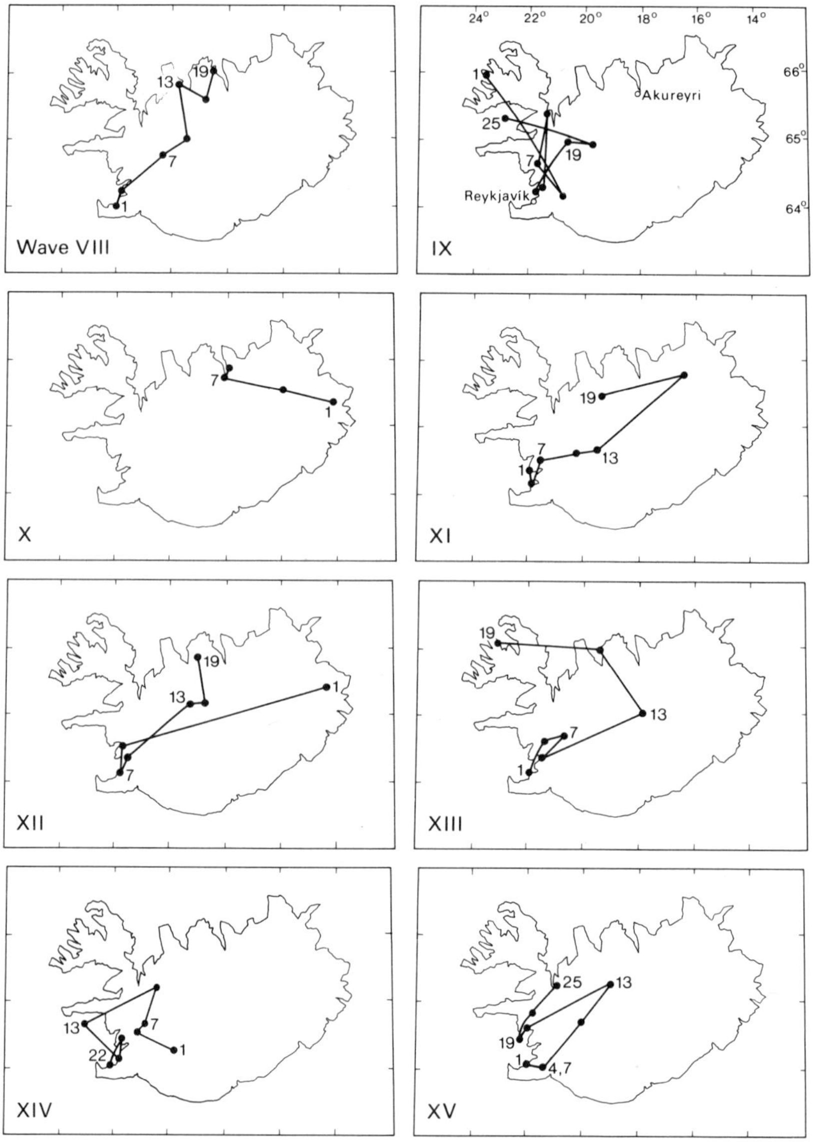

Fig. 5.3 Tri-monthly trajectory of geographical centroid of reported cases, waves VIII to XV.

centroid of outbreaks for the eight measles epidemics occurring between 1945 and 1970. The diagrams show the trajectories for each of the waves. The first (wave VIII) has the simplest structure, moving from Reykjavíkur to Dalvíkur. Note the contrast between waves IX and X; the former was a large outbreak of over 6,000 cases concentrated in the western part of Iceland, whereas the latter was smaller (fewer than 1,900 cases). It followed rapidly after wave IX and was confined to the eastern half of the island. Arguably, wave X exhausted the susceptible population missed by wave IX. In general, outbreaks seem either to start in the Reykjavík area or to reach it very quickly. A general north-easterly drift tends to occur after the seventh month of each wave

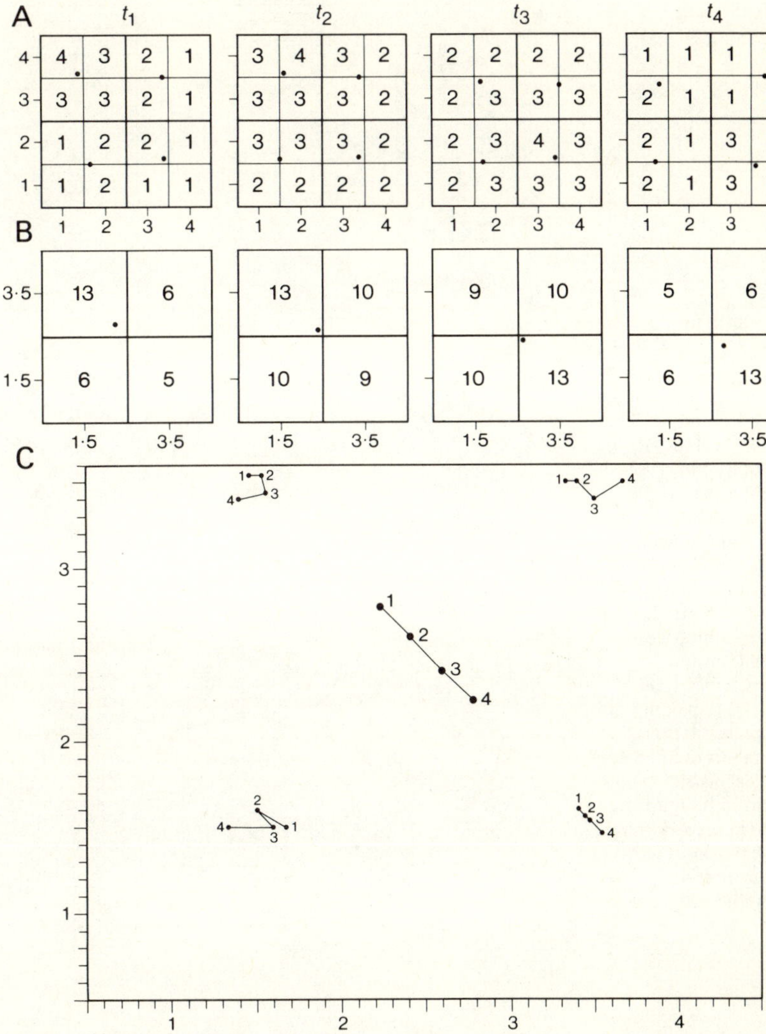

Fig. 5.4 Hypothetical example of centroid trajectories. (A) Maps at four successive time periods, $t_1 - t_4$, with county values as shown and cartesian co-ordinates of cell centres marked. Dots give centroid positions for each group of four cells. (B) as (A), with larger regions obtained by aggregating cells on (A). (C) Trajectories of centroids, $t_1 - t_4$, for maps (A) – tracks in the four corners – and maps (B) – centre.

and, with the exception of wave XIV, the trajectory terminates at the end of each epidemic in the north or north-west corner of Iceland.

One of the advantages of plotting centroids to show flow lines for viral movements through a population is that the problem can be disaggregated to any required level of spatial detail. Figure 5.4 shows such disaggregation for a hypothetical example. Note from Figure 5.4C that, while the regional centroid (calculated for all areas) shows a steady drift towards the south-east, the four local centroids (calculated for each of the four sub-populations) display more complex patterns. In practice, centroid shifts can be plotted not only for different geographical levels but also for cases stratified on a characteristic of clinical interest (e.g., age, sex).

5.3.3 Diffusion on graphs

One approach to the spatial spread of an epidemic is to treat the area over which spread is occurring as a graph (Haggett, 1976; Cliff and

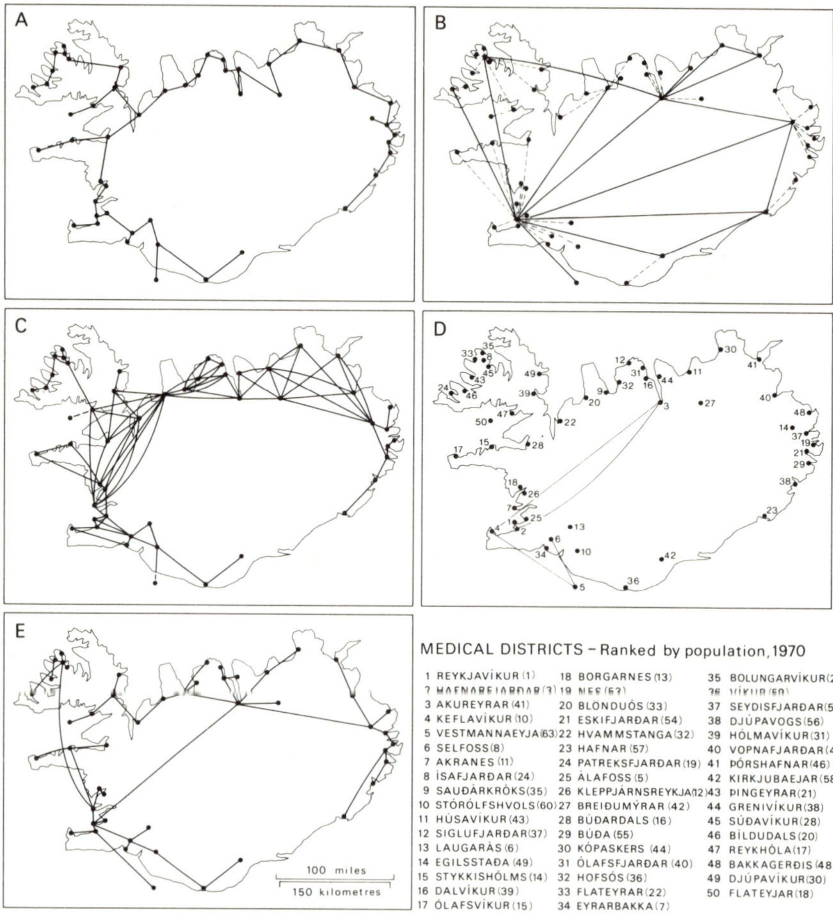

Fig. 5.5 Medical districts of Iceland reduced to graphs corresponding to various hypothetical diffusion processes. Dots indicate main settlement in each medical district; lines give the links in each graph. (A) minimum spanning tree, (B) domestic airline network, (C) 1970 road network, (D) population size, (E) nearest larger place. Numbers in brackets after medical district names correspond with Figure 4.2. On (D), links are drawn for illustrative purposes only between the first six districts on the size scale.

Haggett, 1980). Thus, we can view Iceland as a graph consisting of a set of nodes (the medical districts) and the links between them. Theoretically, each of the 50 Icelandic districts could be linked to any other to give a graph with 2,450 links. In practice, however, we can limit the number of links to give a graph which corresponds as closely as possible with a hypothetical diffusion process. Consider Figure 5.5A which shows Iceland as a minimum spanning tree (MST), which is the simplest network configuration such that all nodes are linked (see Haggett, Cliff and Frey (1977, p. 82) for formal definitions of network elements). Such a network would imply a highly localised spread process around the coast with each centre being open to infection from its neighbour. While this spread model might be appropriate to nineteenth-century conditions, it is less plausible when transport developments in the present century are taken into account (see section 5.5.2). Thus, the remaining graphs in Figure 5.5 take more realistic spread patterns into account. An airline graph (Figure 5.5B) shows scheduled domestic airline links in the 1970s; communities without airline links are joined to the nearest centre on the airline graph (pecked on Figure 5.5B). A road graph (Figure 5.5C) gives links via the 1970 road network. A pure population-size graph (Figure 5.5D) links each district to its next largest and next smallest district in terms of the rank order of the population size of each medical district in 1970. Finally, a modified population-size graph (Figure 5.5E) links districts to the next largest *and* nearest neighbour.

To discriminate between the five graphs, each of the 139 monthly maps was translated into binary 'outbreak/no outbreak' terms. Vertices on each of the 695 (that is, 139 × 5) graphs so defined were coded black (B = outbreak) or white (W = no outbreak) and the Moran BW statistic under non-free sampling (see Cliff and Ord, 1973, pp. 4–7) was computed for each to measure the degree of contagion present. We define BW as

$$BW = \tfrac{1}{2}\sum_{i=1}^{n}\sum_{\substack{j=1 \\ i\neq j}}^{n} w_{ij}(x_i - x_j)^2, \tag{5.5}$$

where $w_{ij} = 1$ if a link existed between vertices i and j on the graph in question and $w_{ij} = 0$ otherwise; $x_i = 1$ if vertex i was colour-coded B and $x_i = 0$ if the vertex was coded W. The sampling distribution of BW under the null hypothesis of no contagion in outbreaks on the graph is approximately normal for the number of vertices (50) considered here, and we may test BW for significant departure from its null value as a standardised normal (z) score. The expectation and variance of BW under H_0 are given in Cliff and Ord (1973, chapter 1). The greater the degree of correspondence between any graph and the transmission path followed by the diffusion wave, the larger (negative) should become the standardised score for BW joins. As Haggett (1976, p. 145) has noted, the graphs will not be independent because the same link may appear on more than one graph.

The results of testing the spread pattern on the five different graphs are shown in Figure 5.6. Results for the five graphs are plotted down the page in the sequence (A) MST, (B) airline, (C) highway, (D) urban size, and (E) urban size and distance. If we take values above the 95 per cent significance level (one-tailed test for positive autocorrelation) shown by a z-score $[\times(-1)]$ of 1.64 or greater, then the most effective spread mechanism appears to be the simplest, i.e., the MST. This shows nearly one third of the 139 monthly maps to be significant. The only other graphs of interest are those modelling the road network (C) and the urban size and distance (E).

Two other relationships should be noted. First, when the eight oubreaks are plotted across Figure 5.6 in time sequence, there is a slight reduction in the proportion of significant maps with time, suggesting that the later epidemics may spread by more complex movements than the earlier ones. Second, a distinction may be drawn (see vertical broken line) between the 'waxing', or build-up stage of the epidemic, and the 'waning' stage. Haggett (1976) found distinctive behaviour between the two epidemic phases when working on measles outbreaks in Cornwall. The Icelandic results do not confirm the sharp differences

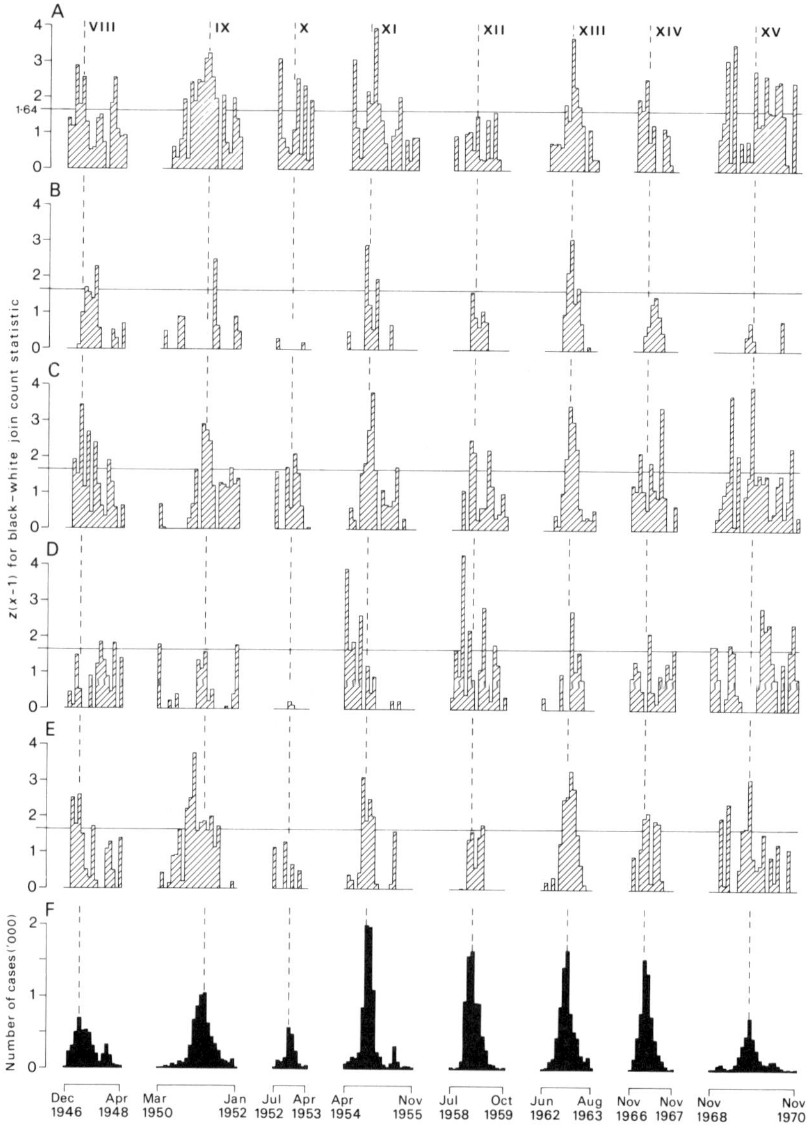

Fig. 5.6 Values of BW join count statistic as standardised score for each month of waves VIII to XV on graphs A – E (defined in Figure 5.5). F gives reported number of cases. Vertical pecked lines correspond with epidemic peaks. The $\alpha = 0.05$ significance level ($z = 1.64$) in a one-tailed test of positive spatial autocorrelation is marked.

observed there, but it is of interest that, in the three most plausible graphs (Figure 5.6A, C and E), the proportion of significant maps is higher in the waxing than in the waning phase. This is consistent with the suggestion that the build-up of an epidemic is spatially more ordered than is the fade-out; the fall-off of intensity in the decline phase is not associated with a corresponding reduction in geographical area, so that the epidemic appears to decay spatially *in situ*.

5.3.4 Regression models of waves

It is argued throughout this study that knowledge of the spatial behaviour of one epidemic may provide clues to the behaviour of subsequent epidemics. One simple test of this hypothesis is provided by the regression model

$$I_{ij} = b_0 + b_1 I_{i,j-1} + e_{ij}, \tag{5.6}$$

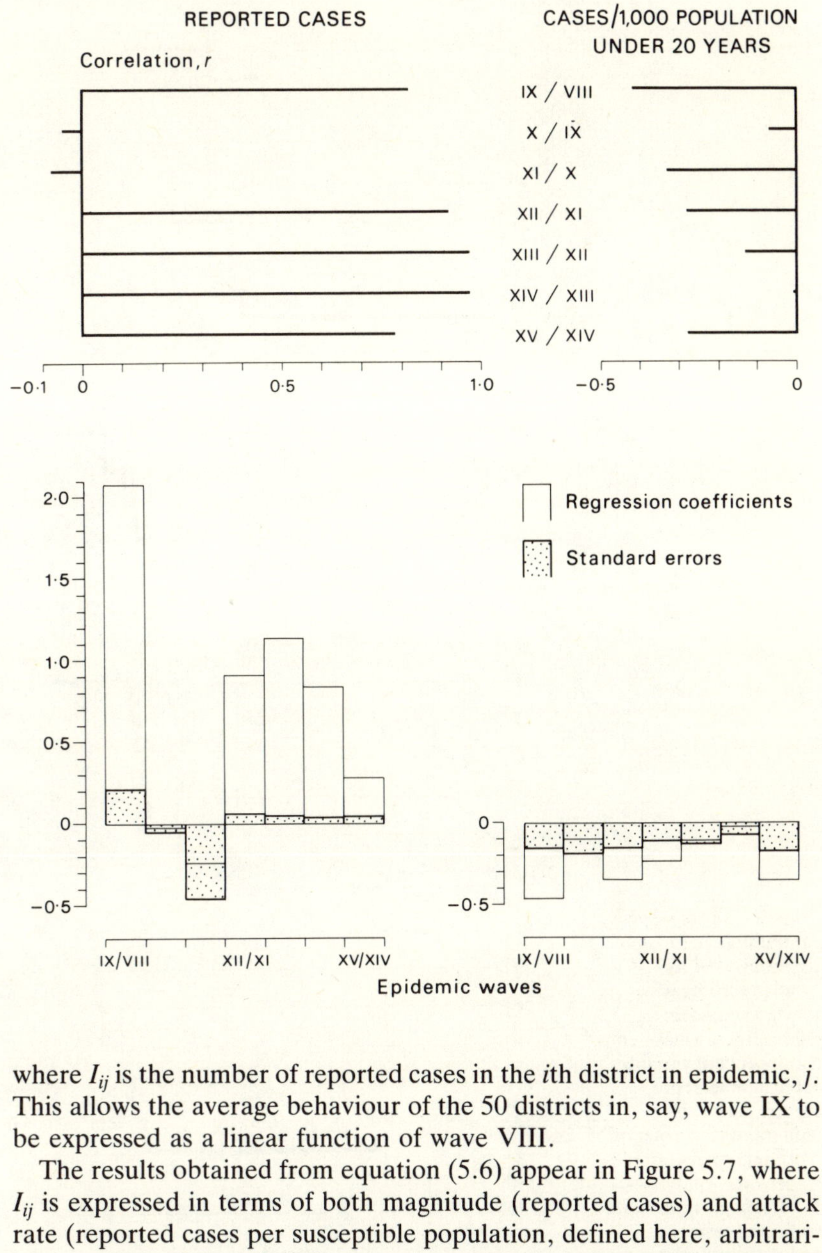

Fig. 5.7 Results of simple linear regression analysis of each wave upon its immediate predecessor. Note that standard errors are, by definition, all positive, but have been superimposed on the regression coefficients for convenience. Analysis has been carried out using reported cases and cases per 1,000 population under 20.

where I_{ij} is the number of reported cases in the ith district in epidemic, j. This allows the average behaviour of the 50 districts in, say, wave IX to be expressed as a linear function of wave VIII.

The results obtained from equation (5.6) appear in Figure 5.7, where I_{ij} is expressed in terms of both magnitude (reported cases) and attack rate (reported cases per susceptible population, defined here, arbitrarily, as under 20 years). The most interesting results are given by the relationships for the attack rate, where the regression coefficients, $\hat{b}_1$, are everywhere negative. This suggests a tendency for a severe epidemic to be followed by a mild one, and vice versa. The coefficients are generally more consistent for the rate data than for the magnitude data.

The simple one-step lag model given in equation (5.6) can be extended to a multiple-step model, viz.:

$$I_{ij} = b_0 + \sum_{k=1}^{h} b_k I_{i,j-k} + e_{ij}. \qquad (5.7)$$

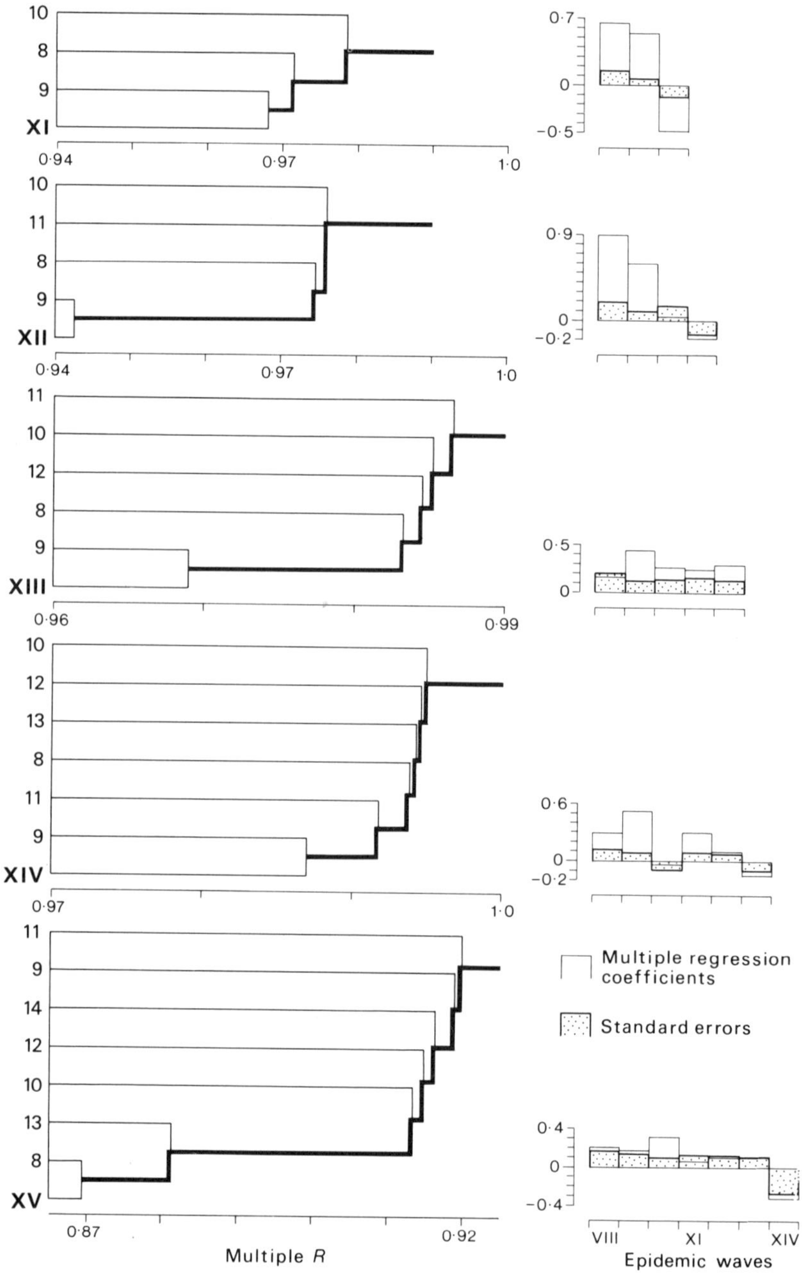

Fig. 5.8 Results of stepwise linear multiple regression analysis of waves XI – XV upon all preceding waves, 1945–70. Dependent variable (Roman numbers) and independent variables (Arabic numbers) are shown on the *y* axis. Dendograms give order of entry of regressor variables (i.e., previous epidemics). Left-hand page of results is for reported cases; right-hand page is for cases per 1,000 population under 20 years. See caption to Figure 5.7.

This incorporates the record of up to *h* earlier epidemics so that, say, wave XV (j) can be expressed in terms of wave XIV ($j - 1$), wave XIII ($j - 2$), wave XII ($j - 3$), etc. Results from application of this model appear in Figure 5.8. This shows some stepwise multiple regressions (using Efroymson's algorithm) of selected epidemics on previous epidemics for all 50 medical districts, based on both the absolute number of reported cases (left part of Figure 5.8) and the number of reported cases per 1,000 population under 20 years (right part of Figure

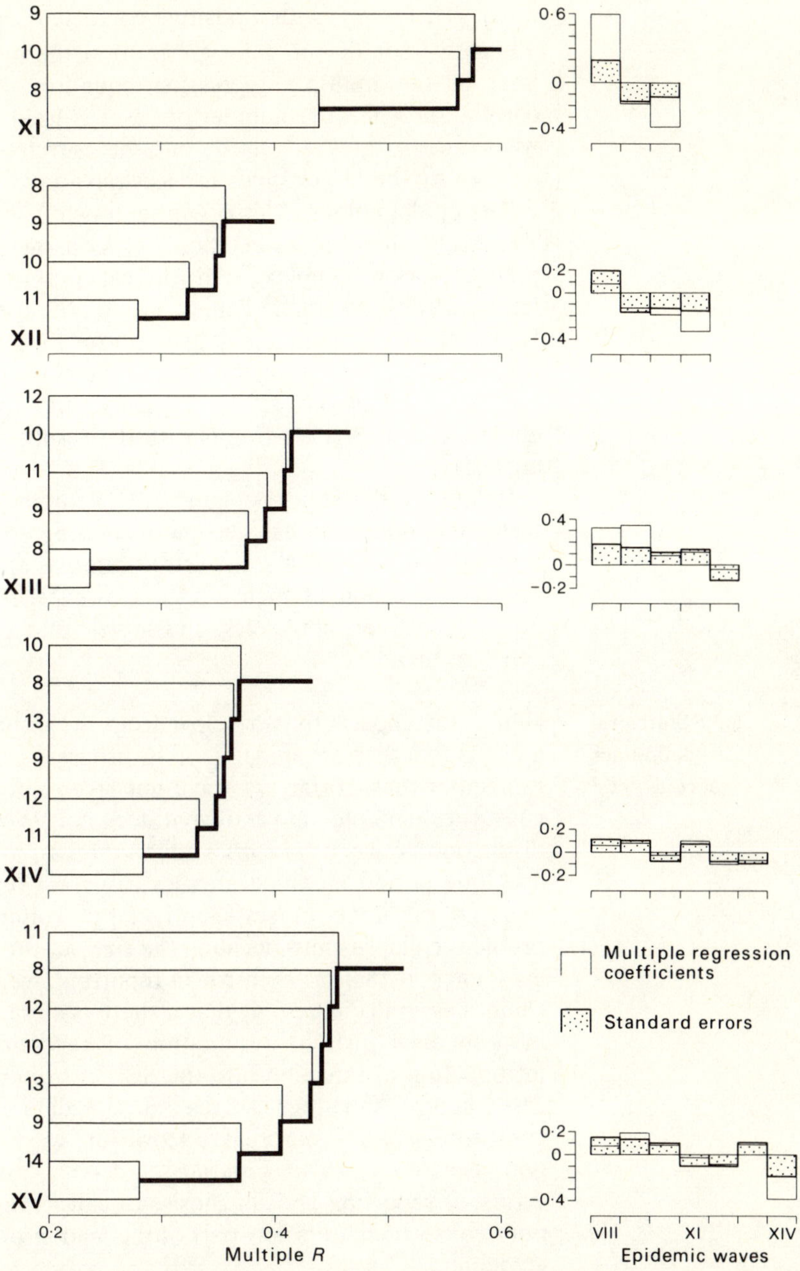

Fig. 5.8 (contd)

5.8). We can understand the structure of Figure 5.8 by looking at the diagram upper right. This shows the attack rates in wave XI as a function of the attack rates in the three preceding waves (VIII, IX and X). The dendrogram traces the way in which the waves enter the equation; wave VIII (the 1946–8 epidemic) is entered first, and it is, thus, a better statistical predictor of attack rates in the 1954–5 outbreak than are the two intervening waves, which are entered later. The regression coefficients and their associated standard errors show that wave VIII ($j-3$), with a positive coefficient, and wave X ($j-1$), with a negative coefficient, are significant at the $\alpha = 0.05$ level (two-tailed test) in the multiple regression equation. Note that the level of correlation when the number of cases is used is generally higher than when attack rates are used, but the correlation coefficients may be inflated by the large values for Reykjavíkur, which acts as an outlier.

The epidemiological lesson to be drawn from the multiple regression analysis is that the association between one epidemic wave and its predecessors is complex. With the exception of wave XII (Figure 5.8, right), there is no simple dependence on the past history of the process. However, the repeating negative sign for the first lag term ($j-1$), and the variations in sign of the other regression coefficients, point to an oscillatory behaviour in the intensity, and therefore in the size, of epidemics which is consistent with the results of the simple regression analysis.

Related to this result is Figure 5.9. We noted in section 3.5.2 that the Icelandic population has become increasingly youthful throughout this century but, despite this, the attack rate has apparently decreased with time (third graph of Figure 5.9). However, if we allow for the time interval between epidemics, the attack rate seems to vary around a constant mean.

5.3.5 Statistical definitions of epidemics[1]

While it is apparently very clear from the visual record of Figures 3.1 and 8.3 whether an epidemic is in progress or not, it is important to remember that, so far, we have not given a formal definition of what constitutes an epidemic and what does not. We need to make a formal distinction between *epidemics* and *outbreaks*. We define an *outbreak* as any time period in which measles cases are reported. An *epidemic* is then an outbreak of sufficiently large volume, and our definition problem collapses into deciding the size cut-off between outbreaks and epidemics. If there is no error in reporting, we know from the measles chain diagram (Figure 3.4) that if there is a break in the cases reported in a medical district, resumption of reporting must imply the re-introduction of infection into the district from outside. Thus, reported cases before and after a break in the data record, however short, constitute separate outbreaks. However, we would not wish to define odd, isolated cases as separate epidemics, and given the inevitable errors of reporting and diagnosis, to call as separate epidemics those outbreaks which are really part of the lead-in or fade-out of an existing epidemic.

Several criteria have been proposed in the literature for deciding when an outbreak is sufficiently large to be called an epidemic (Cliff, Haggett, Ord, Bassett and Davies, 1975, p. 101). All involve monitoring two pieces of information, namely (1) epidemic *size*, as measured by the total number of cases reported in a given length of time; and (2)

[1] This section relies on the work of C. Goodall, now of Harvard University, who was supervised by one of us (A.D.C.) while working as a student on a field project as part of the postgraduate diploma in mathematical statistics at Cambridge University. See Goodall (1978) for details of the project.

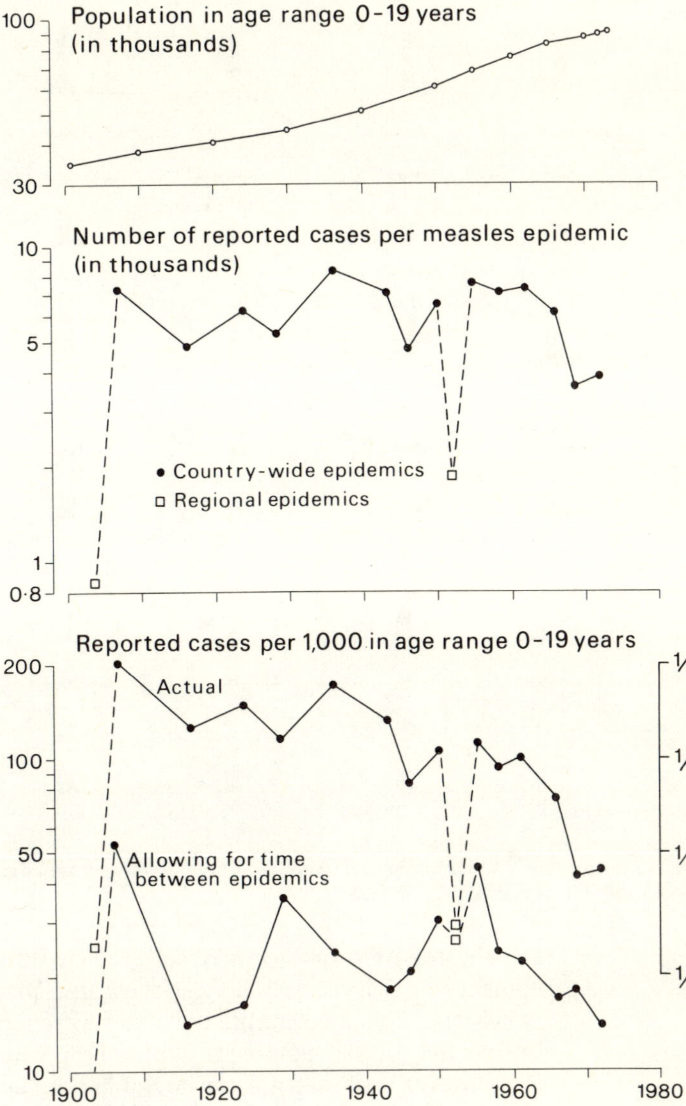

Fig. 5.9 Size of epidemics (waves I to XVI) in relation to population aged 0–19 years.

epidemic *intensity*, as measured by the rate of attack (number of cases per head of population) in a given length of time. In general, we require outbreaks to pass thresholds for both (1) and (2) before they are classified as epidemics. Use of (1) prevents short, sharp bursts of infection being called epidemics, while criterion (2) ensures that long strings of small numbers of cases are not called as separate epidemics. What we wish to do is to establish thresholds which isolate the 'mountain peaks' of cases which most people would agree constitute an epidemic. Inevitably, the procedure is subjective, in that we can vary the number of epidemics defined simply by varying the threshold positions.

To illustrate the issues involved, we consider the three medical districts shown in Figure 5.10. Diagrams A show the number of cases

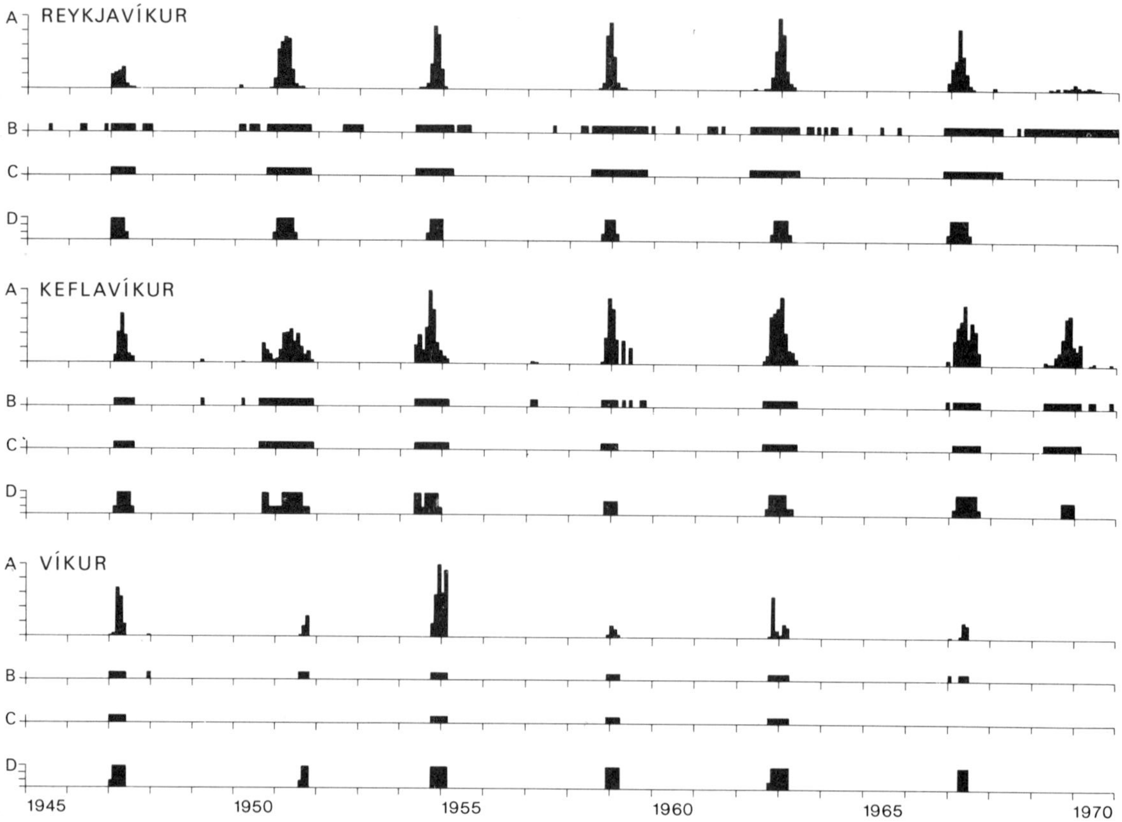

Fig. 5.10. Defining an epidemic. (A) Reported case levels. (B) Columns one unit high if cases reported in a given month. (C) Using model 1 and (D) using model 2 as defined in text.

actually reported in each medical district. Because of the scale, small numbers of cases simply do not show up. Diagrams B show a binary switch; unit columns indicate that cases were reported in a given month, irrespective of the numbers. Notice how small numbers of cases in Reykjavíkur trail on for a considerable time either side of the obvious epidemic peaks shown in Figure 5.10A. This does not happen in Keflavíkur and Víkur.

To determine whether an outbreak should be classified as an epidemic, two models were tried.

Model 1. Let I_t be the number of cases reported in month t of an outbreak in a given medical district, and let P_t be the population of the medical district in month t. Suppose that the outbreak lasts T months. An outbreak may be called an epidemic if

$$\sum_{t=1}^{T} I_t \Big/ \sum_{t=1}^{T} P_t \geq 1/C_1 \qquad (5.8)$$

where C_1 is a constant to be determined empirically. Equation (5.8) is a size criterion. We found that $C_1 = 250$ in order to separate out waves XIV (1968) and XV (1970) in Reykjavíkur. However, in smaller medical districts where epidemics tend to be shorter and more sharply peaked (see Víkur in Figure 5.10), this meant that any isolated knot of cases was called an epidemic, and so we imposed the additional requirement that $T > 3$. Application of model 1 to the three medical districts is shown in Figure 5.10C. In the case of Reykjavíkur, it allows epidemics to trail on a little beyond the obvious peaks shown in Figure 5.10A, but it is much more restricted than the binary switch (Figure 5.10B). For the other medical districts, the criterion corresponds almost identically with the main epidemic blocks.

Model 2. Both intensity and size criteria were incorporated within this model.

(a) *Intensity.* An epidemic is declared in a medical district from the month in which

$$I_t / P_t \geqslant 1 / C_2 \tag{5.9}$$

and terminated when

$$I_t / P_t \leqslant 1 / C_3 \tag{5.10}$$

(b) *Size.* Let J be the set of months for which

$$I_t / P_t > 1 / C_4 \tag{5.11}$$

The months are declared an epidemic if

$$\sum_{j \in J} I_j > P / C_5 \tag{5.12}$$

where P is the average population of the medical district over the outbreak. Values of the constants $C_2 - C_5$ were determined empirically. In Figure 5.10D, where an outbreak met criterion (a) above, columns two units high have been drawn; $C_2 = 250$, $C_3 = 400$ were found to yield the best results. If criterion (b) above was met, columns one unit high have been drawn; $C_4 = 500$, $C_5 = 18$. If criteria (a) and (b) *both* have to be satisfied before an epidemic is called, columns three units high have been drawn.

As Figure 5.10D shows, epidemics are called slightly earlier on the basis of (b) than (a). In addition, model 2 cuts off the long tails of the outbreaks in Reykjavíkur much more effectively than does model 1; it also declares the 1951 (wave IX) and 1967 epidemics (wave XIV) in Víkur which are missed by model 1.

In defining epidemics in the remainder of this book for modelling purposes, we have taken model 2 and required that both (a) and (b) be met. On this basis, over the 50 medical districts, 1945–70, a total of 242 epidemics may be identified.

The analysis described in this section naturally raises the question of whether a criterion such as: 'If

$$I_t / P_t > k, \tag{5.13}$$

an epidemic is expected', can be used to provide a brief warning of the approach of an epidemic. We are monitoring the monthly rate of reporting and, as the attack rate goes up, becoming more and more

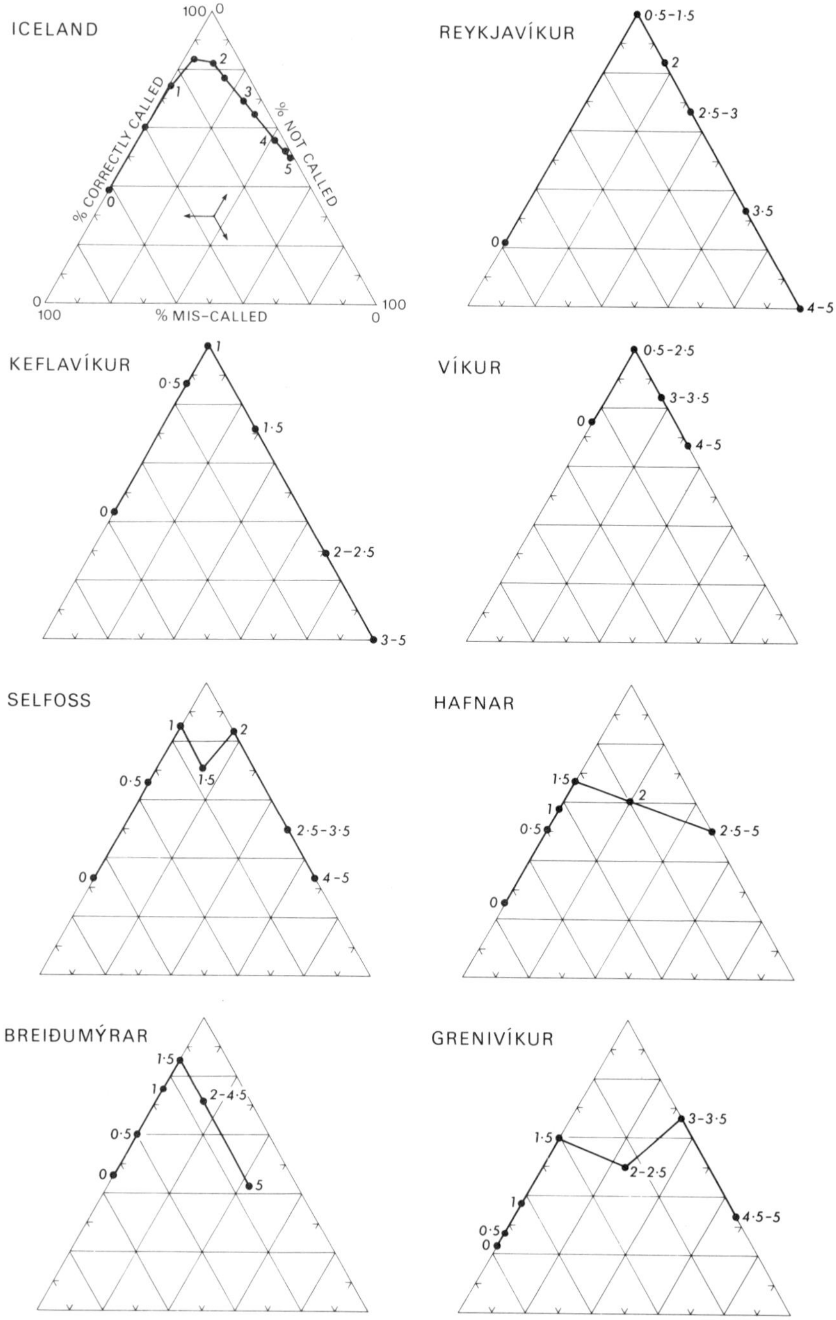

Fig. 5.11 Percentage of epidemics in Iceland and medical districts shown, 1945–70, correctly called, not called and mis-called if an epidemic is declared when reported cases/ population reach percentage levels shown by dots.

certain that an epidemic is about to begin. For any given value of k, three things can result from application of rule (5.13): (1) some epidemics will be called and actually occur (a correct call); (2) some epidemics will occur but not be recognised by the rule (not called); (3) some epidemics will be called by the rule but not, in fact, occur (a mis-call). In Figure 5.11, we indicate what percentage of the 242 epidemics identified in Iceland, 1945–70, would fall into categories

(1)–(3) for various values of k. The curve for values of k peaks quite sharply at 1.5–2.0 per cent; that is, once the ratio, cases/population, reaches 1.5 per cent in a given month, we can be about 85 per cent certain that an epidemic is at hand. Applying (5.13) to individual medical districts, we find, from Figure 5.10, that the k curves are all reasonably well behaved, and that an attack rate of 1.5 per cent of the population in any month gives good warning of an epidemic. Indeed, we can view lower attack rates as providing different levels of alert and read off the probability of being right or wrong from the chart. Obviously, this approach is not foolproof; its merit is that it is not data-demanding and that it is simple to apply from a public-health viewpoint.

5.4 Diffusion at the macro-scale: statistical reconstruction at the regional level

The third level of analysis moves above that of the individual medical districts to that of the region. In the first study described below, a simple distinction is made between Reykjavíkur and the rest of Iceland; in the second, six separate regions are defined. In order to define regions in the Icelandic context, two factors had to be considered; first, the conventional regional distinctions recognised in the standard geographical works (Preusser, 1976; Schutzbach, 1976) and in the statistical accounts of Iceland, and second, the need to recognise and contain the shifts in medical district boundaries described earlier (section 4.2) so as to preserve comparability over time.

5.4.1 Variations in epidemic velocity

The concept of epidemic velocity has attracted theoretical attention because of its importance for possible preventive measures. Where we are dealing with a simple spatial process with a well-defined wavefront, (as in the case of the studies by Mollison (1977) described in section 2.3.1), then the physical concept of distance travelled over time may be appropriate. However, where the wavefront is not a well-defined line, and where the susceptible population through which the epidemic moves is both discontinuous in space and has sharp variations in intensity, then an alternative definition must be sought. We have chosen to adhere to classical statistical measures, and to use the higher moments of the frequency distribution of cases measured in the time domain. These are defined in equations (4.1)–(4.4) and Table 4.1.

The simplest measure, the arithmetic mean, $\bar{t}$, indicates the lag in months between the start of the epidemic (the month in which the first case was recorded) and the average time at which cases occur. Thus, in the case of wave I, the first cases occurred in April 1904; if we measure from the start of the month and ignore the three-day variation in length over the standard month of 30.44 days, the average case falls in August 1904 ($\bar{t} = 4.53$). Where we have separate data for Reykjavíkur, the top part of Figure 5.12 plots the comparative means for the capital medical district and for the rest of Iceland excluding Reykjavíkur. Note that, in all but two cases, the Reykjavíkur mean is less than that for the rest of Iceland, suggesting that the epidemic moves more quickly through the main urban centre.

Since the epidemics studied varied in their duration and intensity, the

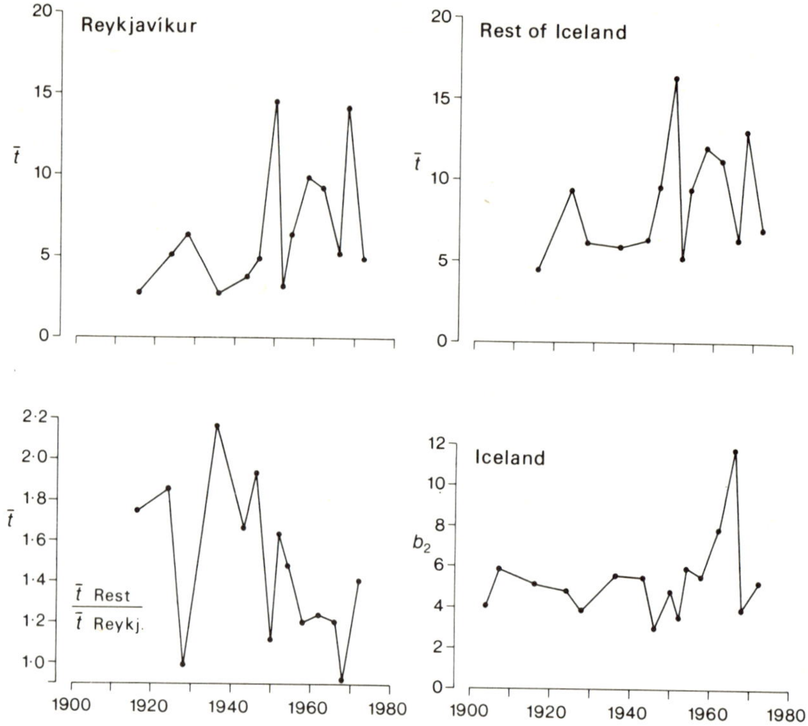

Fig. 5.12 Average time, $\bar{t}$, in months when cases occurred for each wave, 1916–75, for Reykjavíkur and the rest of Iceland. The sample kurtosis coefficient, b_2, for Iceland for each wave, 1896–1975, is also shown.

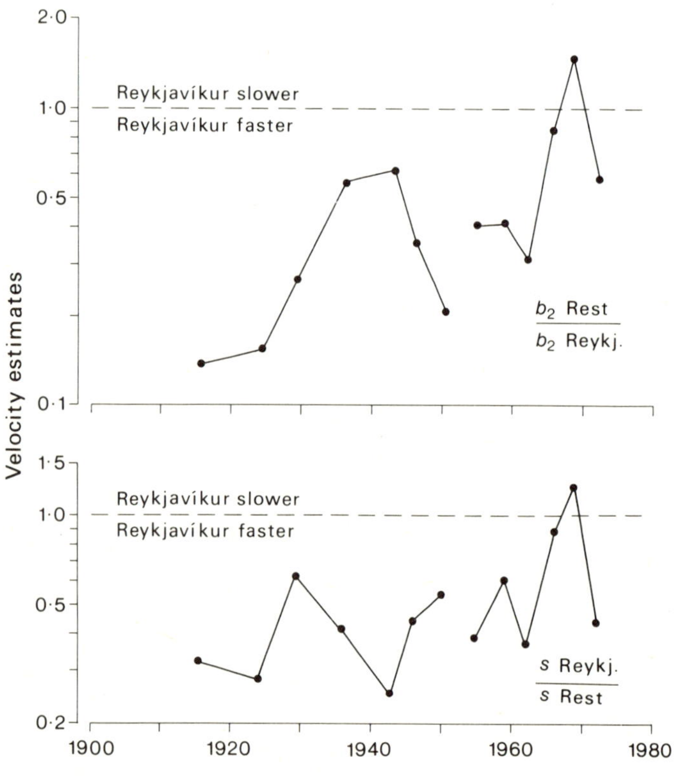

Fig. 5.13 Comparison of velocities of epidemic waves passing through Reykjavíkur and the rest of Iceland, 1916–75. Two estimates of velocity, the kurtosis, b_2, and the sample standard deviation, s, are used (see equations (4.1) – (4.4)).

values of $\bar{t}$ must reflect that variation, thus invalidating comparisons of velocities *between* epidemics. To overcome this problem, parts of Figure 5.12 and Figure 5.13 use the dimensionless measure of kurtosis (b_2) defined in equation (4.4). In terms of an epidemic wave, kurtosis measures the extent to which cases are concentrated into the peak period of an epidemic, and thus its speed in infecting a population. Waves with high kurtosis have a high velocity, and vice versa.

In Figure 5.12, b_2 shows a weak tendency for the measles waves in Iceland as a whole to increase in velocity. If, however, we separate the waves into those for Reykjavíkur and those for Iceland minus Reykjavíkur (Figure 5.13), we see that the overall increase is made up of two countervailing trends: (1) a decreasing velocity for Reykjavíkur, and (2) an increasing velocity for the rest of the country. If we compare the ratios for the two velocities as measured by b_2 and the sample standard deviation, s, we see a convergence, with the velocity of the rest of Iceland approaching that of Reykjavíkur, and in one epidemic (wave XV) even surpassing it. It would be tempting to associate the increased velocity within the rest of Iceland with improved internal transport links, while the relative slowdown in Reykjavíkur itself might be seen in terms of improved public health control within the urban community. We consider these propositions further in sections 5.5 and 5.5.3.

5.4.2 Variations in regional incidence rates

Given the existence of neighbourhood effects in the measles diffusion process, it is clear that the outbreak pattern in one medical district will be strongly linked to those of adjacent areas. It is economical, therefore, to group districts together into regions to allow analysis of coarser-grained trends within the country. The regional boundaries adopted in Figure 5.14 take into account the traditional provincial divisions of Iceland, together with the stability of the medical district boundaries over our study period. Six regions are recognised: Reykjavíkur, and the rest of Iceland divided into SW, NW, N, E and S sectors.

From the regional distribution of cases, it is possible to build up a picture of variation in the regional intensity of each outbreak. Figure 5.14 shows (lower left) variations in the size, spread and intensity of the 15 measles outbreaks from 1904 to 1970 on a national basis. It emphasises the large size of the 1936 outbreak, the wide spread of the 1916 outbreak and the high intensity of the 1907 outbreak. The graph on the lower right of Figure 5.14 shows the regional intensity of each outbreak as a biproportionate score within a 14 (epidemics) × 6 (region) matrix.

Biproportionate matrices (Bacharach, 1970) form one way of disentangling the relations between changes in incidence within individual regions and changes in the whole country of which they form a part. In biproportionate matrices, the values $\{x_{ij}\}$ in an $m \times n$ matrix are scaled so that each row sum is equal to n. Then the columns are scaled so that each column sum is equal to m. This process of column and row adjustment is repeated successively until adequate convergence to an

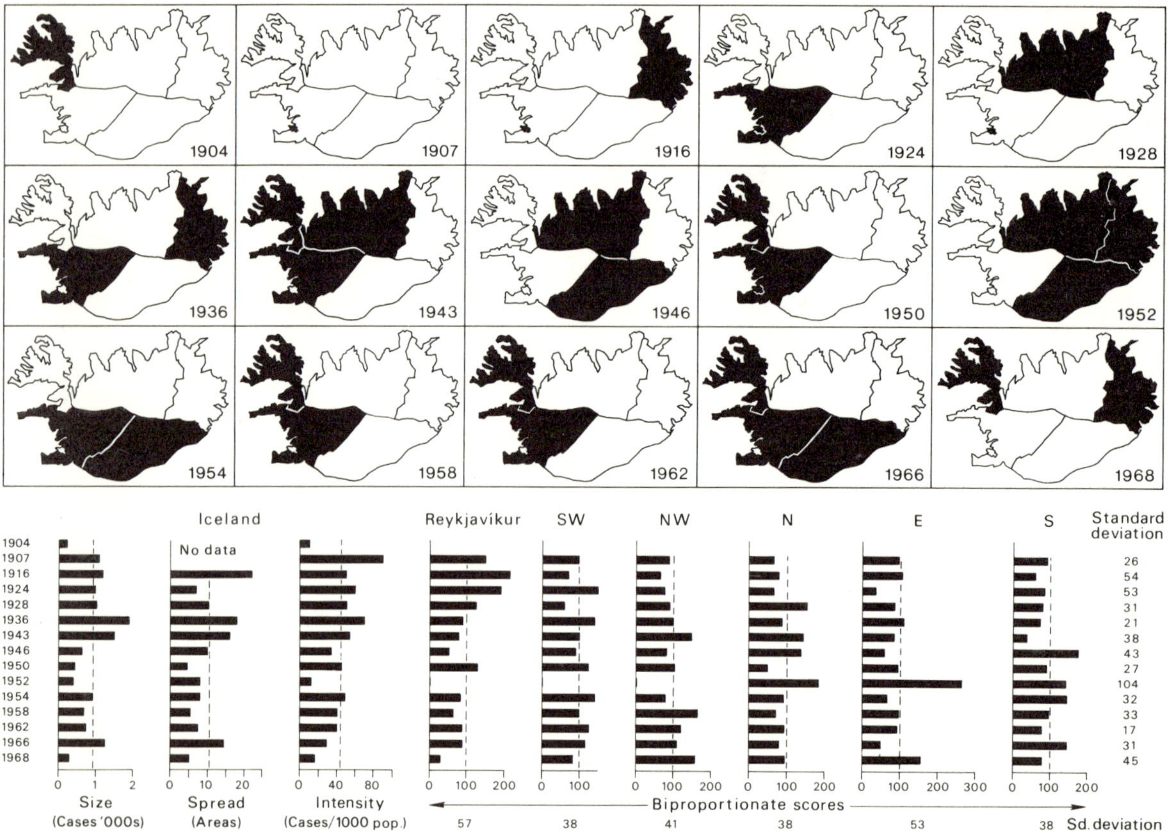

Fig. 5.14 Measures of regional concentration of epidemics in parts of Iceland. On maps, areas are shaded black if they have biproportionate scores in excess of 100. For size, spread and intensity, vertical pecked lines mark averages; for biproportionate scores, 100 denotes equal concentration over the regions.

equilibrium solution is obtained. We can express this process more formally as

$$\begin{bmatrix} x_{11} & x_{12} & \ldots x_{1j} & \ldots x_{1n} \\ x_{21} & x_{22} & \ldots x_{2j} & \ldots x_{2n} \\ \cdot & \cdot & \cdot & \cdot \\ \cdot & \cdot & \cdot & \cdot \\ \cdot & \cdot & \cdot & \cdot \\ x_{i1} & x_{i2} & \ldots x_{ij} & \ldots x_{in} \\ \cdot & \cdot & \cdot & \cdot \\ \cdot & \cdot & \cdot & \cdot \\ \cdot & \cdot & \cdot & \cdot \\ x_{m1} & x_{m2} & \ldots x_{mj} & \ldots x_{mn} \end{bmatrix} = \begin{bmatrix} n+e \\ n+e \\ \cdot \\ \cdot \\ \cdot \\ n+e \\ \cdot \\ \cdot \\ \cdot \\ n+e \end{bmatrix}$$

$$\parallel$$

$$[m+e \ldots\ldots\ldots\ldots m+e] \tag{5.14}$$

where e is an allowable tolerance term. The procedure produces a standardisation of the matrix values over the rows and columns of the matrix.

In Figure 5.14, the matrix values have been multiplied by 100. Reading down the columns shows the *relative* change in each region over time. Thus, the eastern region (E) plays an important role in the 1916, 1936, 1952 and 1968 outbreaks but has biproportionate scores below 100 in the other 10 outbreaks. Reading along the rows shows the regional distribution in each epidemic. Note the difference between the intense regional contrasts of the 1952 epidemic, and the relatively low regional variation within the 1962 epidemic. The maps above the matrix in Figure 5.14 highlight these patterns by having regions with biproportionate scores of 100 or more coloured black.

5.5 Diffusion processes in a context of change

The 16 measles epidemics whose spread is studied in this volume span a period of eight decades. During this time, Iceland moved from its role as an isolated province of Denmark with a population of only 78,000 and very limited external contact, to one of an independent state of over 205,000 people and strong international contacts. This section looks at the environment of change within Iceland over two generations and comments on its role in interpreting the spatial diffusion processes examined.

5.5.1 Demographic change

The 1901 census shows Iceland as a country of exceptionally low population density (0.76 per km^2). Its 78,000 people were concentrated on small pockets of land around the perimeter of the island. Reykjavík, the capital, had 6,700 people (about one twelfth of the total population); only two other towns had more than 1,000 inhabitants (Akureyri and Isafjörður); 80 per cent of the population was classified as rural; 80 per cent of the workforce was engaged directly in agriculture and fishing.

By 1970, many elements in the demographic picture had changed. The population total had multiplied by 2.6 to a density of 1.97 people per km^2. Its population of 205,000 remained scattered around the perimeter of the island but was now more heavily concentrated into fewer centres, in particular Reykjavík which, with 82,000 people, housed two-fifths of the population. Twelve other towns had passed the 1,000 bench-mark; only 14 per cent of the population was classified as rural; the proportion in agriculture and fishing had fallen by three-quarters to around 20 per cent.

From the viewpoint of the spread of measles three aspects of this demographic change are important:

(1) *Changing age structure.* The 1901 census showed that 38 per cent of the total population was under 20 years. By 1970, this proportion had increased to 42 per cent. Iceland has had high birth-rates during this century. The birth-rate of 28.7 per 1,000 in the first decade fell to 22.5 in the 1930s but rose again to 28.6 in the late 1950s. This was followed by a subsequent fall to below the 1930s level. The increased proportion of young people has been due partly to the fall in still-births (from 33 to 1 per 1,000 total births, 1901–70) but even more to the decline in infant mortality (Baldursson, 1975, p. 31). All other things being equal, these facts imply a general growth in the population susceptible to measles over the study period (cf. section 3.4.2). Yet, as noted in the discussion

on Figure 5.9, the attack rate has not increased over the study period. This may reflect, in part, the improvements in medical care to be discussed in section 5.5.3.

(2) *Changing spatial structure.* At the beginning of the century, the bulk of Iceland's population was distributed in isolated farmsteads or small fishing villages. Black (1966) and Haggett (1975) have demonstrated that we should expect the transmission of measles epidemics through such low-density populations to be, *ceteris paribus*, a significantly slower process than in concentrated populations. We should expect the switch to a more clustered demographic pattern by 1970 to lead to a faster diffusion rate, but tests of this supposition are likely to be confounded by a reduced attack rate due to vaccination and improved public-health measures. However, as we saw in section 5.4.1 and Figure 5.13, there is some evidence of an increase in the velocity of measles waves in parts of Iceland over this century.

(3) *Size of Reykjavík.* Bartlett (1957) indicates that the minimum size of a city in which measles will be endemic is approximately 250,000. Although the size of Reykjavík was well below this threshold throughout the study period, it has been increasing steadily (Figure 3.8). In terms of Figure 3.3, Reykjavík moved from being a type III city to a type II city, 1900–70, so that in each epidemic we may expect measles cases to occur in the capital. Given the bond structure of Figure 4.19, Reykjavík is then likely to act as a diffusion pole for the spatial transmission of the disease in most epidemics.

5.5.2 Transport change

Both the introduction of measles virus into Iceland and its subsequent spread through the island are assumed to be wholly dependent on international and internal movement of the human population. We look at these two levels of spatial interaction in turn.

(1) Iceland's contacts with the rest of the world

The fragmentary Irish contacts with Iceland from the end of the fifth century and permanent Norwegian settlement from AD 874 were both reflections of the prevailing technology of sea transport. The sea link remained the only avenue for man-borne disease for the next 1,000 years; it was 1919 before the first aeroplane contact added a second transport mode to Iceland's external links.

Data are not available for the whole of the study period. From the fragments obtainable, we can see something of Iceland's increasing level of contact with the outside world. In 1918 the number of foreign ships arriving in Reykjavík harbour averaged 13 each month, a figure which had increased more than tenfold by 1941, the peak year of the Allied occupation. Post-war figures on passenger movement (Figure 5.15) show the exponential growth in contact was due not to sea transport, where numbers in 1970 were around the same as a quarter of a century before, but to air transport, where they had increased sixteenfold.

The eclipse of sea transport by air movement has had important epidemiological implications, since all international air movements terminate at a single airport (Keflavík, 50 km west of Reykjavík); in contrast, sea contacts may be spread around a number of major

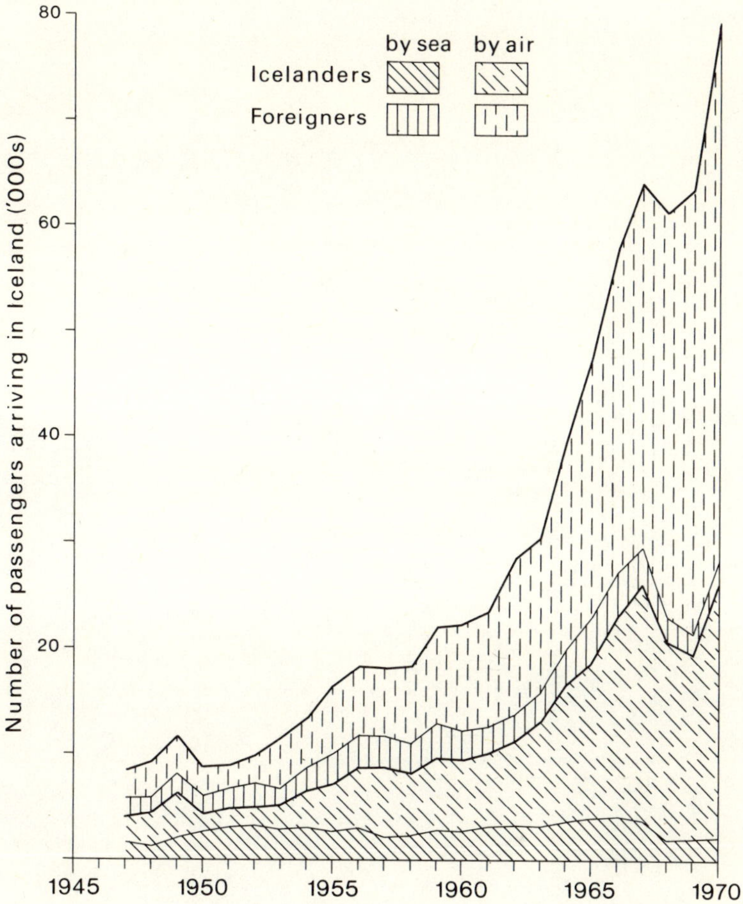

Fig. 5.15 Passenger arrival by sea and air in Iceland, 1947–70. *Source: Tölfræðihandbók* (1974, p. 149).

harbours. It may not be without significance that, since 1945, all epidemics with known sources of origin have started in the south-west corner of Iceland (see Figure 4.20). Study of the origin of foreign passengers arriving in Iceland (Figure 5.16) shows that 80 per cent of all passengers come from just four countries. The share of the United States has increased steadily over the 1960s and now accounts for around 40 per cent of all foreign passengers.

From the viewpoint of spatial diffusion, the potential importance of the United States as a virus source is reduced by the high proportion of United States arrivals who are either (a) in transit to Europe and do not move outside the Keflavík international airport during their very brief stay in Iceland, or (b) are service personnel or dependents bound for the United States base at Keflavík. Contact between the Keflavík base and the adjacent Icelandic population is low, and the children of servicemen in the critical under-15 age group attend a separate school within the base.

It is worth noting that, of the 16 epidemic waves, 1896–1975 (see Table 4.1), 7 occurred in the 50 years from 1896 to 1945 and 9 in the 30

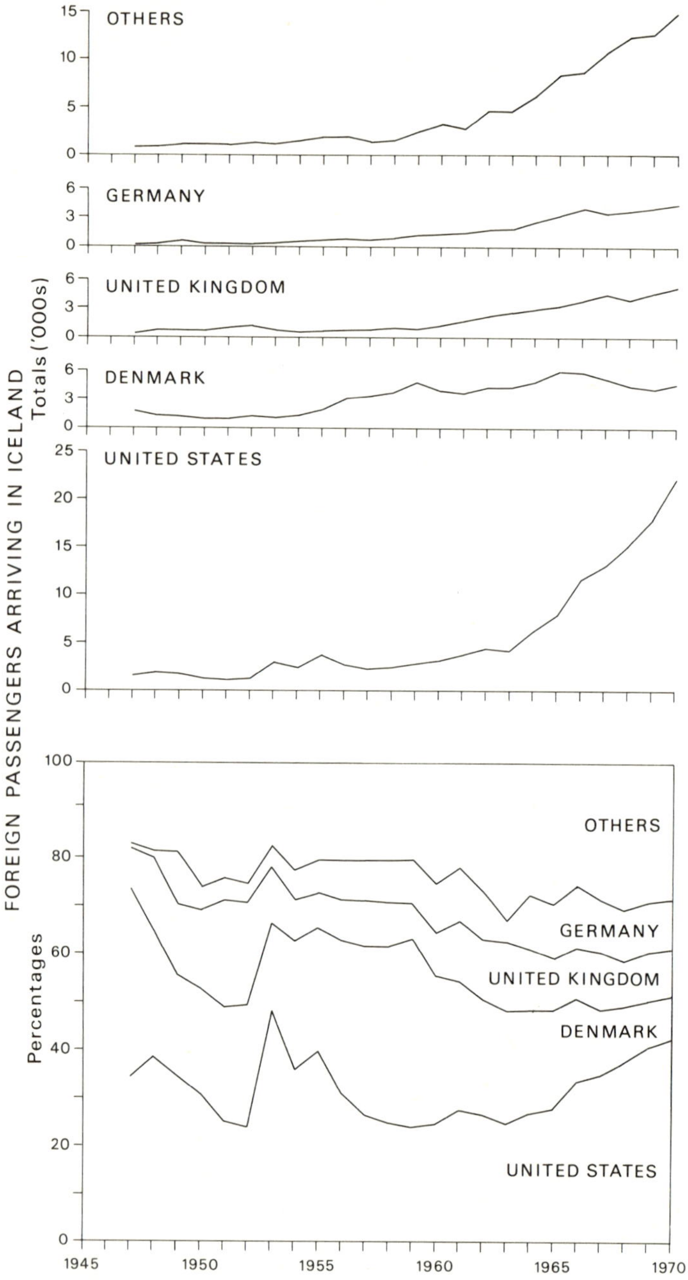

Fig. 5.16 Country of origin of foreign passenger arrivals in Iceland, 1947–70. *Source: Hagtíðindi* (publication of Statistical Bureau of Iceland, Reykjavík).

years afterwards. This increased epidemic frequency also probably reflects Iceland's increasing external contacts.

(2) Internal contacts within Iceland

At the beginning of this century, travelling conditions in the rural areas of Iceland were little different from those at the time of first settlement: movement on horseback was the only way of getting about overland. As Kristinsson (1975, p. 231) comments, 'Communications by land were extremely difficult and it is hardly going too far to say that virtually

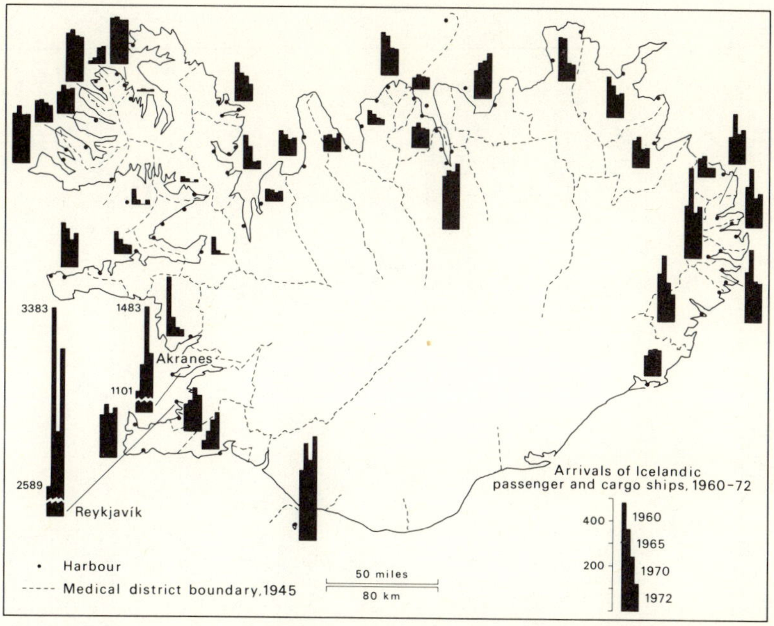

Fig. 5.17 Arrivals of Icelandic passenger and cargo ships in Icelandic ports, 1960–72. *Source: Tölfræðihandbók,* (1974, pp. 136–7).

nothing was done to improve them in the first thousand years of the nation's existence.' Route improvements had begun in the late nineteenth century, and the first large bridge was opened in 1891. The first major boost to road-building came in the 1910s when the first motor vehicle was imported into Iceland (in 1913) and the present network of gravel roads began to emerge. A second major boost to both road- and bridge-building came with the Allied occupation during World War II, and there has since been a sharp increase in motor vehicles: from 11,000 in 1950 to 47,000 in 1970. Even today, the only asphalt roads outside the major towns are from Reykjavík (1) west to Keflavík and (2) south-east to Selfoss, about 150 km in all.

Given the difficulty of overland movement, contacts between the coastal settlements have been traditionally reliant on coastal shipping. As Figure 5.17 shows, Iceland has a comprehensive network of small harbours, with the only major gap being along the south-east coast. The more remote rural areas in the north-west and north-east used to be wholly dependent on coastal shipping for contact with the rest of Iceland, and even this link could be cut in severe winters by pack ice (see section 5.5.4). Coastal passenger services were established after World War I and, from 1929, were organised by a State Shipping Department (Skipaútgerð ríkisins). However, we note that passenger traffic by coastal shipping, and thus the possible sea-borne movements of index cases, has been falling since 1960.

An increasingly extensive and regular bus service now links the main centres (Figure 5.18). This has been supplemented, and to some extent superseded, by the growth of a rapid and relatively cheap airline network (Figure 5.19). The rapid growth of internal air travel is shown by the fact that, in 1955, the number of passengers (44,512) represented

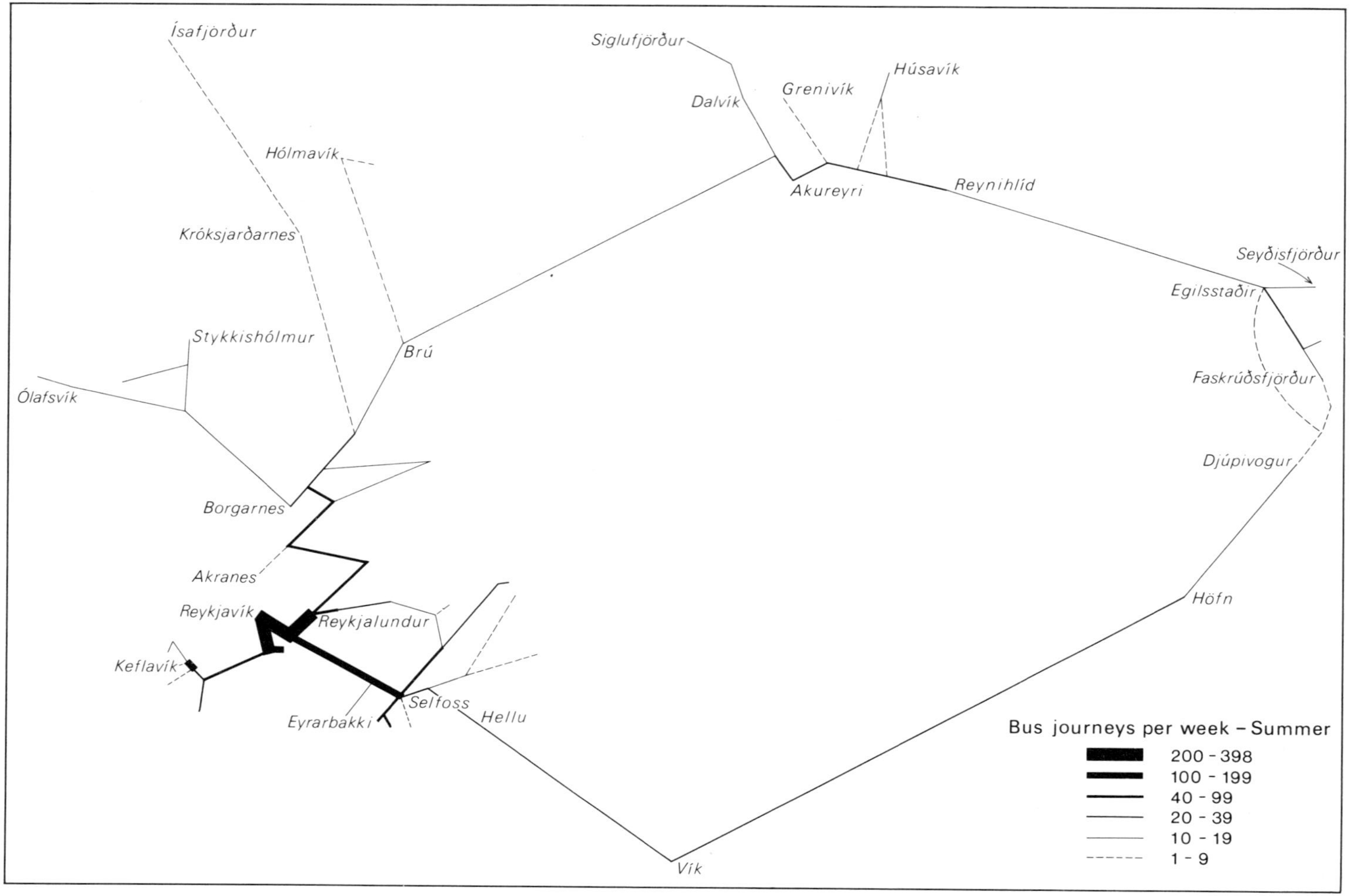

Fig. 5.18 Summer and winter bus journeys per week on all routes, 1978. *Sources:* Local bus timetables.

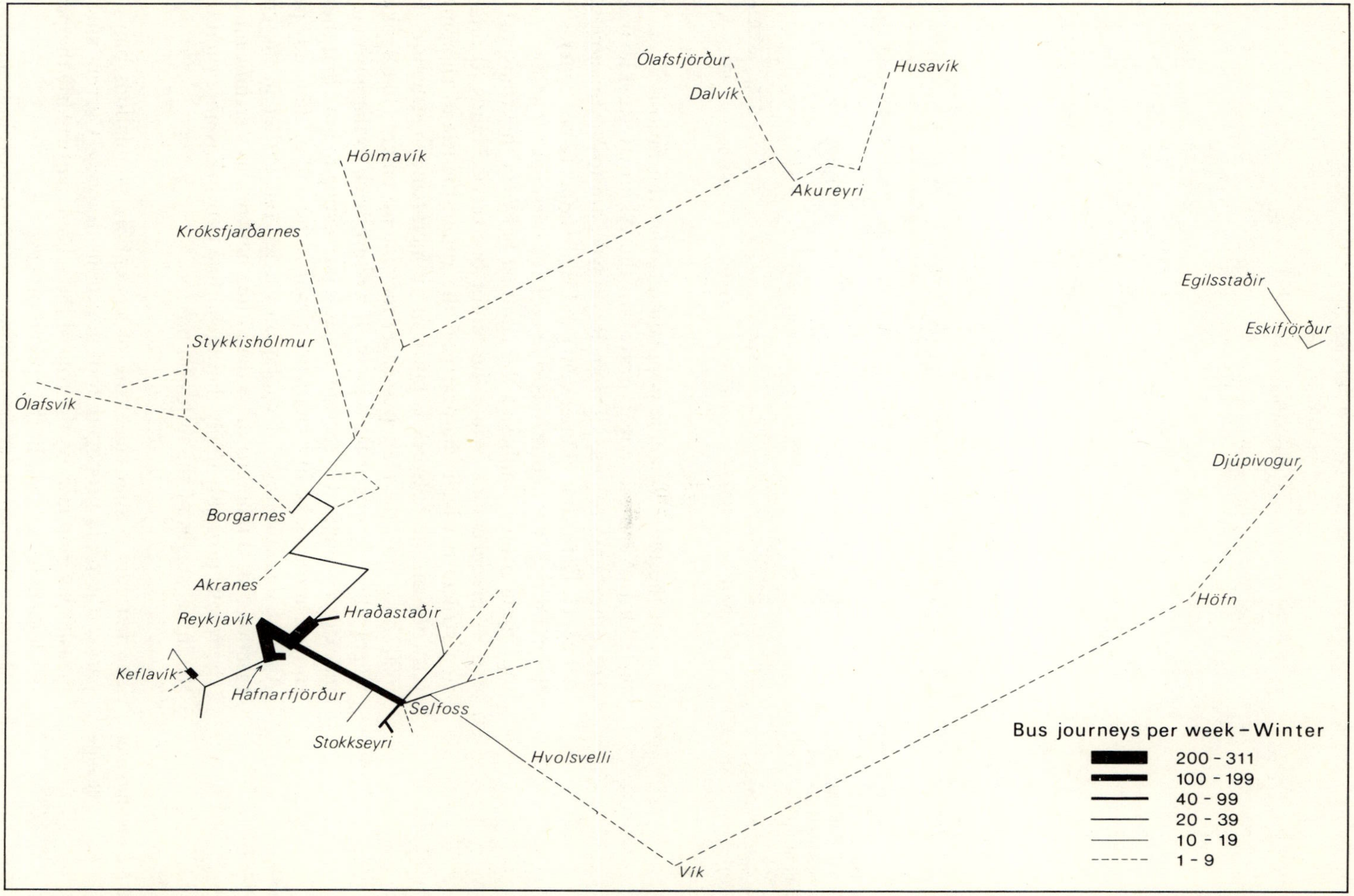

Fig. 5.18 continued

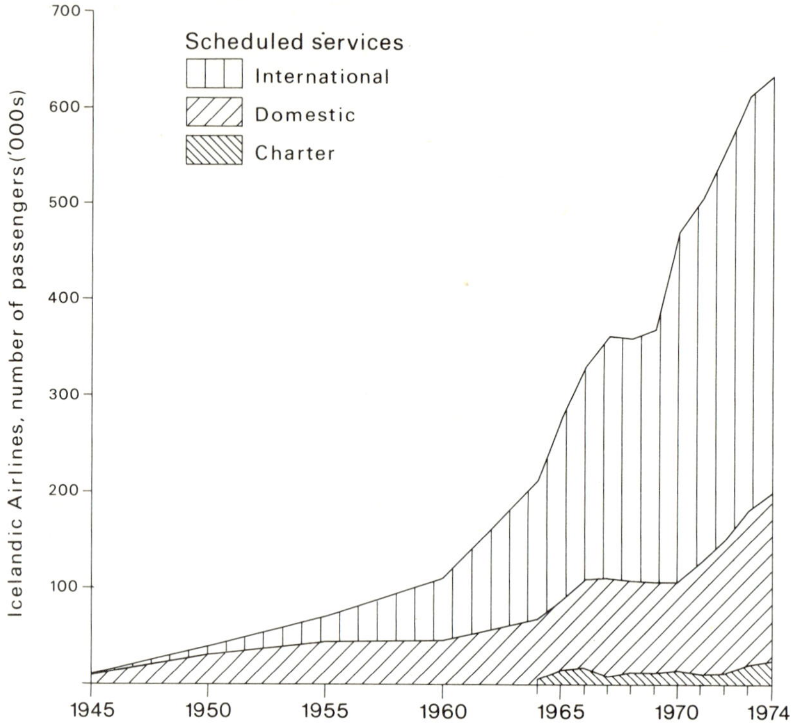

Fig. 5.19 Number of international, domestic and charter passengers carried by Icelandic airlines, 1945–74. *Source: Tölfræðihandbók* (1974, pp. 139–40).

1 : 4 of the then Icelandic population; today the ratio is 1 : 1. About one third of the passengers travel on the Akureyri–Reykjavík route. The other main routes, all from Reykjavík, are to Vestmannaeyja (19 per cent), Ísafjörður (13 per cent) and Egilsstaða (12 per cent) – that is, the main regional centres. The figures for passenger loadings on these four main routes emphasise the contrast between this transport mode and its predecessors. While the motor bus service tends to retain the ring structure which characterised the round-the-island shipping pattern, the airline network is much more hierarchic in structure. Figure 5.20 shows how the main passenger movements emerge like spokes in a wheel whose hub is at Reykjavík. If we turn back to the movements of index cases mapped in section 4.3, it is interesting to note that these too show a more spoke-like character towards the end of the study period. Against this, the tests of contagion carried out earlier in the chapter (section 5.3.3) failed to show the airline network as a significant graph. The results probably imply that the airline network is important only in the initial stages of the diffusion process.

5.5.3 Institutional change

(a) Education

The periodic spatial clustering of susceptible populations plays some part in the rapid propagation of infectious diseases. Current studies of measles lay emphasis on the role of the school, particularly the primary or elementary school, in the spread process.

Despite a Royal order establishing primary schools in Iceland in 1542 and the founding of a school on Vestmannaeyja in 1745, the Icelandic school system dates effectively from 1880 when the first permanent

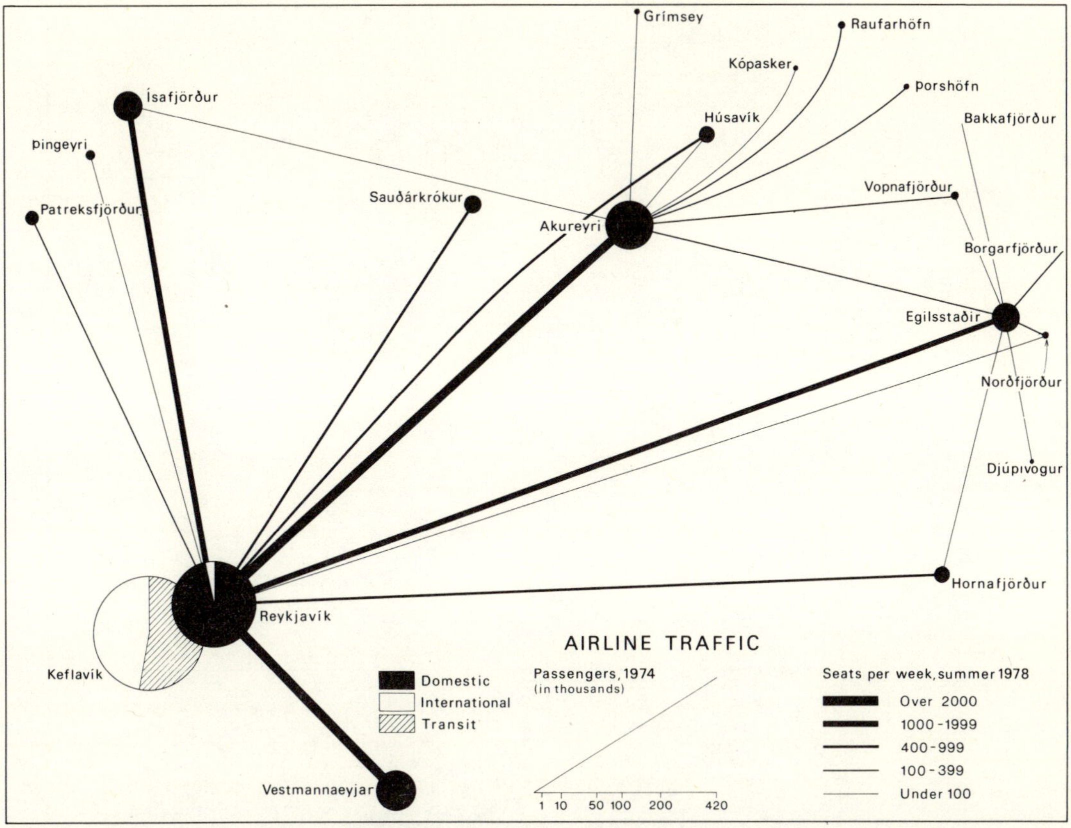

Fig. 5.20 Airline traffic. Passengers carried, 1974, and passenger seats per week on all scheduled internal airline flights, Iceland, summer 1978. *Sources: Tölfræðihandbók* (1974, p. 141); Icelandair Domestic Schedule (1978).

school was established in Reykjavík (Elíasson, 1967, p. 290). In 1907, the state took over responsibility for providing schools and made attendance compulsory for children between 10 and 14 years of age. Up to age 10, teaching was provided at home. Subsequent Education Acts (in 1926, 1936 and 1946) widened the age band for attendance from 7 to 15 years of age, with the last 2 years being spent in a secondary school (*gagnfraeöaskóli*).

In the towns, villages, and thickly populated rural counties, schools are run as day schools in the conventional manner with a nine-month session extending from 1 September to 1 June. School buses are used to move children in from outlying settlements. But in the more sparsely populated rural districts other solutions have had to be found. One early solution was the use of travelling teachers who spent one to three weeks on different farms, with children from nearby farms coming over to join the small class. These 'ambulatory' country schools operate over a much shorter term than the permanent schools (four to six months, as against nine). A second solution was to create small boarding schools with two or three teachers. Children who attend such boarding schools commonly switch their location, spending two to four weeks alternately at school and at home.

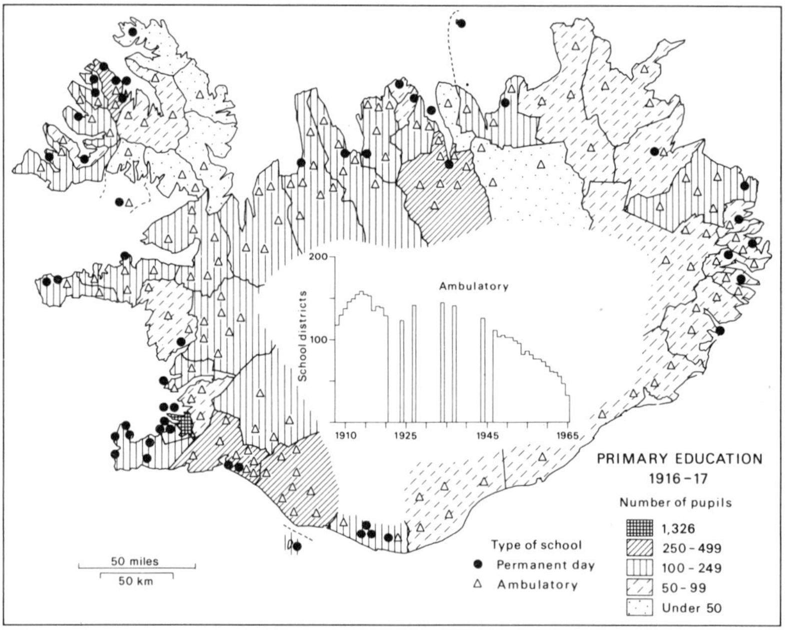

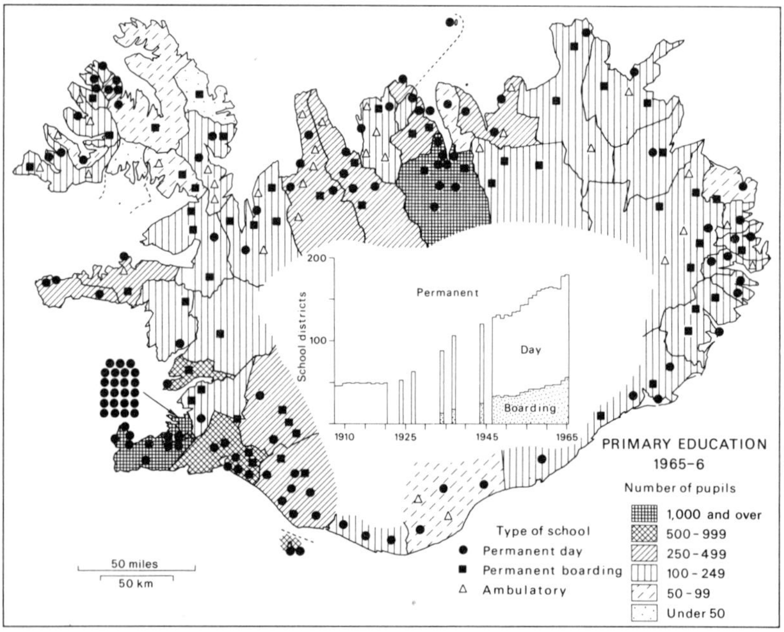

Fig. 5.21 Number of pupils in primary education, 1916–17, and 1965–6, by type of school. On the 1965–6 map, the category, 1,000 and over, is 1,000–2,000 for all places except Reykjavík, where it is 11,784. Graphs show changes in numbers of ambulatory and permanent schools, 1905–66. *Sources: Barnafræðsla* (1916–20; 1920–66), supplemented by unpublished data supplied by the Statistical Bureau of Iceland.

The changing structure of the Icelandic school system over two generations is shown in Figure 5.21. At the start of the period, two-thirds of school districts were served by ambulatory country schools; the remaining one third was split between permanent day schools and those with no teaching. The 1920s saw the beginning of a system of permanent boarding schools while, by the 1930s, the districts with no teaching had shrunk to insignificant proportions. By the end of the period, the permanent day school was the dominant form in over half the school districts, with the remainder split between the ambulatory and boarding schools.

The epidemiological significance of this change in school organisation is brought out in Figure 5.21. The map for 1916–17 shows a situation in which the rural settlements in most parts of the island were served by ambulatory teachers; the fewer permanent schools were confined to the Reykjavík area and to the major towns and fishing villages. By the school year of 1965–6, the permanent boarding school had taken over from the ambulatory teacher in the remote rural areas. Meantime, the shift of population into the towns in general, and to the Reykjavík area in particular, had been matched by a major increase in urban day schools. Over this period, most children of primary school age had been 'institutionalised' into much larger units. The impact of large units of susceptibles is twofold: (a) it enables wholesale measures to be taken over isolation or immunisation procedures, but (b) it increases the likelihood of rapid spread within the school once an infective has been introduced. The role of schools in the mixing process of susceptibles and infectives has been summarised by Fox, Elveback, Scott, Gatewood and Ackerman (1971, p. 183) as follows:

> The schools serve to bring together sub-groups of the population defined by age, by broad area of residence and in many cases, by socioeconomic status. They bring together children from different families and different immediate neighbourhoods. Further, in rural and suburban areas, the school bus serves as a particularly effective exposure chamber for respiratory agent spread. Since school age children are characterised by high susceptibility rates for many infectious diseases, the schools provide potentially important paths of spread from one part of the population to another. Hence, whether or not the school is open may be of major importance in the occurrence of an epidemic.

(b) Medical care

As one would expect, the standard of medical care in Iceland has improved throughout the century. However, the top graph of Figure 5.22 indicates that this improvement – as measured by number of doctors per 1,000 population – has been concentrated in the Reykjavík area. Although other factors may be involved, this improvement must help to account for the decreased velocity of measles waves in Reykjavíkur noted in section 5.4.3 and the reduced intensity of attack in the capital implied by the lower graph of Figure 5.22.

5.5.4 Environmental change

The Icelandic population occupies an island subjected to an unusually high level of environmental change. The most spectacular of these changes occur suddenly, such as the eruption of Helgafell volcano which led to the evacuation of population from Heimaey in Vestmannaeyja in 1973. Over the period 1896–1975, the more important changes from the viewpoint of measles diffusion have been the less spectacular movements in Icelandic climate. We look here at two aspects, the short-term seasonal rhythm and at longer-term climatic changes.

(a) Seasonal variation

The standard accounts of measles frequently ascribe to it a strong seasonal pattern. Thus, Ball, A. P. (1977, pp. 245–6) describes measles as

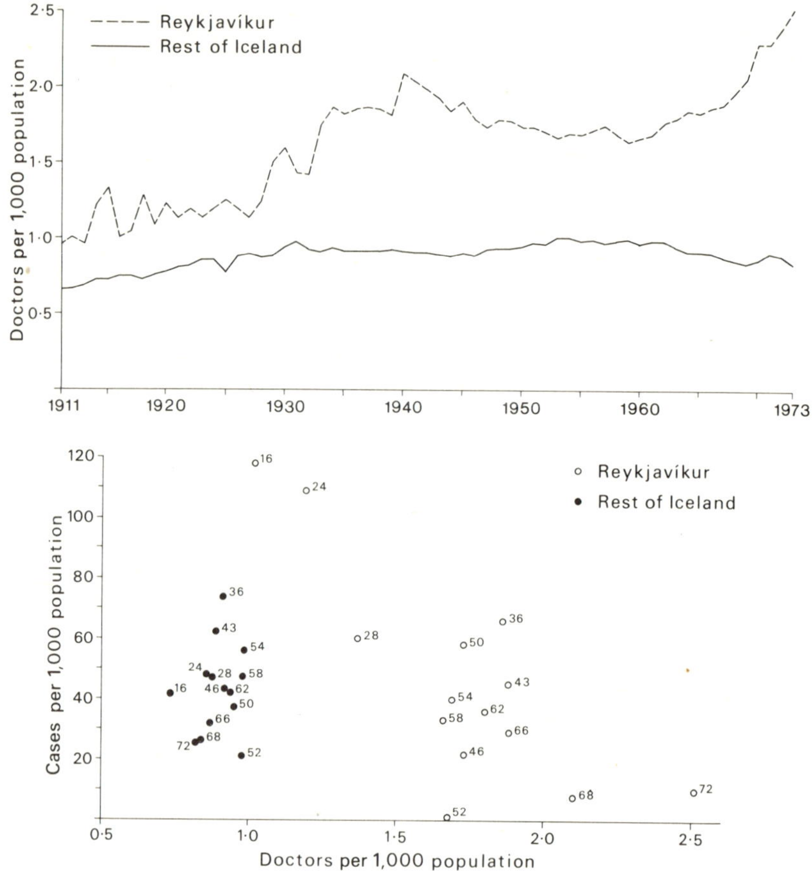

Fig. 5.22 Medical care in Iceland. Change in doctors per 1,000 population and relationship of attack rate from measles to doctors per 1,000 population. On the lower graph, the last two digits of the date of the wave are given. Thus, 16 denotes 1916, etc. *Sources: Heilbrigðisskýrslur* (1911–70).

having 'a higher incidence in the colder months, reaching a peak in January and February which is most marked in an epidemic year'. This generalisation is based on northern temperate countries and we should expect the corresponding months to be July and August in the southern temperate countries. Ball notes a less regular pattern in tropical countries. In India, for example, the peak incidence is in the hot, dry period from March to June.

Variations in infection rates are *not* generally ascribed to the primary effects on the measles virus of temperature and humidity fluctuations, but rather to the secondary effects of such fluctuations on the susceptible population. Thus, in the United Kingdom, the January–February epidemic peak may relate to the opening of schools in early January after the Christmas holiday (itself a period of high contact between members of families) plus the two- or three-week lag while index cases are incubating and spreading the disease.

The monthly distribution of measles cases in Iceland is an interesting one. For the period since 1945 (including waves VIII to XV), Figure 5.23 shows a seasonal pattern much like that suggested by Ball, with a January peak and a marked concentration of cases in the winter half of the year. The period 1900–44 is, however, strongly contrasting (Figure

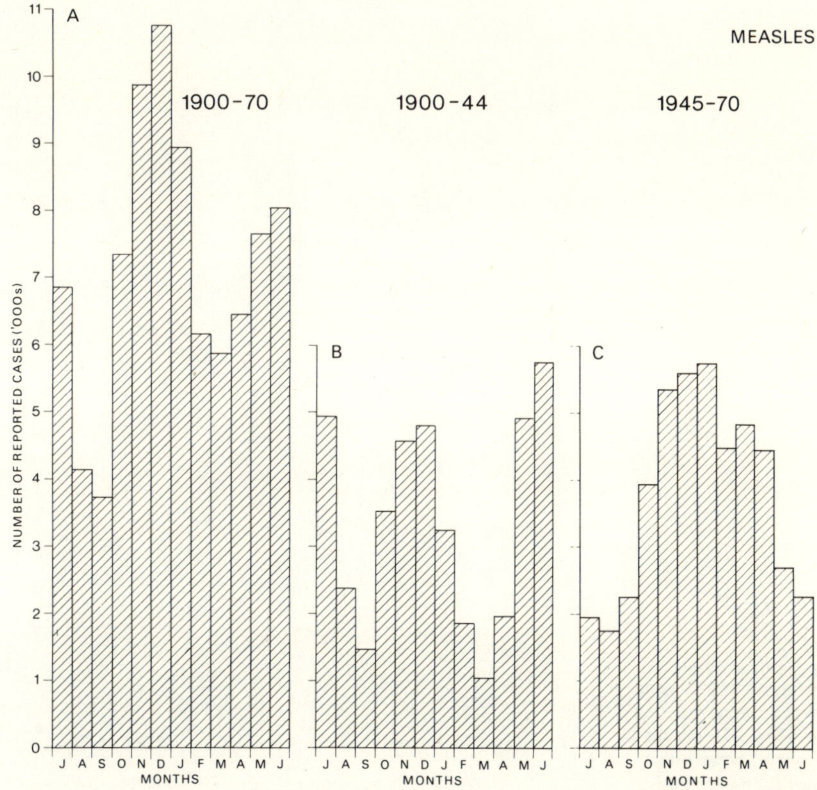

Fig. 5.23 Monthly distribution of measles cases. (A) 1900–70, (B) 1900–44, (C) 1945–70. *Sources:* as for Figures 4.3–4.18.

5.23): the seasonal distribution is bi-modal with the two distinct peaks in December and June.

Any explanation of the Icelandic pattern must begin with the reminder that, since measles are not endemic in Iceland, the seasonal distribution will reflect the starting date on which an epidemic begins. Of those waves before World War II, all but one started in the first half of the year, so that a mid-year peak would not be unexpected. In contrast, the post-war waves have starting months more randomly spread through the year. The haymaking season in Iceland peaks in June and this communal activity would be important in spreading the virus through a farm community, particularly in the earlier half of the century when farming families would form the most important segment within the susceptible population. The persistent winter peak over the whole period probably reflects levels of crowding within school classrooms and the rapid spread within such institutions. If contacts at this micro-spatial level were accelerated by the winter weather, then contacts at the meso-level between districts would be retarded. Figure 5.18 shows the substantial cutback in bus journeys in Iceland during the winter. Note that, not only is the level of service reduced, but the network is dismembered, so that both north-west Iceland and north-east Iceland are cut off from the rest of the country. In considering the seasonal differences for Iceland, it is important to recall the extreme

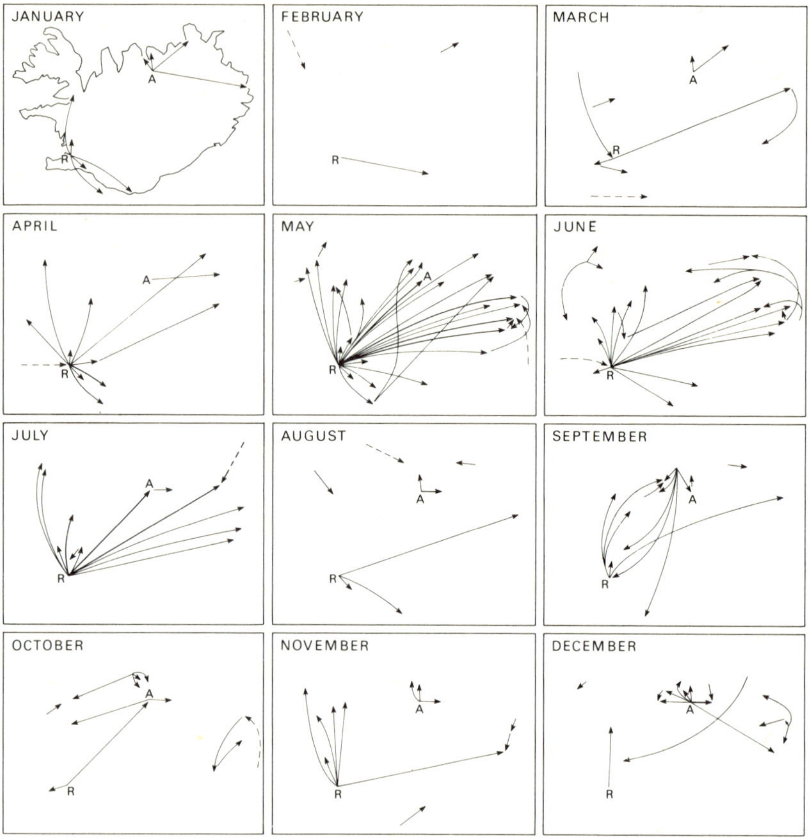

Fig. 5.24 All known movements of index cases between medical districts, 1896–1975, as recorded in chapter 4, shown on a month-by-month basis. A = Akureyrar, R = Reykjavíkur. *Sources:* as for Figures 4.3–4.18.

contrasts between winter and summer due to the climatic elements (e.g., the blocking of roads by snow) and also the effect of Arctic Circle location on day length: Reykjavík, the world's most poleward capital city, has less than six hours of daylight in mid-winter.

Figure 5.24 illustrates the seasonal effect in another way. On this diagram, all the bonds showing movements of infected index cases recorded on the maps of chapter 4 have been ordered on a monthly basis. The mushrooming of contacts in May is striking. These fall steadily throughout the summer and autumn to a winter quiet period. Bearing in mind that most of the bond information is for the period 1896–1944, Figure 5.24 must reflect, in part, the improved transport during the summer months (see, for example, Figure 5.18), and the May peak is consistent with the June maximum of cases, 1900–44, shown in Figure 5.23.

(b) Long-term climatic swings

The work of Thorarinsson (1961) has made Iceland a classic area for the study of long-run climatic changes. Study of the snow-line in South Vatnajökull and the persistence of drift ice shows a steady worsening of Iceland's average climate from AD 930 up to the last decades of the nineteenth century. Over the years critical to our own study (1896–1975), the growing network of climatic stations points to a generally

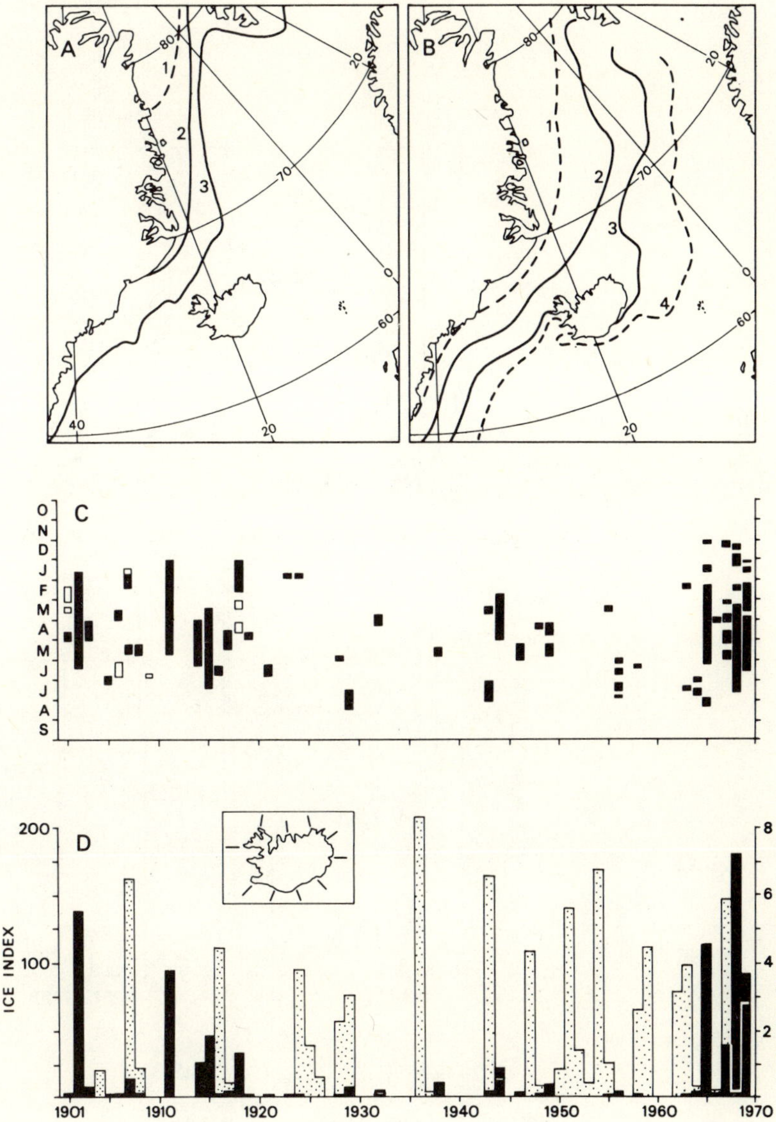

Fig. 5.25 Severity of winters as measured by limits of sea ice near Iceland. (A) Early October; 1 = minimum, 2 = normal, 3 = maximum. (B) March–May; 1 = recent minimum, 2 = recent normal, 3 = recent maximum, 4 = estimated maximum in historical times. (C) Periods when ice observed around the coast this century. (D) Ice index (product of number of weeks with ice per year and the number of coastal areas near which it was observed) shown in black, and reported measles cases (stippled). Inset map shows coastal areas. The outline ice periods on (C) are not included in the index. *Source:* Eythorsson and Sigtryggsson (1971, pp. 46–7).

ameliorating situation, with short-run regression to colder conditions. Analysis of the drift-ice conditions around Iceland indicates that, even in the most severe winter (Figure 5.25), Iceland generally was not completely ice-surrounded (as it had been in 1964). Over the 80-year study period, a cold spell for the first two decades gave way to 40 years of relatively ice-free conditions until the situation worsened again in the 1960s (Figure 5.25D). The main measles waves have been added in Figure 5.25 for convenience. We do not wish to argue for any strong connection between environmental change and epidemics, but would like to note that the persistence and areal extent of drift ice would inevitably restrict the number of ports into which index cases could be brought.

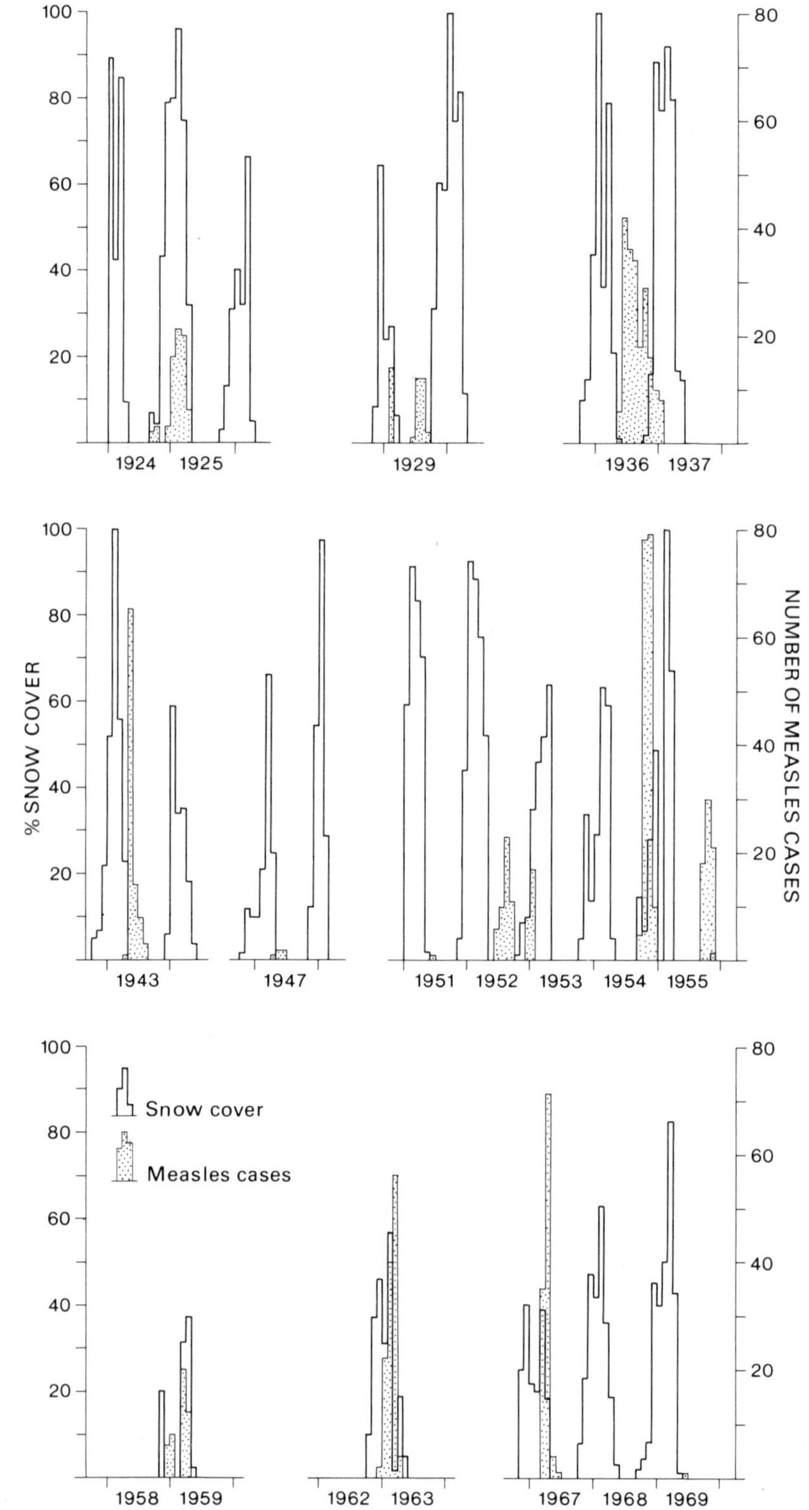

Fig. 5.26 Percentage snow cover reported by month, 1924–70, at Stykkishólms for epidemic years. *Source:* Volumes of *Veðráttan* (1924–70).

Inland communications would be affected by other climatic elements, notably snow. Figure 5.26 gives the record for one climatic station (Stykkishólms) since the 1920s to show the wide seasonal incidence of epidemics with peaks in spring (1925), summer (1936), autumn (1955) and winter (1963). Snow conditions vary sharply over short distances and we have not attempted to pursue this line of investigation further.

5.6 Conclusion

In this chapter, we have used a series of elementary methods of statistical analysis to unravel the broad patterns in the main measles epidemic waves to affect Iceland in this century. The analysis has been undertaken at micro-(doctor), meso-(district) and macro-(regional) scales, and an attempt has been made to relate the main empirical regularities identified to changes in the socio-economic conditions in Iceland since 1900. In Table 5.1, we summarise these patterns and their related explanations. The results of this chapter form the backcloth against which the formal modelling of chapters 6 and 7 is undertaken.

Table 5.1. *Epidemic characteristics and possible related explanations*

Characteristic	Possible explanation	Chapter sections
Spatial transmission with hierarchic and contagious components.	Decrease in population size with distance from Reykjavíkur.	5.3.1 – 5.3.3
Oscillatory behaviour of epidemic size (large followed by small, etc.).	Large epidemic severely depletes susceptible population.	5.3.4
Increasing velocity of spread in Iceland, excluding Reykjavíkur, since 1900.	Increasing youthfulness of population, increase in urbanisation, internal transport improvements, shift from ambulatory to fixed schools.	5.4 – 5.5
Decrease in velocity in Reykjavíkur.	Improved medical care in the captital; larger susceptible population distributed at increasingly lower residential densities since 1945.	5.4.1
Increase in frequency of epidemics since 1945.	Increasing contact of Iceland with rest of world.	5.5.2
June and December peaks of reported cases, 1896–1944; January peak, 1945–70.	Transport improvement in summer as opposed to winter months and increased communal farming activity in summer, 1896–1944. Winter peak because of concentration of children in schools.	5.5.4

6 Diffusion models, 1: time series approaches

6.1 Introduction

In this and the next chapter, we consider and illustrate the use of various kinds of models of spatial diffusion processes. For convenience, we have divided the methods to be discussed into two broad categories, namely (1) time series approaches of the sort considered by Box and Jenkins (1970) and Kalman (1960), and (2) stochastic process models of the Hamer–Soper and chain binomial kind (Bailey, 1975). The division is a natural one. Box–Jenkins methods have been discussed widely in geography as ways of modelling and forecasting economic time series (see, for example, Cliff, Haggett, Ord, Bassett and Davies (1975), Hepple (1978a) and Bennett (1979)). However, the number of successful empirical applications in geography is low, and it therefore seemed appropriate to give them an extended trial on a large spatial data set of the sort considered here. The Hamer–Soper and chain binomial models, in contrast to those of Box and Jenkins, have been classically used to examine epidemic diffusion processes – purpose-built for that particular application. While the theory of these models has been developed over the last 70 years, they, like the Box–Jenkins methods, have similarly not been subjected to extensive field trials with space–time data sets. They do, however, form an obvious bench-mark against which to assess the performance of other models not specifically designed to handle diffusion processes, but which can be adapted for the purpose. We consider time series methods in this chapter, and stochastic process models in chapter 7.

6.2 Box–Jenkins methods

6.2.1 Types of models

The basic philosophy underlying the so-called 'Box–Jenkins models' is that the past behaviour of regional systems provides the key to how they will act in the future, and that this can be modelled using *autoregressive* and *moving average* components. Let $x_{i,t}$ denote the value of a variate in region i at time t – for example, the number of measles cases reported in Akureyrar in October 1958. We know from the discussion of that epidemic wave in section 4.3.2 that the disease arrived in Akureyrar from Reykjavíkur two months previously, and that it moved on from Akureyrar to Ólafsfjarðar, Grenivíkur and Kópaskers in subsequent months. A distinct space–time transmission process is involved. We index time periods earlier than t by $t-k$, and periods later than t by $t+k$. Akureyrar is our reference medical district, i, and we use j to denote other medical districts. The pattern of dependencies among medical districts outlined above may thus be formulated as shown in Figure 6.1.

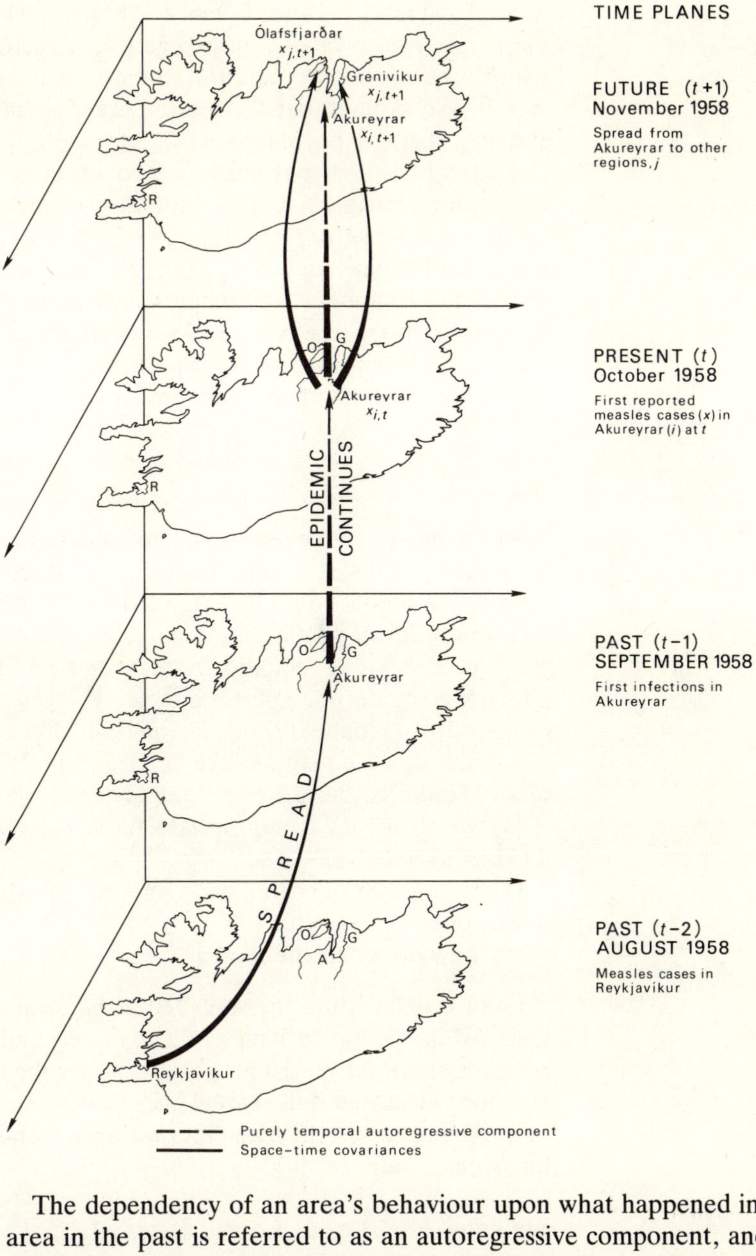

Fig. 6.1 Pattern of dependencies among medical districts for part of the 1958–9 measles epidemic (wave XII) in Iceland.

The dependency of an area's behaviour upon what happened in that area in the past is referred to as an autoregressive component, and the dependency upon other areas as space–time covariances. In an extension of the Box–Jenkins notation proposed in Cliff, Haggett, Ord, Bassett and Davies (1975, chapter 10), we may refer to such models as *s*pace–*t*ime *a*uto*r*egressive (STAR) models and write

$$E(X_{i,t}|\text{past history}) = b_1 x_{i,t-1} + b_2 \sum_j w_{ij} x_{j,t-1}$$

$$i = 1, 2, \ldots, n \qquad (6.1)$$

$$j = 1, 2, \ldots, n, \quad j \neq i$$

as a typical model. Here, b_1 and b_2 are parameters to be estimated, the $\{w_{ij}\}$ are pre-specified, non-negative, structural weights indicating which areas, j, affect i, and the summation is over all areas j for which $w_{ij} \neq 0$. We assume that there are n areas of interest in the space–time system. There is no reason why the temporal dependency should be restricted to a single past map, and equation (6.1) could be extended to earlier time periods (that is, time lags of order $k=2, 3, \ldots$). As it stands, equation (6.1) is said to be of order 1 in time and n in space.

It often happens that change over time cannot be accounted for solely in terms of systematic components such as those in equation (6.1), and we may envisage random 'shocks' arriving in a region both from other areas and from within itself on past maps. Thus, we might postulate a *s*pace–*t*ime random shocks, or *m*oving *a*verage, model (STMA) as

$$x_{i,t} = \varepsilon_{i,t} + b_1\varepsilon_{i,t-1} + b_2 \sum_j w_{ij}\varepsilon_{j,t-1}, \tag{6.2}$$

where b_1 and b_2 are parameters, and the epsilons (ε) are random shocks with zero means, constant variances and zero intercorrelations. As before, the model could be extended to cover more than one time lag and any order of spatial interaction. Additionally, there is nothing to stop us combining equations (6.1) and (6.2) to define a general STARMA model (see, for example, Haggett, Cliff and Frey (1977, chapter 16), Hepple (1978a), Bennett (1979)).

Writing down equations like (6.1) and (6.2) is the easy part of our task. The difficulties arise in three areas:

(1) which model is appropriate for the problem in hand – STAR, STMA, STARMA?

(2) what order of spatial and temporal lags should be included in the model once it is selected?

(3) how do we fit the model?

(1) and (2) constitute the so-called *identification* or *specification* problems, while (3) raises issues of *estimation*, and, in turn, whether the assumptions of the model proposed hold for the data set being analysed. It is quite clear that if the model is incorrectly specified, there is no hope of obtaining consistent parameter estimates, and so we now turn to the question of identification.

6.2.2 Model identification

We know from Figure 3.4 and section 3.3.4 that the average length of time between an infected individual contacting a person at risk and the emergence of symptoms is 14 days, and that chain lengths range between about 7 and 21 days. Given that the Icelandic data are recorded on a monthly basis, we are unlikely to need to include temporal lags greater than one when considering any single epidemic, but a lagged term of the order of about 48 might be necessary on the basis of Figure 3.1 to model epidemic recurrences. Spatially, we have suggested localised contagious diffusion is important, but that inter-regional transmission is effected largely by contacts between the main urban centres of Reykjavík, Ísafjörður, Akureyri and Seyðisfjörður (Figure 4.19 and section 4.4). These findings imply that low-order spatial lags will be necessary to handle local disease spread, but higher-order ones will be needed for any inter-regional modelling. Finally, since the process of spread seems fairly well documented and structured, AR models seem more reasonable than MA models.

While we have been able to suggest a specification for a model on *a priori* grounds, methods of model identification do exist which are based upon an analysis of the data series – here, of reported cases of measles in each medical district for each time period. The theory involved is described in Martin and Oeppen (1975) and Bennett (1979, chapter 3). Briefly, in our notation, we define the spatial lag operator

$$L^0 x_{i,t} = x_{i,t} \tag{6.3}$$

and

$$L^s x_{i,t} = \sum_j w_{ij} x_{j,t}, \quad s > 0, \tag{6.4}$$

where s denotes the spatial lag which is s steps away from area i and the summation is over the j areas at spatial lag s from i. An estimator of the autocorrelation between the spatially and temporally lagged terms, $L^g x_{i,t-k}$ and $L^s x_{i,t-l}$, is the quantity

$$r = \frac{\sum_{i=1}^{n} \sum_{t=v+1}^{T} L^g z_{i,t} L^s z_{i,t-v}}{\left[\sum_{i=1}^{n} \sum_{t=1}^{T} (L^g z_{i,t})^2\right]^{\frac{1}{2}} \left[\sum_{i=1}^{n} \sum_{t=1}^{T} (L^s z_{i,t})^2\right]^{\frac{1}{2}}}. \tag{6.5}$$

Here, $v = l - k (l > k)$, either g or s is zero, T is the number of time periods and

$$L^s z_{i,t-k} = L^s (x_{i,t-k} - \bar{x}_i) \tag{6.6}$$

where $\bar{x}_i = \frac{1}{T} \sum_t x_{i,t}$.

Identification then consists, first, in evaluating the autocorrelations and partial autocorrelations using (6.5) for all values of g, k, s and l. The autocorrelations define the relationship between values of a variate in a reference area, i, at a given time and values of the variate in other areas at different time periods (i.e., at different temporal and spatial lags). The partials define this relationship for a given temporal and spatial lag with the effect of intervening areas and time periods held constant. The second step is to examine the plots of levels of (partial) autocorrelation against time/space lag. These plots have a characteristic form depending on the underlying process model:

(1) for an STAR (p,q) process of order p in space and q in time, the level of autocorrelation should fall off exponentially in time and space, while the partial autocorrelations should be approximately zero after lag p in space and q in time;

(2) for an STMA (r,u) process of order r in space and u in time, the autocorrelations are zero after lags r and u, while the partials decay exponentially in time and space;

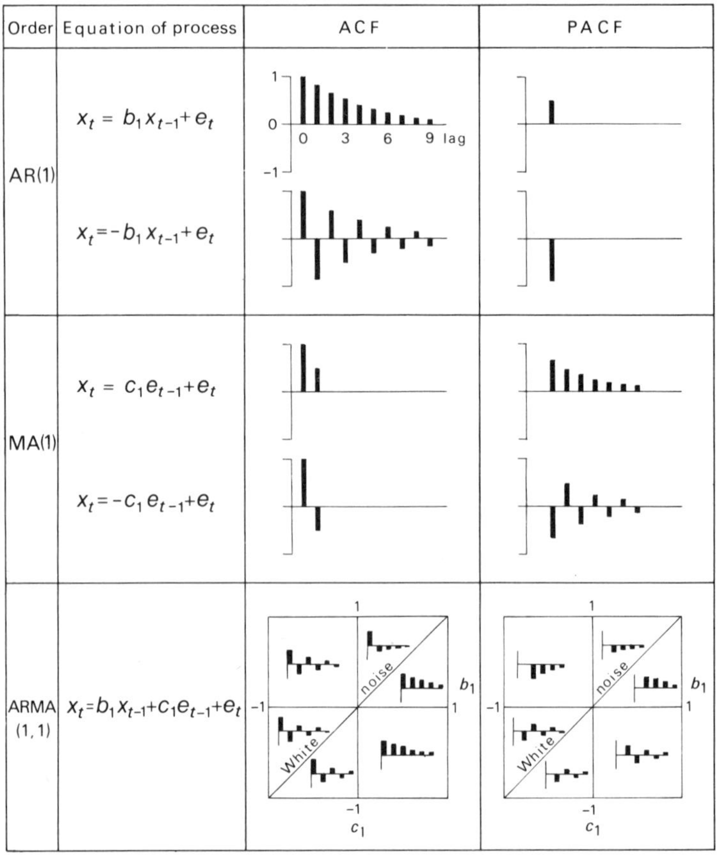

Fig. 6.2 The autocorrelation function (ACF) and partial autocorrelation function (PACF) for various low-order single-region ARMA models. *Source:* Bennett (1979, p. 152).

(3) STARMA (p,q,r,u) processes display autocorrelations and partials which fall off as a mixture of exponential curves and damped sine waves. The autocorrelations exhibit this tailing off after the first $(r-p)$ and $(u-q)$ lags in time and space respectively, and the partials after the first $(p-r)$ lags in space and $(q-u)$ in time, taking only positive order lags into account in each case.

The features described are illustrated in Figure 6.2 for various *single-region* ARMA models.

The autocorrelation (ACF) and partial autocorrelation (PACF) functions have been evaluated for each of the 50 medical districts for the modelling period 1945–70. Nearly all produced ACF and PACF plots which were very similar in form, and we reproduce six in Figure 6.3 for the capital medical district, Reykjavíkur, the three regional centres of Akureyrar, Ísafjarðar and Seyðisfjarðar, and the smaller districts of Breiðumýrar (north Iceland) and Laugarás (south-west Iceland).

Comparison of Figures 6.3 and 6.2 suggests that, with the exception of Breiðumýrar, the process is low-order autoregressive (AR(2)) in time, with higher-order cyclical components corresponding to the periodicity between epidemic recurrences (note, for example, the renewed levels of positive autocorrelation at lag 48, 96, etc. for Reykjavíkur). The negative autocorrelations in the ACFs are due to non-stationarities in the data, a

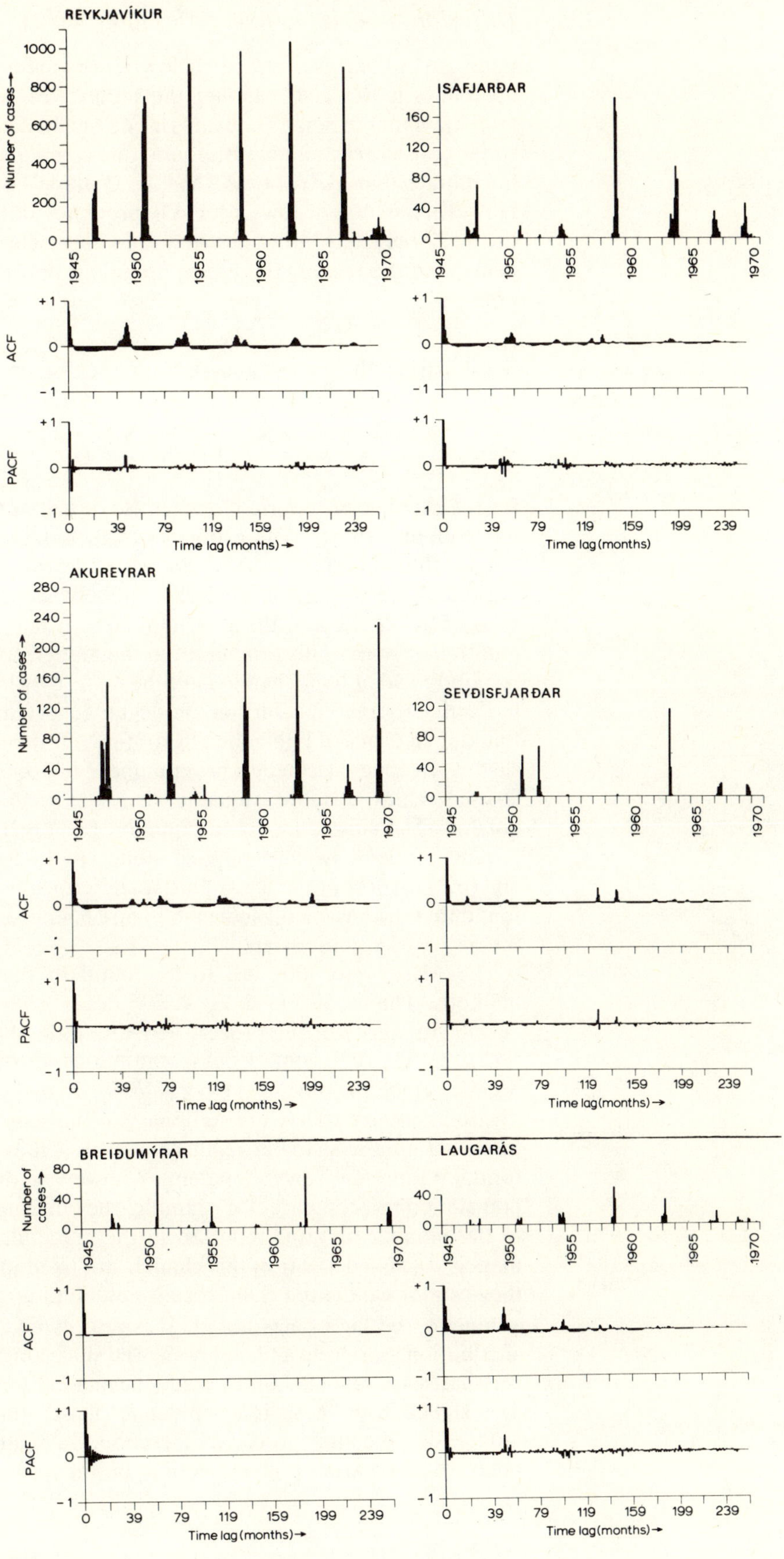

Fig. 6.3 Some sample ACFs, PACFs and time series plots for reported cases of measles in six medical districts in Iceland, 1945–70.

point to which we return below. The main periodicity between epidemics is detected whether the number of cases reported is large (Reykjavíkur) or small (Laugarás). For the medical district we have not so far considered, namely Breiðumýrar, comparison of Figures 6.2 and 6.3 implies that MA(1) or ARMA (1,1) models would be worth trying. However, as noted, low-order AR processes dominate in the medical districts; only one other district, Bíldudals, clearly had MA components, and the results, therefore, broadly support our *a priori* specification.

6.2.3 Model fitting

To illustrate the fitting and performance of an AR model, we have calibrated, using ordinary least squares (OLS), the simple form

$$x_t = b_1 x_{t-1} + e_t \tag{6.7}$$

for the number of reported cases in Reykjavíkur for waves IX and XII (cf. equation (6.1)). The estimates of b_1 obtained were then used to obtain the one-month-ahead forecasts shown in Figure 6.4. While reasonable correspondence is achieved between the forecast and actual sizes of the epidemics, the striking feature is that the forecasts run one month in arrears. This is inherent in the model structure; (6.7) can only respond to what happened in t at time $t+1$, by which time the epidemic has either burgeoned further or begun to decline. Clearly, if one is thinking in terms of public-health strategies for controlling an epidemic, say by selective vaccination programmes, an accurate forecast of phase characteristics is more valuable than an accurate forecast of total volume. The simple model in equation (6.7) is unacceptable on these grounds. Indeed, we have applied models of the form of equations (6.1) and (6.2) to most of the Icelandic data described in this volume and have found that the basic fault shown in Figure 6.4 persists whatever model of the STARMA genre is applied.

The reasons for this are to be found in the assumptions of the methods. The models assume:

(1) stationarity of the process generating the data series,
(2) that the data come from a continuous distribution.

Measles epidemic waves have been described by Bartlett (1957) as being 'quasi-stationary'. They are stationary in the sense that the waves tend to repeat a basic shape at regular intervals – they have a cyclical wave form. Within any given epidemic, however, the process is clearly non-stationary; compare, for example, the build-up and fade-out phases in the number of cases reported in the epidemics of Figure 6.4. The models discussed so far in this chapter are fixed in the parameters, and they cannot handle the changes between build-up and fade-out without producing the lag effects noted. It is also evident that the underlying distribution is discrete and highly skewed since long runs of months when zero cases are reported (inter-epidemic phases) separate each epidemic. The signal from these inter-epidemic phases tends to dominate the model identification procedure described in section 6.2.2 and contributes to a persistent identification of the process operating in the

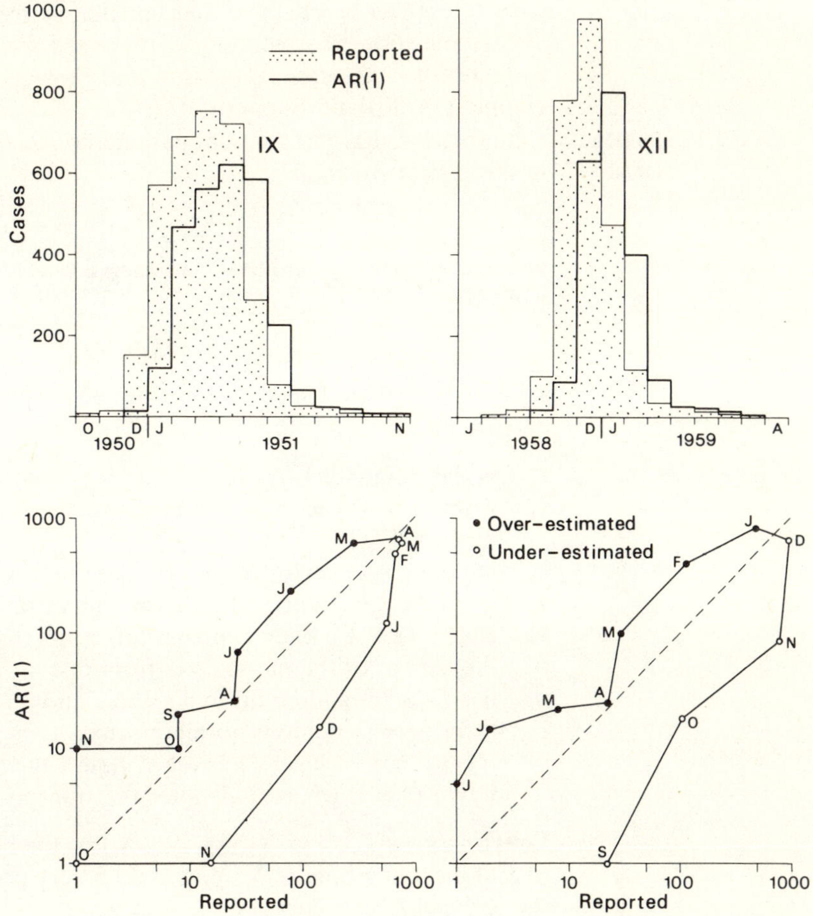

Fig. 6.4 Reported measles cases and one-month-ahead forecasts from AR(1) model for Reykjavíkur, waves IX and XII. The graphs show reported cases against forecasts. Pecked line denotes coincidence of reported and forecast cases; letters indicate months of the wave. The graphs show vividly how the AR(1) model under-estimates cases up to the epidemic peak and over-estimates thereafter.

medical districts as being AR in character. This finding suggests that the models are being applied outside the province for which they were designed. We have described and fitted them here for both positive and negative reasons; first, to illustrate the dangers involved in ignoring under-pinning assumptions, and secondly, because they form the basis for extended models which overcome the problems noted. We now turn to these extensions.

6.3 Kalman filtering[1]

An obvious way of overcoming the lack of stationarity in the data is to formulate a model which is dynamic in its parameters; that is, whose

[1] This section relies on the work of F. Ball, now of Sussex University, who was supervised by one of us (A.D.C.) while working as a student on a field project as part of the postgraduate diploma in mathematical statistics at Cambridge University. See Ball, F. (1977) for details of the project.

parameters can be changed and updated as fresh information arrives. The framework most commonly proposed for this updating uses the *Kalman filter algorithm* (Harrison and Stevens (1976), Martin (1978), Hepple (1978b) and Bennett (1979)).

6.3.1 Definition of model

Suppose we have a system of parameters, $\boldsymbol{\theta}_t$, evolving through time as in the *system equation*

$$\boldsymbol{\theta}_t = \mathbf{G}\boldsymbol{\theta}_{t-1} + \boldsymbol{\eta}_t \tag{6.8}$$

where $\boldsymbol{\eta}_t \sim N(\mathbf{0}, \mathbf{V}_t)$, and that we observe $\mathbf{y}_t$ according to the *observation equation*

$$\mathbf{y}_t = \mathbf{X}_t\boldsymbol{\theta}_t + \boldsymbol{\varepsilon}_t, \tag{6.9}$$

where $\boldsymbol{\varepsilon}_t \sim N(\mathbf{0}, \mathbf{U}_t)$. In equations (6.8) and (6.9) we make the following definitions:

- t is the time index, $t = 1, 2, \ldots,$
- $\mathbf{y}_t$ is the $(n \times 1)$ vector of observations (the dependent variable) made at time t,
- $\boldsymbol{\theta}_t$ is the $(k \times 1)$ vector of process parameters at time t,
- $\mathbf{X}_t$ is the $(n \times k)$ matrix of independent variables known at time t,
- $\mathbf{G}$ is the $(k \times k)$ known matrix of structural weights defining the movement of the parameters from one moment to the next,
- $\boldsymbol{\eta}_t$ is a $(k \times 1)$ random normal vector, and
- $\boldsymbol{\varepsilon}_t$ is an $(n \times 1)$ random normal vector; $\boldsymbol{\eta}_t$, $\boldsymbol{\varepsilon}_t$ are taken to have zero means and variances known at time t, given by $\mathbf{V}_t = E(\boldsymbol{\eta}_t\boldsymbol{\eta}_t^T)$ and $\mathbf{U}_t = E(\boldsymbol{\varepsilon}_t\boldsymbol{\varepsilon}_t^T)$, where T denotes the transpose operator.

Let $\mathbf{H}_t = (\mathbf{y}_1, \mathbf{y}_2, \ldots, \mathbf{y}_t, \mathbf{X}_1, \mathbf{X}_2, \ldots, \mathbf{X}_t)$ be the history of the process up to and including time t. We now state a very powerful result known as the *Kalman filter* algorithm.

Suppose that, at time $t = 0$, the prior distribution of $\boldsymbol{\theta}_0$ is $N(\mathbf{m}_0, \mathbf{C}_0)$. Then the posterior distribution of $\boldsymbol{\theta}_t$ given $\mathbf{H}_t$ is also normally distributed; that is, $(\boldsymbol{\theta}_t | \mathbf{H}_t) \sim N(\mathbf{m}_t, \mathbf{C}_t)$, where $\mathbf{m}_t$, $t = 0, 1, \ldots,$ are $(k \times 1)$ column vectors and $\mathbf{C}_t$, $t = 0, 1, \ldots,$ are $(k \times k)$ positive definite matrices calculated from the following recursion. Let

$$\left.\begin{array}{ll} \hat{\mathbf{y}}_t = \mathbf{X}_t\mathbf{G}\mathbf{m}_{t-1}, & \mathbf{e}_t = \mathbf{y}_t - \hat{\mathbf{y}}_t, \\ \mathbf{R}_t = \mathbf{G}\mathbf{C}_{t-1}\mathbf{G}^T + \mathbf{V}_t, & \hat{\boldsymbol{\Sigma}}_t = \mathbf{X}_t\mathbf{R}_t\mathbf{X}_t^T + \mathbf{U}_t, \\ \mathbf{A}_t = \mathbf{R}_t\mathbf{X}_t^T(\hat{\boldsymbol{\Sigma}}_t)^{-1}. & \end{array}\right\} \tag{6.10}$$

Then

$$\mathbf{m}_t = \mathbf{G}\mathbf{m}_{t-1} + \mathbf{A}_t\mathbf{e}_t, \quad \text{and} \quad \mathbf{C}_t = \mathbf{R}_t - \mathbf{A}_t\hat{\boldsymbol{\Sigma}}_t\mathbf{A}_t^T. \tag{6.11}$$

For one-step-ahead forecasting we proceed as follows:

$$(\boldsymbol{\theta}_{t-1} | \mathbf{H}_{t-1}) \sim N(\mathbf{m}_{t-1}, \mathbf{C}_{t-1}),$$

and

$$\boldsymbol{\theta}_t = \mathbf{G}\boldsymbol{\theta}_{t-1} + \boldsymbol{\eta}_t,$$

where $\boldsymbol{\eta}_t$ is independent of $(\boldsymbol{\theta}_{t-1}|\mathbf{H}_{t-1})$. Therefore, from equations (6.10)

$$(\boldsymbol{\theta}_t|\mathbf{H}_{t-1}) \sim N(\mathbf{Gm}_{t-1}, \mathbf{GC}_{t-1}\mathbf{G}^T + \mathbf{V}_t)$$
$$\sim N(\mathbf{Gm}_{t-1}, \mathbf{R}_t).$$

Now, as given in equation (6.9),

$$\mathbf{y}_t = \mathbf{X}_t\boldsymbol{\theta}_t + \boldsymbol{\varepsilon}_t,$$

where $\boldsymbol{\varepsilon}_t$ is independent of $(\boldsymbol{\theta}_t|\mathbf{H}_{t-1})$. Thus, from equations (6.10)

$$(\mathbf{y}_t|\mathbf{H}_{t-1}) \sim N(\mathbf{X}_t\mathbf{Gm}_{t-1}, \mathbf{X}_t\mathbf{R}_t\mathbf{X}_t^T + \mathbf{U}_t)$$
$$\sim N(\hat{\mathbf{y}}_t, \hat{\boldsymbol{\Sigma}}_t).$$

Hence the quantities in (6.10) have the following meaning:

$\hat{\mathbf{y}}_t$ is the one-step-ahead forecast of $\mathbf{y}_t$,
$\mathbf{e}_t$ is the one-step-ahead forecast error,
$\mathbf{R}_t$ is the variance of $\boldsymbol{\theta}_t$, and
$\hat{\boldsymbol{\Sigma}}_t$ is the variance of the one-step-ahead forecast, all conditional on $\mathbf{H}_{t-1}$ and $\mathbf{X}_t$.

Finally, an application of Bayes' Theorem yields the posterior distribution for $\boldsymbol{\theta}_t$, given

$$\mathbf{H}_t = (\mathbf{H}_{t-1}, \mathbf{y}_t, \mathbf{X}_t),$$

as

$$(\boldsymbol{\theta}_t|\mathbf{H}_t) \sim N(\mathbf{m}_t, \mathbf{C}_t).$$

In turn, this distribution acts as the prior for time period $(t+1)$.

6.3.2 Application to Reykjavíkur, 1945–70

To illustrate the algorithm, we consider a modification of the simple AR model given in equation (6.7), namely the observation equation

$$y_t = b_{1t}y_{t-1} + \varepsilon_t,$$

where $\varepsilon_t \sim N(0, y_{t-1}\sigma^2)$ and $y_t (t = 1, 2, \ldots, 312)$ is the number of cases reported in Reykjavíkur in each month, 1945–70. The model assumes that each infected individual at $t-1$ transmits the disease independently to a normally distributed number of susceptibles (who become infected) during month t; he then ceases to be an infective. This simplification is not unreasonable given the discussion in section 3.3.4. Using the Kalman approach, the model can be written in the form

$$\left.\begin{aligned} y_t &= b_{1t}y_{t-1} + \varepsilon_t & \varepsilon_t &\sim N(0, y_{t-1}\sigma^2) \\ b_{1t} &= b_{1t-1} + \eta_t, & \eta_t &\sim N(0, V). \end{aligned}\right\} \quad (6.12)$$

Because no constant is fitted, b_{1t} may be interpreted as the 'rate of infection' at time t (cf. Cliff and Ord, 1971, p. 63), and this rate is now

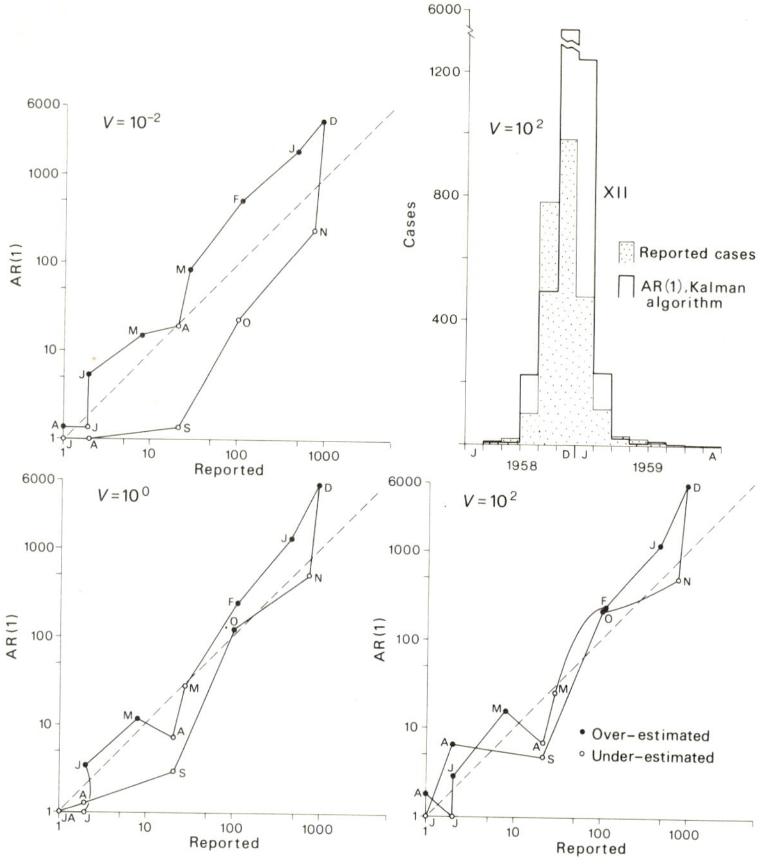

Fig. 6.5 Reported measles cases and one-month-ahead forecasts from AR(1) model fitted by the Kalman algorithm to Reykjavíkur, wave XII. Pecked line denotes coincidence of reported and forecast cases; letters indicate months of the wave. V is defined in equation (6.12).

allowed to vary through time. Application of equations (6.10) and (6.11) yields the recursion

$$\left.\begin{aligned} m_t &= m_{t-1} + A_t(y_t - y_{t-1}m_{t-1}) \\ C_t &= A_t\sigma^2 \\ A_t &= (C_{t-1} + V)/[y_{t-1}(C_{t-1} + V) + \sigma^2]. \end{aligned}\right\} \tag{6.13}$$

Note that the matrices of recursion in (6.10) and (6.11) have now become scalars because we are treating a single region and have only one independent variable.

Initial parameter estimates

We treated the months of 1945–7 (i.e., $t = 1$–36), which includes wave VIII, as a calibration period to calculate initial values for m_0, C_0 and to estimate σ^2. For the calibration period, we took $b_{1t} = b_1$, a constant, and ignored those t in which zero cases were reported. We can then rewrite (6.11) as

$$\frac{y_t}{\sqrt{(y_{t-1})}} = b_1\sqrt{(y_{t-1})} + \varepsilon_t', \quad \varepsilon_t' \sim N(0,\sigma^2). \tag{6.14}$$

We assumed a uniform prior for b_1 on $(0, \infty)$, and using Bayesian least

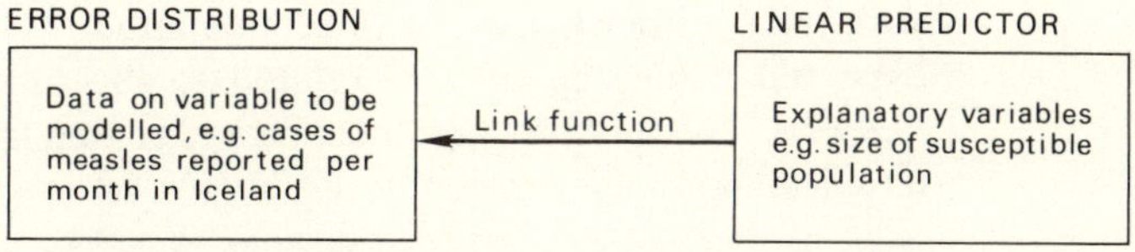

Fig. 6.6 Structure of the GLIM

squares methods (Lindley, 1965 and section 6.7), we obtained the posterior distribution of b_1 and estimates as

$$m_0 = 0.7997; \quad C_0 = 0.0183; \quad \hat{\sigma}^2 = 17.94.$$

Results (Figure 6.5)

The model was then used to forecast the number of cases reported in Reykjavíkur in wave XII. Various values of V were tried, to allow the parameters to 'wobble' through time. Notice, as we would expect, that as V increases (i.e., we move further away from fixed parameters through time) the 'one-month-in-arrears' forecasts noted with the simple AR model begin to disappear. The model is able to lock on more rapidly to change because of the adaptive parameter structure, but a price is paid in the vast over-estimate of the magnitude of the epidemic. That is, the fixed-parameter AR model is poor at predicting arrival but provides reasonable estimates of numbers of reported cases; conversely, the adaptive parameter form can detect change from non-epidemic to epidemic more easily, but it is grossly in error as a predictor of epidemic size. We thus return to the point discussed in section 6.2.3; from a control point of view, is it better to be able to forecast correctly the phase characteristics or the ultimate size of an epidemic? In terms of modelling, the results so far suggest that the next logical extension is to consider (1) combinations of two (or more) models, designed specifically to handle the non-epidemic and epidemic phases respectively, of the recurrent waves; (2) the development of a trigger mechanism to switch models when an epidemic appears to be starting. We discuss this possibility in the next two sections.

6.4 Mixed-state models: generalised linear integrated models (GLIM)[2]

6.4.1 The class of models

This class of models was proposed by Nelder and Wedderburn (1972), where statistical details are given. The structure of the models is summarised in Figure 6.6. We envisage a set of observations $\{y_t\}$, namely the number of cases of measles reported in a given medical district at time t, whose variability we wish to model. The $\{y_t\}$ are assumed to have come from the exponential family of distributions. Secondly, we have a set of known variables (such as the size of the susceptible population or population at risk, the number of people who contracted measles in earlier time periods), $\{x_{jt}\}$, which we are going to use to model the variability in the $\{y_t\}$. These known variables are combined to form a *linear predictor*,

$$\xi_t = \sum_j \beta_j x_{jt}, \tag{6.15}$$

[2] This section relies on the work of A. Sutherland who was supervised by one of us (A. D. C.) while working as a student on a field project as part of the postgraduate diploma in mathematical statistics at Cambridge University. See Sutherland (1979) for details of the project.

with the β_j either known or to be estimated. Then the model is that the expected value, μ_t, of y_t is related to the linear predictor by a *link function.* The link function must be a specified monotonic differentiable function, so that

$$\mu_t = h_t(\xi_t) \quad \text{or} \quad \xi_t = g_t(\mu_t). \tag{6.16}$$

It is this link function which can be modified between epidemic and non-epidemic phases to enable model switching to occur. Thus, a generalised linear model is

$$y_t \sim F[h_t(\Sigma\beta_j x_{jt})], \tag{6.17}$$

where F is some exponential family of distributions, indexed by the values of the mean. The model is specified by stating the family of distributions, F, the link function, h_t, and the composition of the linear predictor. Models are fitted to data by iterative solution of the maximum likelihood equations; a standard package program is available from the Numerical Algorithms Group (NAG) to do this.

6.4.2 Choosing a model

GLIM allows its user considerable choice in the model to be fitted to the observations. In particular, the following must be specified:

(1) the family of distributions from which we suppose our $\{y_t\}$ observations to have come (the 'error distribution');

(2) the link function, giving the expected value of the observation from the linear predictor;

(3) the composition of the linear predictor – which of the many possible variables do we suspect of having an effect on the observations? We take each of these in turn.

The 'error distribution'

As noted in section 6.3.2, a reasonable assumption is that measles cases arise independently; that is, the catching or non-catching of measles by person A during month t depends only on some specified set of conditions prevailing during month t and not on whether persons B, C, D, . . . also catch measles during the same month. This suggests the use of a Poisson distribution for the number of cases occurring in month t; that is, independently at some specified rate. An assumption of this type has been made for the stochastic process models of measles epidemics (see chapter 7).

The link function

Given a Poisson error distribution, the main functions available are the *log link*, $\mu = e^{\xi}$, where μ is the expected value of the observation and ξ is the value of the linear predictor, and the *linear link*, $\mu = \xi$. The linear link was found to be more useful.

The linear predictor

As we know from the Appendix to the book, the following data are available for each of the 50 medical districts, 1945–70:

I_t: the number of infectives reported in month t,

S_t: the number of susceptibles in month t.

Various combinations of these variables were tried in the linear

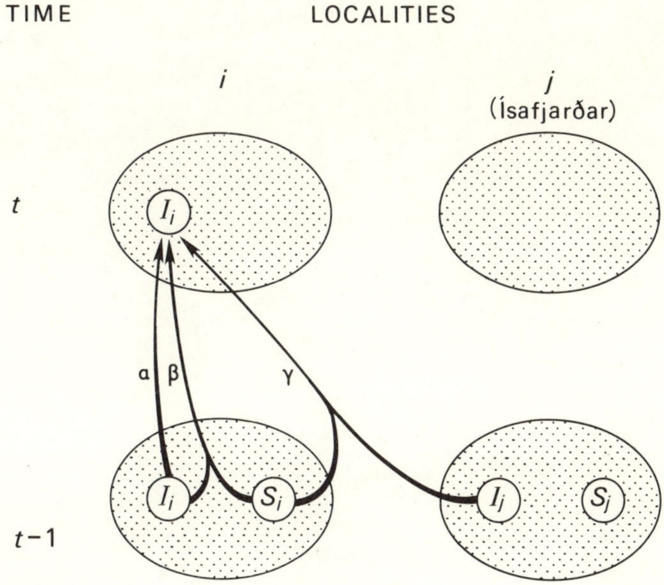

Fig. 6.7 Form of regional model (6.18) for measles transmission. Terms are defined in text.

predictor, and again precise forms will be outlined in the discussion of the results in section 6.4.3.

6.4.3 Regional application

Since measles is not endemic in Iceland, an epidemic must necessarily begin by the introduction of infection from abroad. Similarly, at a local level, infection must come from elsewhere in the country for an epidemic to occur. In order to produce a model which stands some chance of predicting the start of an epidemic in a given locality (that is, of avoiding the 'one-month-in-arrears' problem noted earlier), we must move from the single-region models considered so far in this chapter to a multi-region version which takes into account the links between districts we know to exist from chapter 4. The north-west fjords, centred on Ísafjarðar, suggest themselves as a natural choice for a test area. As discussed in chapter 4, they operated in a totally 'closed' way in the epidemic of 1904 (wave I); in general (Figure 4.19), the diffusion structure in the area is straightforward – consisting of initial introduction of the disease into Ísafjarðar from elsewhere in Iceland, and then localised spread to other medical districts in the area.

Since new infectives are created by contact between existing infectives and susceptibles, a simple random mixing argument suggests the use of a Poisson model with a linear link function, that is,

$$I_{i,t} \sim P[(\alpha I_{i,t-1} + \beta I_{i,t-1} S_{i,t-1} + \gamma I_{j,t-1} S_{i,t-1})] \qquad (6.18)$$

to model the number of new cases in medical districts in the north-west fjords area, *other than Ísafjarðar*. Here, $I_{i,t}$ is the number of cases of measles reported in region i at time t, $S_{i,t}$ is the number of susceptibles, i is used to index medical districts other than Ísafjarðar and j denotes Ísafjarðar. α, β and γ are unknown parameters in the linear link function. The term in α is the familiar AR component; β measures the

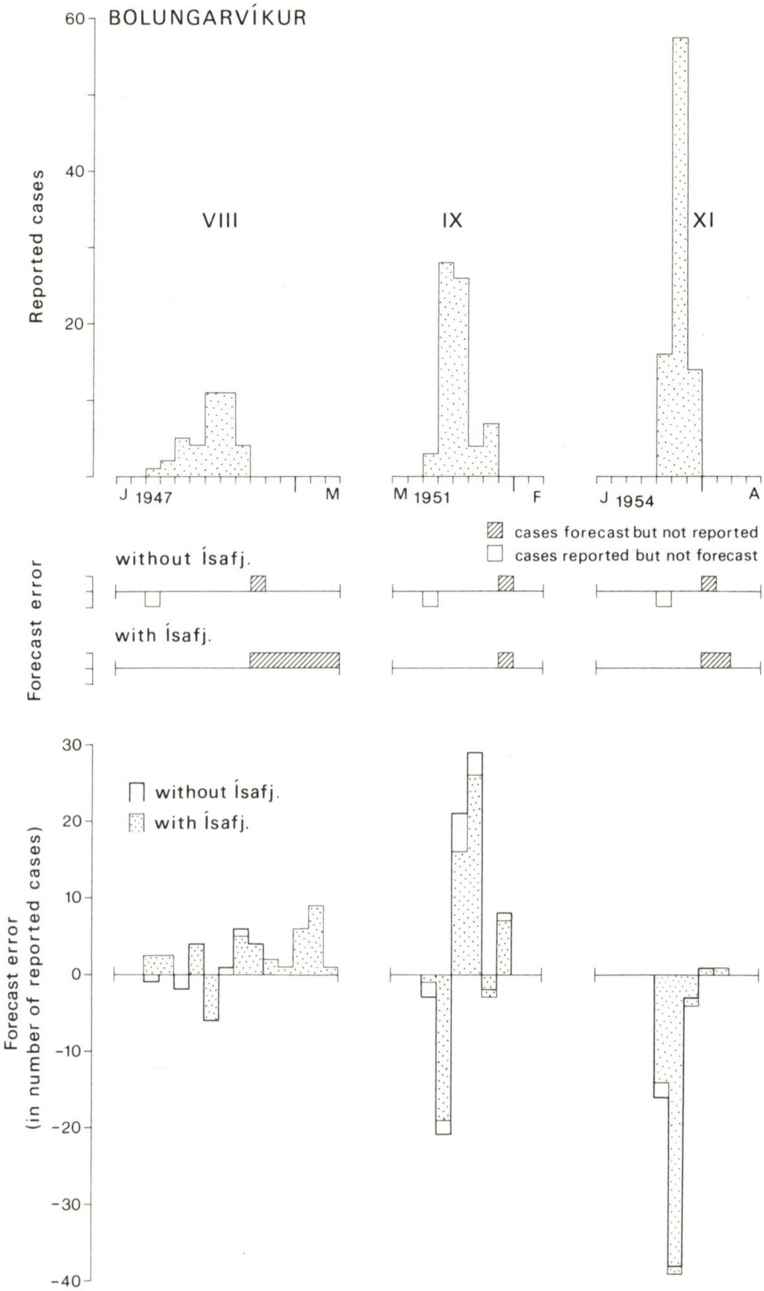

Fig. 6.8 Application of GLIM to waves VIII, IX and XI in Bolungarvíkur and Flateyrar, north-west Iceland. Results are for model (6.18) calibrated (1) with term for Ísafjarðar, thus allowing impulse transmission from this regional centre to lower-order districts, and (2) without term for Ísafjarðar. The one-month-ahead forecast errors are given both in indicator random variable and interval scaled random variable forms.

proportion of new cases created by within-area contacts between susceptibles and infectives in i; and γ measures the proportion of new cases created by contact between infectives in Ísafjarðar and susceptibles in i (see Figure 6.7).

Perhaps we might consider that the arrival of infection from Ísafjarðar in other areas is important only if there is no local source of infection within the community, thus suggesting a revised term in γ as

$$\gamma I_{j,t-1} S_{i,t-1} \delta_{(I_{i,t-1}<a)} \qquad (6.19)$$

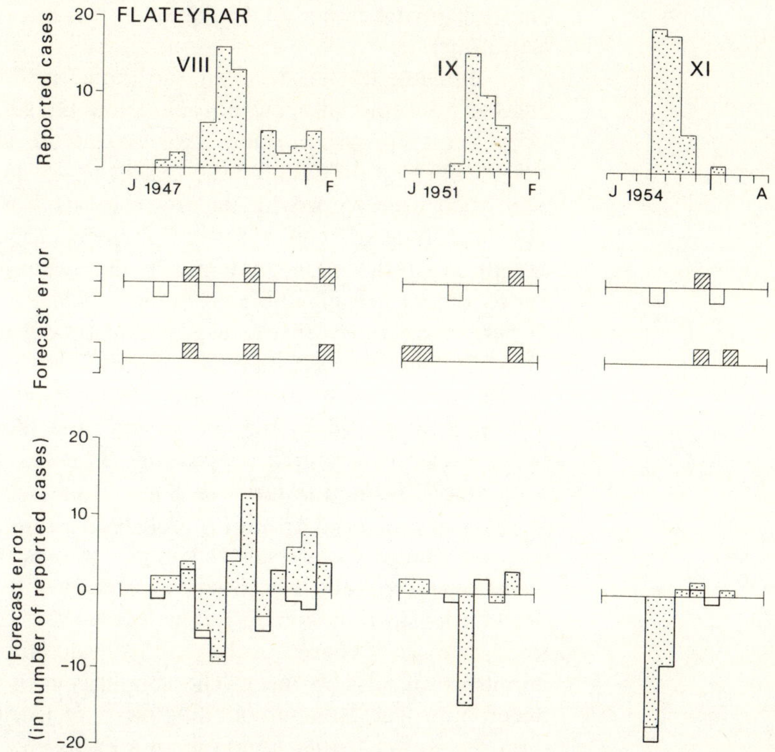

Fig. 6.8 (contd)

where $\delta_{(I_{i,t-1}<a)} = 1$ if $I_{i,t-1}<a$
$= 0$ otherwise.

Here, a is a pre-specified constant, and we 'import' infection from Ísafjarðar only when $I_{i,t-1}<a$. Alternatively, we might use

$$\gamma S_{i,t-1}\delta_{(I_{j,t-1}>0)} \tag{6.20}$$

where $\delta_{(I_{j,t-1}>0)} = 1$ if infection is present in Ísafjarðar in $t-1$
$= 0$ otherwise,

or

$$\gamma\delta_{(I_{j,t-1}>0)} \tag{6.21}$$

with the delta (δ) function defined as in (6.20). The term (6.20) suggests that there is a risk of infection in i from Ísafjarðar, and that its size will be governed by the size of the susceptible population able to receive it; (6.21) implies only that infection can arrive from Ísafjarðar, and it is a simple trigger for starting epidemics in other areas, i.

The various models (6.18)–(6.21) have been applied to the number of measles cases reported, 1945–70, in the medical districts which are adjacent to Ísafjarðar (see Figure 4.1). We note that the rate of spread from Ísafjarðar to other areas can be slowed down by using $I_{j,t-2}$ rather than $I_{j,t-1}$. Inevitably, problems were encountered with the small number of cases reported in some districts (see book Appendix), and we give in Figure 6.8 the results for two of the larger districts, Flateyrar (22) and Bolungarvíkur (25). For comparison, the model has also been fitted omitting any term in γ (that is, ignoring any inter-area transmission from Ísafjarðar).

In applying the models, all the data for 1945–70 were taken and divided into epidemic and non-epidemic phases. We consider first the 'epidemic in progress' data. Two tasks were attempted. The models were calibrated on data for the period, 1945–56, and the fitted models were then used to provide *ex post* forecasts for the period thereafter. The modelling of inter-epidemic phases is considered later. With the exception of the 1954 epidemic in the calibration period, a marked improvement in our ability to model epidemic starts was provided by (6.18), compared with the use of that model omitting the term in γ. Thus, the binary forecast error graphs in Figure 6.8 indicates that model (6.18) never failed to forecast cases when measles were actually reported. If anything, the model over-reacted to the stimulus from Ísafjarðar; for example, reporting of cases in Ísafjarðar between November 1947 and January 1948 meant that cases were still forecast by (6.18) in Bolungarvíkur until March 1948 – long after the epidemic had died out there. Conversely, the same graphs indicate that, when the term in γ is omitted, the model consistently fails, as we would expect, to detect the start of epidemics; it has no information upon which to forecast cases. These results confirm the importance of the spatial impulse transmission term. The simplifications (6.19)–(6.21) also produced improvements in modelling phase characteristics. However, they required so much fine tuning from area to area to fix the value of the cut-off constant a and to adjust the lag regulating the rate of spread from Ísafjarðar (see discussion below equation (6.21)) that we found it simpler to use the general model (6.18) throughout. The 1954 epidemic proved problematical because of the extremely rapid take-off of infection; there was virtually no lead-in period as was the case with the other epidemics. In practical terms, the availability of weekly data would probably suffice to overcome this problem. If we consider the number of cases reported in each epidemic, as opposed to stressing phase characteristics, it is clear from the graphs in Figure 6.8, which give forecast error in number of reported cases, that both models are ineffective.

The estimates of the coefficients of the model appear in Table 6.1. The small size of $\hat{\gamma}$, compared with $\hat{\alpha}$ and $\hat{\beta}$, reflects the relative lack of importance of inter-area transmissions in following the actual course of an epidemic in an area; once an epidemic is established in a medical district, within- rather than between-area effects dominate. However, as we have seen, the spatial term is crucial as a trigger mechanism to model epidemic starts. This parallels the result Cliff, Haggett, Ord, Bassett and Davies (1975, chapter 10) found in modelling the inter-regional transmission of business cycles in south-west England.

The difficulty we have continually experienced in modelling the phase characteristics of epidemics probably reflects, in part, the fact that our data are monthly, whereas the serial interval of the disease is approximately two weeks (section 3.3.4). This means that the number of reported cases tends to climb very rapidly when an epidemic arrives.

Table 6.1. *Values of parameters for model (6.18) for Flateyrar and Bolungarvíkur, based on measles epidemic data, 1945–56*

	Model				
	(6.18) without inter-area transmission term		(6.18) including spread from Ísafjarðar		
Area	$\hat{\alpha}$	$\hat{\beta}$	$\hat{\alpha}$	$\hat{\beta}$	$\hat{\gamma}$
Flateyrar	−5.2	0.016	−3.5	0.011	0.00049
Bolungarvíkur	−3.2	0.027	−2.9	0.024	0.00089

Standard errors all approximately 0.1 of estimated coefficients.
Note: In the 'spread from Ísafjarðar' model, best results were obtained with $I_{j,t-1}$ for Flateyrar, but using $I_{j,t-2}$ for Bolungarvíkur. The $\hat{\gamma}$ values refer to these terms.

Less advance warning can be given by the monthly data record in Iceland as compared with data collected say, weekly, as in the United Kingdom.

The one-month-ahead forecasts from model (6.18) – allowing for spread from Ísafjarðar – were obtained using the estimated values of α, β and γ given in Table 6.1; applying them to the epidemics between 1957 and 1970 gave the results shown in Figure 6.9. Disappointingly, the one-month time lag in forecasts has reappeared in some cases, and there is gross over-estimate of the size of epidemics. As we know that susceptible population in Flateyrar and Bolungarvíkur increased between 1945 and 1970, these inflated estimates may partly reflect the use of parameters calculated from relatively smaller susceptible populations than existed in the forecast period. Since we are back again with a stationarity problem, we can hold out little hope of using these models with parameters fixed through time for other than short-term (a few months ahead) forecasting.

Returning to Table 6.1, we note that $\hat{\alpha}$ is negative. In applying models of this kind to many of the medical districts in Iceland, we found that this was nearly always the case. From (6.18)

$$\begin{aligned}\hat{\alpha}I_{i,t-1} + \hat{\beta}\, I_{i,t-1}S_{i,t-1} &= \hat{\beta}I_{i,t-1}(S_{i,t-1} + \hat{\alpha}/\hat{\beta}) \\ &= \hat{\beta}I_{i,t-1}(S_{i,t-1} - M),\end{aligned} \tag{6.22}$$

where $M > 0$ if $\hat{\alpha} < 0$ and $\hat{\beta} > 0$. Equation (6.22) suggests that we should perhaps be considering a susceptible population somewhat smaller than that actually projected by the cohort model (Appendix to book). One way of arriving at too large an estimate of the S population is if under-reporting of cases occurs. On the basis of the values of M that we obtained in our analyses, it would seem that the reporting rate would have to be about 40 per cent of the true rate of attack. This is of the same order of magnitude as Black (1966) found (see Figure 3.7 and the discussion on this figure).

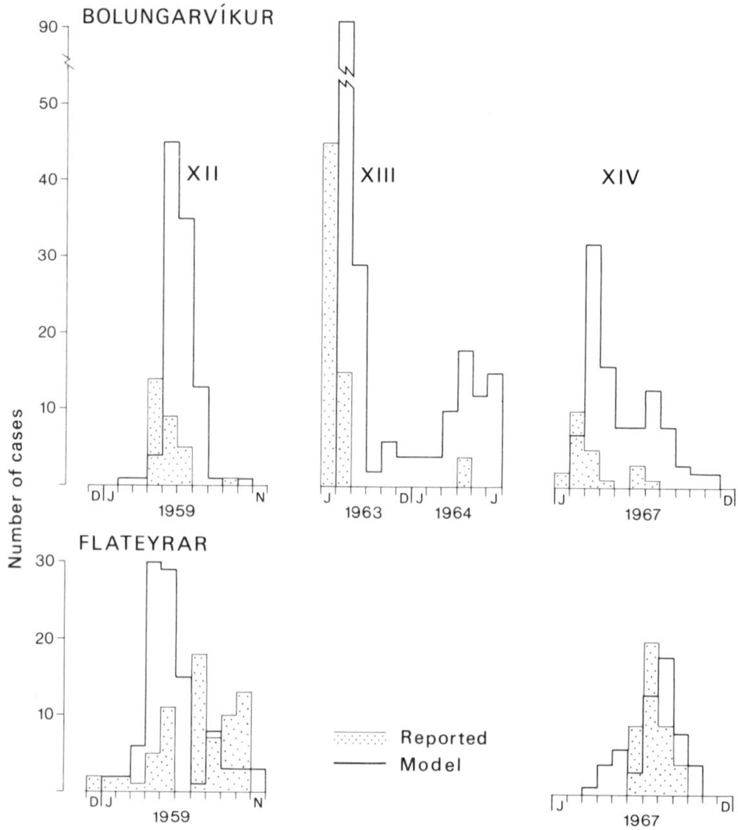

Fig. 6.9 Forecasts of reported measles cases in Bolungarvíkur and Flateyrar, 1959–67, obtained from GLIM (6.18) calibrated on data for 1945–56.

If we consider the inter-epidemic phases, 1945–70, the simple model

$$I_{i,t} \sim P[(\alpha I_{i,t-1})] \tag{6.23}$$

works satisfactorily – as we would expect, since we are tracking low, virtually constant levels of activity. We may combine the models for the epidemic/inter-epidemic phases (relationships (6.18) and (6.23) respectively) by the simple specification

$$K = (1-\delta)E + \delta(NE), \tag{6.24}$$

where K is the combined model, E denotes model (6.18), and NE model (6.23). Set $\delta = 0$ when an epidemic starts in the 'lead' area appropriate for the medical district to which K is applied. For example, Reykjavíkur may be regarded as a national lead indicator, or Ísafjarðar for the north-west fjords. Put $\delta = 1$ in the inter-epidemic phases.

6.5 Mixed-state models: Bayesian-entropy methods[3]

6.5.1 Theory

As we have seen in the preceding pages, our modelling problems arise from two main sources:

(1) the non-stationarity of the process and, in particular, how to handle epidemic/no-epidemic changes to avoid lagged forecasts;

(2) growth/decline in the S population due to changes in birth-rates and/or net migration.

[3] This section was contributed by Dr R. C. Souza (see Preface).

Of these, (1) is by far the more significant.

The combined model (6.24) considers two different states of the generating process:

state I: no epidemic
state II: epidemic

to overcome this difficulty, and we here put the approach within a Bayesian framework.

Assume that, for a particular study area affected by an epidemic, we observe a Poisson process, I_t, for the number of infectives at time t, with mean level θ_t which depends upon past levels of the process. We suppose that, at any time t, the generating model is a random choice between two models (that is, two states) where:

$$M_t^{(1)}: \text{ Model 1: (no epidemic); } \theta_t = \theta_c; \quad \theta_c \text{ is a small positive constant;} \tag{6.25}$$

$$M_t^{(2)}: \text{ Model 2: (epidemic); } \theta_t \text{ is a gamma-distributed random variable.} \tag{6.26}$$

Equation (6.25) states that when there is no epidemic, the observations come from a Poisson process with a constant, low-valued rate ($\theta_t = \theta_c$). This implies the assignment of a high probability to the occurrence of small-valued observations (depending on the selected value for θ_c), and almost zero probability to the occurrence of high-valued observations. On the other hand, with $M_t^{(2)}$ in (6.26), θ_t is a gamma-distributed random variable, and the model itself corresponds to the single steady-state Poisson–gamma BEF (Bayesian-entropy forecasting) model described in Souza (1978).

The various components of the model are as follows:

(1) initial (possibly subjective) estimates for the parameters at the start (time $t=0$);

(2) a probabilistic description of the state of the model at time $(t-1)$ given $\mathbf{H}_{t-1}$ (the information in the system at time $(t-1)$ (see section 6.3.1));

(3) an updating procedure for the description in (2) which takes into account the new information on infectives, I_t, whence $\mathbf{H}_t = (\mathbf{H}_{t-1}, I_t$, plus any new subjective information).

The model at time $(t-1)$ is described in the first section of Table 6.2 in terms of the expressions (A1–A4) which give: (i) the probability of being in either the no-epidemic or the epidemic state at time $(t-1)$, (ii) the summary of information about the parameter θ at that time, and (iii) the appropriate transition probabilities between states.

Given a complete specification for time $(t-1)$, we can evaluate the one-step- (generally, m-step-) ahead predictors for θ_t and I_t. These will depend upon both the past history, $\mathbf{H}_{t-1}$, and upon the states of the system at times $(t-1)$ and t. The results are summarised in section B of Table 6.2. The updating procedure identifies the entropy maximising predictive distribution for θ_t (or I_t); Souza (1978, 1980) gives fuller details. In particular, the function g_t can be regarded as a discount factor

Table 6.2. *The structure of the Bayesian-entropy mixed-state model*

A Model at time $(t-1)$

(A1) Probability that model j was operating at time $(t-1)$:

$$p_{t-1}^{(j)} = \text{Prob}\,(M_{t-1}^{(j)} \mid \mathbf{H}_{t-1}), \quad j = 1, 2.$$

(A2) Parameter distribution conditional on model j at time $(t-1)$:

$$(\theta_{t-1} \mid M_{t-1}^{(1)}, \mathbf{H}_{t-1}) \sim \theta_c \text{ (constant)}$$

$$(\theta_{t-1} \mid M_{t-1}^{(2)}, \mathbf{H}_{t-1}) \sim \text{gamma}\,[\alpha_{t-1}(2), \beta_{t-1}(2)].$$

(A3) Transition probabilities for movement between states:

$$\pi_{kj} = \text{Prob}\,(M_t^{(j)} \mid M_{t-1}^{(k)}, \mathbf{H}_{t-1}).$$

(A4) From (A1) and (A3) it is evident that:

$$\text{Prob}(M_t^{(j)} \text{ and } M_{t-1}^{(k)} \mid \mathbf{H}_{t-1}) = \pi_{kj} \cdot p_{t-1}^{(k)}; \quad k,j = 1, 2.$$

B One-step-ahead prediction

(B1) for $j = 1$ and $k = 1, 2$:

$$(\theta_t \mid M_{t-1}^{(k)}, M_t^{(1)}, \mathbf{H}_{t-1}) \sim \theta_c$$

$$(I_t \mid M_{t-1}^{(k)}, M_t^{(1)}, \mathbf{H}_{t-1}) \sim \text{Poisson}\,(\theta_c).$$

(B2) for $j = 2$ and $k = 1, 2$:

$$(\theta_t \mid M_{t-1}^{(k)}, M_t^{(2)}, \mathbf{H}_{t-1}) \sim \text{gamma}\,(\alpha_t^*, \beta_t^*)$$

$$(I_t \mid M_{t-1}^{(k)}, M_t^{(2)}, \mathbf{H}_{t-1}) \sim \text{negative binomial}\,[(1+\beta_t^*)^{-1}, \alpha_t^*]$$

$$[= \text{Prob}\,(i_t \mid M_{t-1}^{(k)}, M_t^{(2)}, \mathbf{H}_{t-1})],$$

where $\alpha_t^* \equiv \alpha_t^*(k, 2) = 1 + g_{t-1}(\alpha_{t-1} - 1)$,

$\beta_t^* = \beta_t^*(k, 2) = g_{t-1}\beta_{t-1}(S_{t-1}/S_t)$,

and $g_t = [1 - \exp(-ch_t)]^2$.

$\ln h_t$ is Shannon's entropy measure for the gamma distribution, given by

$$\ln h_t = \ln \Gamma(\alpha_{t-1}) + \alpha_{t-1}[1 - \psi(\alpha_{t-1}) + \ln \beta_{t-1}],$$

where $\psi(\alpha_{t-1}) = \Gamma'(\alpha_{t-1})/\Gamma(\alpha_{t-1})$ is the digamma function.

C Posterior distribution given $I_t = i_t$

(C1) for $j = 1$ and $k = 1, 2$:

$$(\theta_t \mid M_{t-1}^{(k)}, M_t^{(1)}, \mathbf{H}_t) \sim \theta_c.$$

(C2) for $j = 2$ and $k = 1, 2$:

$$(\theta_t \mid M_{t-1}^{(k)}, M_t^{(2)}, \mathbf{H}_t) \sim \text{gamma}\,[\alpha_t, \beta_t],$$

where $\alpha_t \equiv \alpha_t(k, 2) = \alpha_t^*(k, 2) + i_t$

and $\beta_t \equiv \beta_t(k, 2) = \beta_t^*(k, 2) + 1$.

D Collapsing procedure

(D1) The gamma distributions in (C2) have means

$$m_t(k, 2) = \alpha_t(k, 2)/\beta_t(k, 2)$$

and geometric means

$$gm_t(k, 2) = \psi[a_t(k, 2)] - \ln[\beta_t(k, 2)]$$

for $k = 1, 2$.

(D2) The corresponding 'collapsed' single gamma distribution has mean

$$m_t(2) = p_{12}m_t(1, 2) + p_{22}m_t(2, 2)$$

and geometric mean

$$gm_t(2) = p_{12}gm_t(1, 2) + p_{22}gm_t(2, 2),$$

where $p_{k2} = p^*_{k2}/(p^*_{12} + p^*_{22})$

and $p^*_{k2} = \pi_{k2}p^{(k)}_{t-1}\text{Prob}(i_t | M^{(k)}_{t-1}, M^{(2)}_t, \mathbf{H}_{t-1})$

(terms given in (A4) and (B2)).

---

which indicates that the predictive probability statements for θ_t given $\mathbf{H}_{t-1}$ will contain more uncertainty than those for θ_{t-1} given $\mathbf{H}_{t-1}$. We also note that the scale parameter of the gamma posterior distribution is modified by the ratio of susceptibles in successive months, S_{t-1}/S_t. A reduction in the number of susceptibles lowers the mean of θ_t. When the predictive distribution is given, an application of Bayes' Theorem enables us to determine θ_t given $\mathbf{H}_t$, as in section C of Table 6.2. Again, details appear in Souza (1978, 1980). However, the process is not yet complete, since closer inspection of the results in Table 6.2 indicates that the single two-stage model at time $(t-1)$ has given rise to two such models at time *t*, depending upon whether $k=1$ or 2 in (C2). Like the hapless sorcerer's apprentice, we find each model splitting into two new ones with each time period that passes. To call a halt to this progression, Souza (1978, chapter 3) makes use of Jaynes' principle of maximum entropy (Jaynes, 1957). If we specify a single desired distribution (the gamma), then it is possible to collapse the mixture of the two alternatives in (C2) into that single form in a 'least-prejudiced' manner by retaining the values of the sufficient statistics. For the gamma distribution, the sufficient statistics are the mean, m_t, say, and the geometric mean, gm_t, say. The collapsing procedure outlined in section D of Table 6.2 shows how these values are preserved, while the two gamma distributions are collapsed into one. In this instance, the two models for state I are identical, so that no collapsing is necessary. Finally, the collapsed gamma distribution serves as input to section A for the next time period. The initial values will depend upon the particular application, and their selection is described in the next section.

6.5.2 Application of model to measles data for Reykjavíkur

The 312 monthly notifications covering the period January 1945 to December 1970 in Reykjavíkur were taken in order to examine a medical district where inputs from other areas in Iceland are of minor importance in generating outbreaks. The constructed series for susceptibles (see Appendix to book) was used to update the parameters in section B2 of Table 6.2.

Table 6.3. *Observed transitions between epidemic and no epidemic states, Reykjavíkur, 1945–70*

	Time t		
Time $(t-1)$	E^c	E	Totals
E^c	252	7	259
E	7	45	52
Totals	259	52	311

E^c = 'no epidemic'
E = 'epidemic',
t = month.

The preliminary parameter values required to start up the model are:

(i) $p_0^{(j)} = \text{Prob}\,(M_0^{(j)} \mid \mathbf{H}_0), \quad j = 1, 2;$

(ii) θ_c, the mean level for model $M_t^{(1)}$;

(iii) π_{kj}; $j, k = 1, 2$, the matrix of transition probabilities; and

(iv) $\alpha_0(2)$ and $\beta_0(2)$, the parameters of the initial gamma distribution for state $M_0^{(2)}$.

To fix these starting values, we examined the transitions which occurred in the series of reported cases. Strictly speaking, such a procedure is invalid, but in an exploratory study of this kind, it seemed a reasonable jumping-off point. If this approach is to be used regularly, then 'dry runs' of this kind help the researcher to assess appropriate ranges for the starting parameters. Thus, to determine the proportion of time spent in the 'epidemic' state, the number of months with more than 25 notifications was recorded. The transitions from 'epidemic' (>25 cases) to 'no epidemic' (≤25 cases) and vice versa may then be estimated from the same data. The results for Reykjavíkur are given in Table 6.3. The number of cases reported during the 'no epidemic' periods was 620. Similar results are obtained with other definitions of the epidemic/no epidemic states.

Using the figures given in Table 6.3 for guidance, we set

(i) $p_0^{(1)} = 0.75$ and $p_0^{(2)} = 0.25$ (these values are not critical when, as here, the model is started up during a 'no-epidemic' phase, which we would recommend);

(ii) $\theta_c = 5$. This was chosen deliberately as non-zero since our 'no epidemic' state really corresponds to two states, namely (i) no infectives at all or (ii) some infectives but no epidemic. The mean for (ii), taken over all cases with infectives >0 but ≤25 is about three times that of the composite state involving both (i) and (ii);

(iii) the transition matrix was set as

$$\Pi = \begin{matrix} & E^c & E \\ E^c & 0.95 & 0.05 \\ E & 0.05 & 0.95 \end{matrix}.$$

Table 6.4. *The state probabilities and one-step-ahead forecasts for the Bayesian-entropy mixed-state model for wave VIII*

Time	Number of cases		State probabilities	Joint probabilities*			
	Observed	Forecast $E(I_{t+1}\|\mathbf{H}_t)$	$p_t^{(1)}(=1-p_t^{(2)})$	$p_t(1,1)$	$p_t(1,2)$	$p_t(2,1)$	$p_t(2,2)$
1946							
October	0	5	1.0	1.0			
November	5	5	1.0	1.0			
December	0	5	1.0	1.0			
1947							
January	221	5	0.0		1.0		
February	244	187	0.0				1.0
March	270	222	0.0				1.0
April	311	250	0.0				1.0
May	79	286	0.0				1.0
June	15	168	0.0			1.0	
July	13	5	1.0	1.0			
August	0	5	1.0	1.0			

* $p_t(k,j) = \text{Prob}\ (M_{t-1}^{(k)} \text{and } M_t^{(j)}|\mathbf{H}_t)$; all omitted entries are zero to two decimal places

These figures are higher than the empirical values for $E^c \to E$, but lower than those for $E \to E^c$. Since, as argued elsewhere, detecting the beginning of an epidemic is more important than highly accurate estimates in mid-epidemic, we feel that these biasses are justified;

(iv) to obtain the initial parameter values of the gamma distribution for model $M_0^{(2)}$, we took the mode to be around 150 cases and the scale parameter to be equal to $1/c$, where c is given in the expression for g_t in (B2) of Table 6.2. After these initial settings, a search was carried out to minimise the sum of the absolute errors

$$\bar{e}(c) = \sum_{t=1}^{312} [i_t - E(I_t|\mathbf{H}_{t-1})]$$

with respect to c, resulting in $\hat{c} \sim 0.02$. This in turn led to $\alpha_0(2) \sim 4$, $\beta_0(2) \sim 50$ [mean ~ 200, variance $\sim (100)^2$].

6.5.3 Discussion of the results

Since most of the results are similar in form to those obtained from the Kalman model in section 6.3.2, we concentrate here upon waves VIII and IX. The findings are summarised in Tables 6.4 and 6.5. For wave VIII, the five cases in November 1946 are properly ignored, but the model confirms the major outbreak beginning in January 1947 (the joint probability of 'no epidemic' in December and 'epidemic' in January being close to unity). Likewise, the end of the epidemic is correctly identified in June 1947. The numerical forecasts are much less satisfactory and tend to show the 'one-month-behind' effect of the AR models, save that the sharp cut-off at the end of June is picked out as the model swings back into the 'no epidemic' state.

Table 6.5. *The state probabilities and one-step-ahead forecasts for the Bayesian-entropy mixed-state model for wave IX*

Time	Number of cases: Observed	Forecast $E(I_{t+1}\|\mathbf{H}_t)$	State probabilities $p_t^{(1)}(=1-p_t^{(2)})$	Joint probabilities*: $p_t(1,1)$	$p_t(1,2)$	$p_t(2,1)$	$p_t(2,2)$
1951							
September	0	5	1.0	1.0			
October	1	5	1.0	1.0			
November	15	5	1.0	1.0			
December	152	5	0.0		1.0		
1952							
January	569	155	0.0				1.0
February	684	469	0.0				1.0
March	752	595	0.0				1.0
April	720	677	0.0				1.0
May	284	702	0.0				1.0
June	80	522	0.0				1.0
July	27	317	0.33			0.33	0.67
August	25	211	0.35	0.03	0.04	0.32	0.65
September	8	5	1.0	0.02		0.98	
October	8	5	1.0	1.0			
November	0	5	1.0	1.0			

* $p_t(k,j) = \text{Prob}\,(M_{t-1}^{(k)} \text{ and } M_t^{(j)}\,|\mathbf{H}_t)$; all omitted entries are zero to two decimal places

For wave IX, the entry month is correctly identified, but the slow fade-out over July–October 1952 leads to some uncertainty. Nevertheless, the end of the epidemic is forecast for September, which is reasonable. As before, the numerical forecasts are unconvincing.

Given our emphasis upon the identification of epidemic starts, the results of the BEF model are mildly encouraging. Indeed, if weekly rather than monthly data were available, we might expect a better all-around performance from the model, as achieved by Souza (1978, 1980) in his study of measles outbreaks in Cornwall.

6.6 Conclusion

In this chapter, we have considered some time series models to forecast recurrent epidemics. We have started with the simplest fixed-parameter ARMA models, and have moved through to models with time-varying parameters and mixed-state models. It is quite clear that the change from epidemic to no-epidemic conditions in medical districts causes difficulties which can be properly tackled only by having separate models for each state, and then switching from one to the other at the appropriate time. One obvious candidate for a trigger is to identify the disease 'lead indicator' areas (e.g., Reykjavíkur, Ísafjarðar and Akureyrar) and to allow the presence of infection in these districts to give the impulse for an epidemic in other areas. Without this spatial trigger, it is doubtful whether it will be possible to forecast epidemic starts with any reliability, although the mixed-state model allows quick identification of a new epidemic. Nevertheless, early warning of the approach of an epidemic is obviously necessary if control is to be effected through vaccination and isolation programmes.

While spatial impulse/response modelling appears necessary to model the phase characteristics when an epidemic passes through a set of areas, information on the size of the S population seems essential if we are to project the ultimate magnitude of an epidemic, that is, the number of people who will contract the disease. As we shall see in section 7.2.1, the size of S also affects the probability of an area starting an epidemic. These conclusions point us in the direction of complex, data-demanding models. On this somewhat sombre note, we move to consider some of these models in chapter 7.

6.7 Mathematical appendix

Bayesian least squares (see Lindley, 1965)

Consider the simple regression model

$$u_i = b_1 x_i + \varepsilon_i \quad i = 1, 2, \ldots, n, \tag{A1}$$

where $\varepsilon_1, \varepsilon_2, \ldots, \varepsilon_n$ are i.d. $N(0, \varphi)$, φ unknown.

Let $\mathbf{u}^T = (u_1, u_2, \ldots, u_n)$ and $\mathbf{x}^T = (x_1, x_2, \ldots, x_n)$.

$$\text{Now } f(\mathbf{u} | \mathbf{x}, b_1, \varphi) = \frac{1}{(2\pi\varphi)^{n/2}} \exp\left\{\frac{-1}{2\varphi}\left[S^2 + Sxx(b_1 - \hat{b}_1)^2\right]\right\}, \tag{A2}$$

where $Suu = \sum_{i=1}^{n} u_i^2, \quad Sux = \sum_{i=1}^{n} u_i x_i, \quad Sxx = \sum_{i=1}^{n} u_i^2$

$$\hat{b}_1 = Sux/Sxx \quad \text{and} \quad S^2 = Suu - (Sux)^2/Sxx.$$

If we assume that the prior distributions of b_1 and $\log \varphi$ are independent and uniform,

$$\text{i.e., } \pi(b_1, \varphi) = \begin{cases} 1/\varphi \text{ if } 0 < \varphi < \infty \text{ and } a < b_1 < c \\ 0 \quad \text{otherwise,} \end{cases} \tag{A3}$$

where a and c are constants satisfying $-\infty \leqslant a < c \leqslant \infty$, then by Bayes' Theorem

$$\pi(b_1, \varphi | \mathbf{u},\mathbf{x}) \propto \begin{cases} \varphi^{-\frac{1}{2}(n+2)} \exp\left\{\frac{-1}{2\varphi}\left[S^2 + Sxx(b_1 - \hat{b}_1)^2\right]\right\} \\ \qquad\qquad \text{if } 0 < \varphi < \infty \text{ and } a < b_1 < c \\ 0 \quad \text{otherwise.} \end{cases} \tag{A4}$$

Integrating (A4) over $(0, \infty)$ with respect to φ yields

$$\pi(b_1 | \mathbf{u},\mathbf{x}) \propto \begin{cases} \left[S^2 + Sxx(b_1 - \hat{b}_1)^2\right]^{-n/2} \text{ if } a < b_1 < c \\ 0 \quad \text{otherwise.} \end{cases} \tag{A5}$$

$$\text{Let } t = (b_1 - \hat{b}_1)/\left[S^2/Sxx(n-1)\right]^{\frac{1}{2}}. \tag{A6}$$

$$\text{Then} \quad \pi(t | \mathbf{u},\mathbf{x}) \propto \begin{cases} (1 + t^2/[1 + t^2/(n-1)] \quad \text{if } a_1 < t < c_1 \\ 0 \quad \text{otherwise,} \end{cases} \tag{A7}$$

where $$a_1 = (a - \hat{b}_1)/[S^2/Sxx(n-1)]^{\frac{1}{2}}$$
$$c_1 = (b - \hat{b}_1)/[S^2/Sxx(n-1)]^{\frac{1}{2}}.$$

That is, the posterior distribution of t, given $\mathbf{u},\mathbf{x}$, is a truncated t distribution with $(n-1)$ degrees of freedom. By making the substitution $t = (n-1)^{\frac{1}{2}} \tan\theta$ we find the mean and variance of t, $(m, v,$ say) are given by

$$m = \frac{1}{I_{n-2}} \frac{(n-1)^{\frac{1}{2}}}{(n-2)} \{\cos^{n-2}\alpha - \cos^{n-2}\beta\}, \tag{A8}$$

$$v = \frac{(n-1)}{I_{n-2}} I_{n-4} - I_{n-2} - m^2, \tag{A9}$$

where $$\alpha = \tan^{-1}(a_1/(n-1)^{\frac{1}{2}}),$$
$$\beta = \tan^{-1}(c_1/(n-1)^{\frac{1}{2}}),$$

and $$I_n = \int_{b_1}^{\beta} \cos^n\theta \, d\theta.$$

I_n satisfies the recurrence relation

$$I_n = \left[\frac{\cos^{n-1}\theta \sin\theta}{n}\right]_\alpha^\beta + \frac{n-1}{n} I_{n-2}. \tag{A10}$$

$S^2/(n-1)$ is an unbiassed estimate of φ, which we used to estimate the variance σ^2. Finally, for b_1 we have the posterior mean and variance as

$$m_0 = gm + \hat{b}_1$$

and $$C_0 = g^2 v,$$

where $$g = [S^2/Sxx(n-1)]^{\frac{1}{2}}.$$

7 Diffusion models, 2: Hamer–Soper and chain binomial

7.1 Introduction

The classic work on models for measles epidemics was undertaken by Hamer (1906) and Soper (1929) for the Hamer–Soper model, and by Reed, Frost (see Abbey, 1952) and Greenwood (1931) on the chain binomial model. A major distinction exists between the two types of model in the level of data grouping at which they were designed to operate. The Hamer–Soper model was constructed for use with aggregated data, and it can be readily adapted to deal with spatial units of the size considered in this book. Conversely, the chain binomial was developed to study chains of measles infection within household groups, school classrooms, etc. – that is, at a micro-level, where individual people can be distinguished. Our approach in this chapter is to outline the structure of the Hamer–Soper model in section 7.2 and to assess its utility when applied to the Icelandic data in section 7.3. In sections 7.4–7.5, this task is repeated for a regional-level version of the chain binomial. Finally, the models are compared with the time series models dealt with in chapter 6.

7.2 The Hamer–Soper model: theory

7.2.1 A single-region model

At any time t, we assume that the total population in the region can be divided into three classes: namely the population at risk or susceptible population of size $S(t)$, the infected population of size $I(t)$, and the removed population of size $R(t)$. Where the sizes of the S, I and R populations can be referred to unambiguously without the (t) notation, it will be dropped for simplicity. The removed population is taken to be composed of people who have had the disease, but who can no longer pass it on to others because of recovery, isolation on the appearance of overt symptoms of the disease, or death. Four types of transition are allowed (see Figure 7.7, later, for examples of the transitions envisaged):

(1) A susceptible being infected by contact with an infective.

(2) An infective being removed. We assume that infection confers life-long immunity to further attack after recovery, which is reasonable in the case of measles.

(3) A susceptible 'birth'. This can come about either through a child growing up into the critical age range (that is, reaching about six months of age), or through a susceptible entering the population by migration into the region from outside.

(4) An infective entering the I population by migration into the region from outside. For simplicity, we assume that there is no migration out of the region.

Table 7.1. *Transition types and rates*

Type of transition	Rate
1. $S \to S-1;\ I \to I+1;\ R \to R$	βIS
2. $S \to S;\ I \to I-1;\ R \to R+1$	μI
3. $S \to S+1;\ I \to I;\ R \to R$	v
4. $S \to S;\ I \to I+1;\ R \to R$	ε

Suppose that transition i occurs at the rate $r_i (i = 1, 2, 3, 4)$; that is, in a small time interval $(t,\ t+\delta t)$ the probability of transition i occurring is $r_i \delta t + o(\delta t)$, where $o(\delta t)$ means a term of smaller order (that is, considerably smaller) than δt. All events are assumed to be independent and to depend only on the present state of the population. The probability density of the time between any pair of successive transitions is

$$r \exp(-rt), \tag{7.1}$$

where

$$r = \sum_{i=1}^{4} r_i, \tag{7.2}$$

and the probability that the next transition is of type i is

$$\frac{r_i}{r}, \quad i = 1, 2, 3, 4. \tag{7.3}$$

We assume, in the transitions 1–4, that the infection rate is proportional to the product SI, that the removal rate is proportional to I, and that the birth- and immigration-rates are constant. We can thus prepare the table of transitions given in Table 7.1. Note that, in contrast to the ARMA approach discussed in chapter 6, the structure of the process is explicitly incorporated in the model.

The model was first put forward in its deterministic form by Hamer (1906) and was studied extensively by Soper (1929). Haggett (1972, 1975, 1978) and Cliff and Murray (1977) have considered the utility of the model in a regional setting. The main drawback of this deterministic model is that it leads to damping of successive epidemic waves which is not observed in practice – see Figure 7.1. Soper erroneously believed that this damping could be eliminated by allowing for the fact that individuals exposed to measles undergo a latent period before becoming infectious, as shown in Figure 3.4, instead of assuming, as in the deterministic model described, that they transmit infectious material for the entire time between initial exposure and isolation or removal. However, even with this change and, in addition, modifications to allow for seasonal variations in the infection rate and for spatial factors, damping still persists, although it is reduced.

We therefore consider the more realistic stochastic formulation. Even

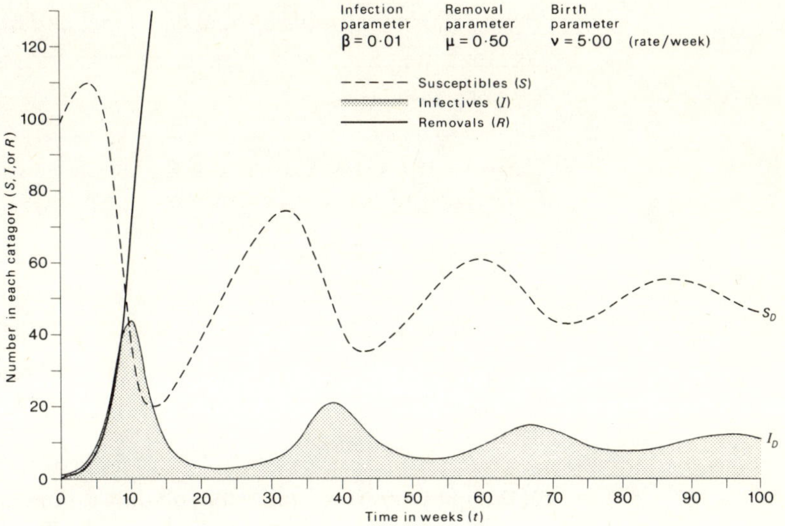

Fig. 7.1 Deterministic form of the Hamer–Soper model for an artificial data set. Note the characteristic damping of the *S* and *I* curves to the levels S_D and I_D respectively.

this relatively simple model is surprisingly intractable analytically and, except in special cases such as $v = \varepsilon = 0$, it is best studied using Monte Carlo techniques. It is, however, possible to see intuitively how the model operates. An infective is isolated after an average period of $1/\mu$ days, and while he is infectious he causes new infections at the rate of βS per day. If we ignore the changes in *S* during this period, one infective infects an average number of $\beta S/\mu$ ($=\varkappa$, say) susceptibles before he is removed. From the theory of the simple birth and death process, we would expect that, when $\varkappa \leqslant 1$, a small epidemic would die out. However, when $\varkappa > 1$, a small epidemic will spark off a major outbreak, although, of course, as the epidemic spreads *S* will fall and $\beta S/\mu$ can become less than unity. Thus, the general pattern will be that the susceptible population will build up (transition type 3) to around the critical population size $S = \mu/\beta$, when an epidemic will continue to spread until the susceptible population falls sufficiently for the epidemic phase to pass (cf. Kendall's (1957) Pandemic Threshold Theorem). The cycle will then repeat itself.

In large communities where measles is endemic, the period between epidemic peaks is of approximate length $\mu/\beta v$, the mean time for the birth of μ/β susceptibles. In smaller communities, where there is fade-out, the period is longer because, once the critical susceptible population size is reached, there is a delay until the disease is introduced again into the region from outside (see Bartlett, 1956). We have noted this contrast in section 3.3.2; the periodicity of epidemics in the United Kingdom is approximately two years, compared with four in Iceland.

7.2.2 A multi-region model

To adapt the model to handle regional interactions, the transitions given in Table 7.1 must be defined for each region. We also wish to allow for the division of the incubation period into latent and infectious components by revising Table 7.1 to define the set of transitions shown in Table 7.2. Each region in an *n*-region system therefore has its own

Table 7.2. *Revised table of transition types and rates*

Type of transition	Rate
1. $S \rightarrow S-1$; $L \rightarrow L+1$; $I \rightarrow I$, $R \rightarrow \mathrm{R}$	βIS
2. $S \rightarrow S$; $L \rightarrow L-1$; $I \rightarrow I+1$; $R \rightarrow R$	ζL
3. $S \rightarrow S$; $L \rightarrow L$; $I \rightarrow I-1$; $R \rightarrow R+1$	μI
4. $S \rightarrow S+1$; $L \rightarrow L$; $I \rightarrow I$; $R \rightarrow R$	v
5. $S \rightarrow S$; $L \rightarrow L$; $I \rightarrow I+1$; $R \rightarrow R$	ε

susceptible (S), latent (L), infectious (I), and removed (R) populations; that is, we have

$$\{(S_i, L_i, I_i, R_i), \quad i=1, 2, \ldots, n\}.$$

Of the parameters, ζ and μ depend only on the nature of the disease and so can be taken to be regionally invariant. Inter-regional interaction is entered into the model by defining the transition rate of infection for region i, β_i, as

$$\beta_i = S_i \sum_{j=1}^{n} \beta_{ij} I_j, \quad i=1, 2, \ldots, n. \tag{7.4}$$

This sum includes the term $\beta_{ii} S_i I_i$, as in the single-region model, and covers the ith intra-regional interaction. The remaining terms handle interactions between region i and other regions j. Again, for simplicity, we assume that there is no migration between regions, although there is no difficulty in adding migration terms to the model. At the aggregate level, distance-decay ideas imply that the probability of contact between a person in I and a person in S will fall off with increasing distance between them. A plausible first step in modelling the $\{\beta_{ij}\}$ is to use the gravity formulation

$$\beta_{\mathrm{ij}} \propto \exp(-kd_{ij}), \quad i \neq j \tag{7.5}$$

where d_{ij} is the distance between the (demographic) centroids of regions i and j.

The diagonal terms $\{\beta_{ii}\}$, the within-region probability interaction rates, represent the proportion of the total population of region i with which a susceptible in region i makes contact. β_{ii} can be taken to be inversely proportional to the total population of region i by the rough argument that any given susceptible might be expected to have approximately the same size of acquaintance and kinship circle (that is, contact group at home, school, etc.), and to have the same level of risk of infection as a result, whatever the population size of the region.

7.2.3 Illustrative example[1]

To illustrate the effect of changes in the crucial parameters, β and ε, upon the model, we have applied the single-region form of section 7.2.1 to Akureyrar in northern Iceland (district 41 on Figure 4.1). The

[1] See footnote to section 5.3.5.

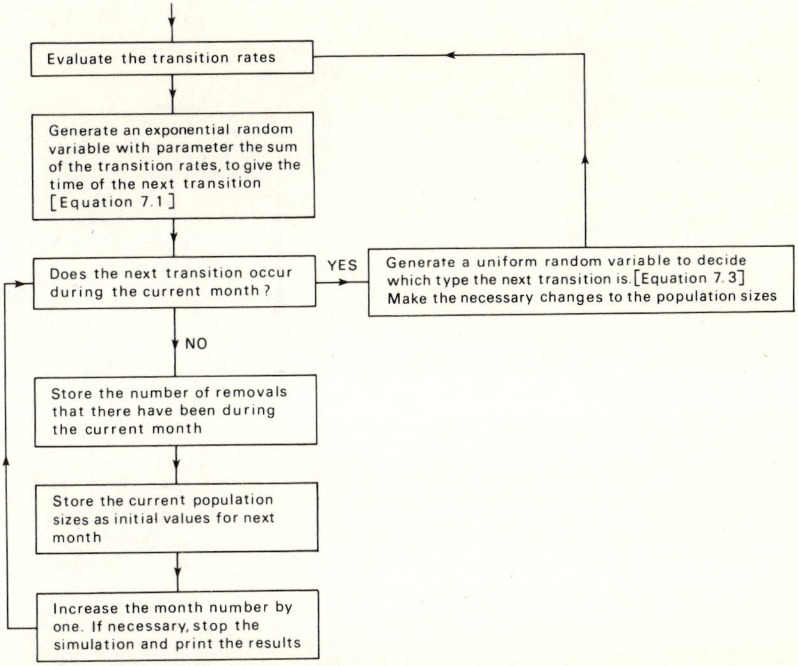

Fig. 7.2 Flow chart of computer program for Hamer–Soper model.

structure of the computer algorithm used to obtain these results and those for the regional applications of section 7.3 is shown in Figure 7.2; the results themselves appear in Figure 7.3, where we define λ as

$$\lambda = \beta I(S/P) \tag{7.6}$$

and P as the total population of medical district i, in addition to notation used previously. In Figure 7.3, the pecked line shows the S population of Akureyrar as estimated from the survival cohort model (see book Appendix), while the solid line gives the estimates of S from the Hamer–Soper model. The lowest line of histograms at the bottom of the figure gives the number of cases of measles actually reported in Akureyrar; all other histograms give the forecast number (I) from the Hamer–Soper model.

To initiate the model in January 1954, we fixed transitions 2 and 3 in Table 7.1 at constant rates. The S population in the Hamer–Soper model was taken as the number of susceptibles given by the cohort model, and I as the number of cases actually reported. The parameter, ε, the rate per day of introduction of new infectives into medical district i (Akureyrar) from other areas j (rest of Iceland), provides the means whereby a new epidemic can be started in i after infection has died out in i. $\varepsilon = 0.0028$ is roughly equivalent to one new infective per year coming into the area. Thus, as shown in Figure 7.3, when other parameters are fixed, the recurrence interval between epidemics *decreases* as ε *increases*. The quantity, λ, may be interpreted as the mixing parameter controlling the rate of interaction between susceptibles and infectives in area i – that is, the mechanism whereby new cases are created within a medical district. As λ increases, so the size of epidemics

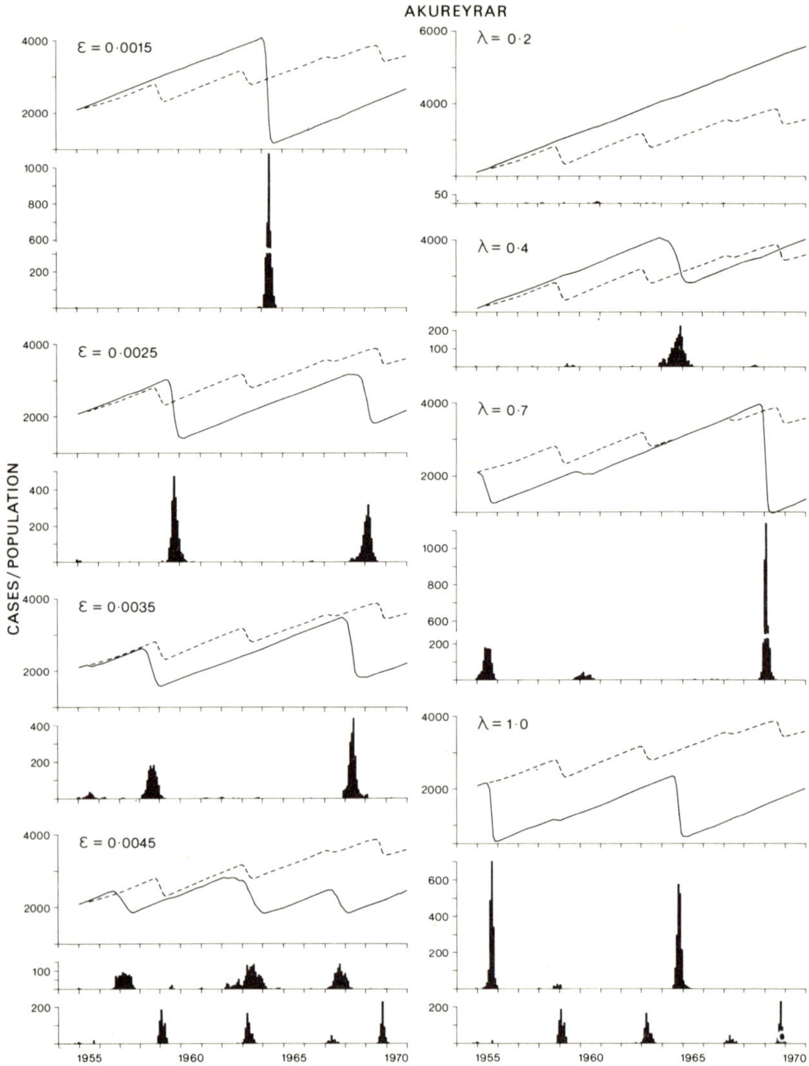

Fig. 7.3 Effects of changes in the parameters ε and λ upon the Hamer–Soper model applied to Akureyrar data. For definitions, see text.

increases, and we see the cyclical behaviour of epidemics by the arguments of section 7.2.1.

The effects of changes in the parameters are not wholly independent. Clearly, if the total population is roughly constant, more epidemics will generally mean smaller epidemics when ε is the only parameter allowed to vary. For λ, large epidemics will mean longer inter-epidemic phases.

7.3 The Hamer–Soper model: application to Iceland[2]

7.3.1 Parameter estimates

The model discussed in section 7.2.1 was fitted separately to each of the 50 medical districts shown in Figure 4.1 (1945) – that is, each medical district was treated as a single-region time series. Starting estimates of the sizes of the S population in each medical district were obtained from the cohort model. The book Appendix indicates that errors in the

[2] See footnote to section 5.3.5.

procedure for obtaining these estimates in the cohort model should have largely worked themselves out by 1954; we therefore chose 1954 as the starting date for the Hamer–Soper model, and ran through to 1970. The reported numbers of measles cases in each district in January 1954 were used to furnish initial estimates of the I populations. The 'death-rate' parameter, μ (transition 2 in Table 7.1), was fixed at the average length of the infectious period from onset of symptoms until isolation when the rash appears – 3.5 days, from Figure 3.4. Thus, $\mu = 2/7$. For the other parameters (β, v, ε in Table 7.1), initial estimates were provided and then adjusted as necessary by direct search until a best-fit model was found. We assessed fit by inspection. For the reasons given in section 6.2.3, we stressed (1) correspondence between projections of the size of the S population from the Hamer–Soper and cohort models, and (2) ability to model the spacing of epidemics (phase characteristics), rather than ability to model ultimate size of epidemics, in deciding what was a good or a bad fit. In general, it was usually clear which was the best combination of parameter values for a given medical district.

In order to facilitate the search procedure, we tried to provide reasonable starting values, namely,

(1) v, the growth rate in the susceptible population, was taken as the average rate of growth given by the cohort model for all inter-epidemic periods, 1954–70;

(2) ε, the rate of introduction of new infectives into a medical district from outside, was taken as 0.0014. From section 3.3.2, we know that measles waves recurred in Iceland about every four years between 1945 and 1970. Since measles is not endemic in any medical district, infection has to be reintroduced from outside; that is, one or two new infectives must come into a medical district during the inter-epidemic period to trigger off the next epidemic when the susceptible population becomes big enough. The value, $\varepsilon = 0.0014$, is roughly equivalent to two new infectives every four years, and can be argued to represent a minimum requirement to start a fresh epidemic. This figure can also be justified from the deterministic theory of the Hamer–Soper model (see Goodall, 1978; Kendall, 1957);

(3) From section 7.2.1, we know that the period between epidemic peaks in any community will not be less than $\mu/\beta v$. Thus, β may be calculated given μ and v (fixed as above), and the need to approximate a four-year epidemic cycle.

The 'best-fit' parameter values obtained for each medical district from application of the Hamer–Soper model are shown in Figure 7.4. λ is defined in equation (7.6). The main contrast between medical districts occurs for v which, as we would expect from Figure 3.12, is substantially higher in the main population growth areas of south-west Iceland, and Akureyrar in the north. It is, effectively, an urban/rural dichotomy.

7.3.2 S and I distributions

In Figure 7.5 we show, for a wide variety of medical districts, the epidemic curves produced by the best-fit Hamer–Soper model for each area. The same cartographic conventions have been followed as in

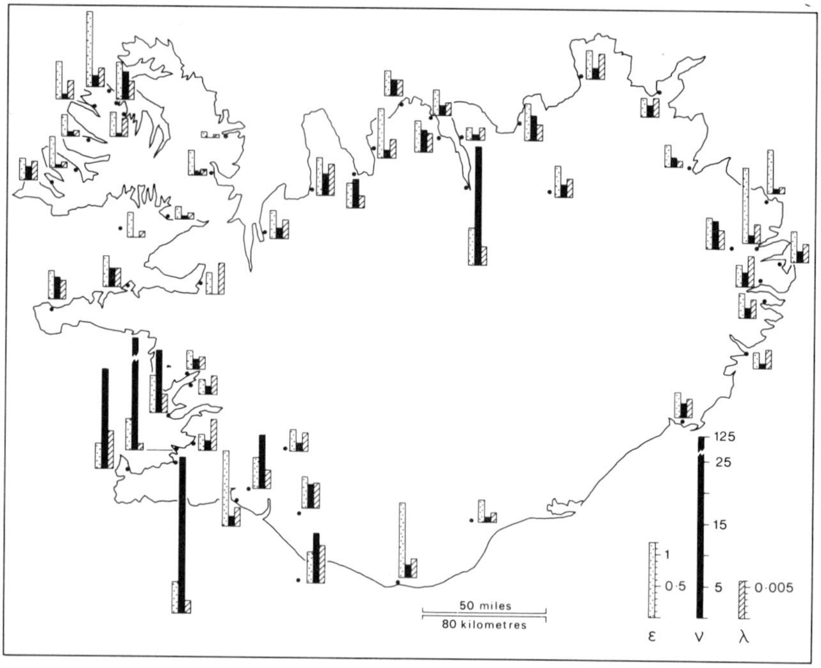

Fig. 7.4 Best-fit parameter values for the Hamer–Soper model for medical districts in Iceland, 1954–70. ε, v, λ are defined in the text.

Figure 7.3.[3] Our time horizons for forecasting are of a totally different order of magnitude from those employed in chapter 6. The model has simply been allowed to run from 1954–70. The effect of incorporating information on the *S* population is clear; the repeating cycles of epidemic/non-epidemic referred to in section 7.2.1 are apparent for all medical districts. Similarly, the need for *S* to reach a critical threshold before an epidemic is triggered in the model is also evident. For example, in Reykjavíkur (Figure 7.5), the model forecast a much larger epidemic than actually occurred in 1954–5. This so depleted *S* in the Hamer–Soper model that the threshold for a major epidemic was next reached only in 1962. In fact, the 1954 epidemic was no larger than the others shown in Figure 7.5 and, as the pecked graph indicates, the actual *S* population was not particularly depleted. It built up again to a critical level by 1958 and produced an epidemic which was detected by the model, but which, unusually, was under-estimated in terms of total size. It is, however, important to note that it is the incorporation of threshold ideas and information on the size of *S* that permits long-term forecasting to be attempted with the Hamer–Soper model in a way that we saw in Figure 6.9 could not be attempted with the ARMA methods. Both modelling approaches seem to share the common fault of over-estimating epidemic size when phase characteristics are stressed. In order to model recurrence properly, it is often necessary to make the

[3] For each medical district, the pecked line shows the *S* population from the survival–cohort model, the solid line gives the estimates of *S* from the Hamer–Soper model; the bottom line of histograms gives the number of measles cases reported, the upper line of histograms gives the forecast number from the Hamer–Soper model.

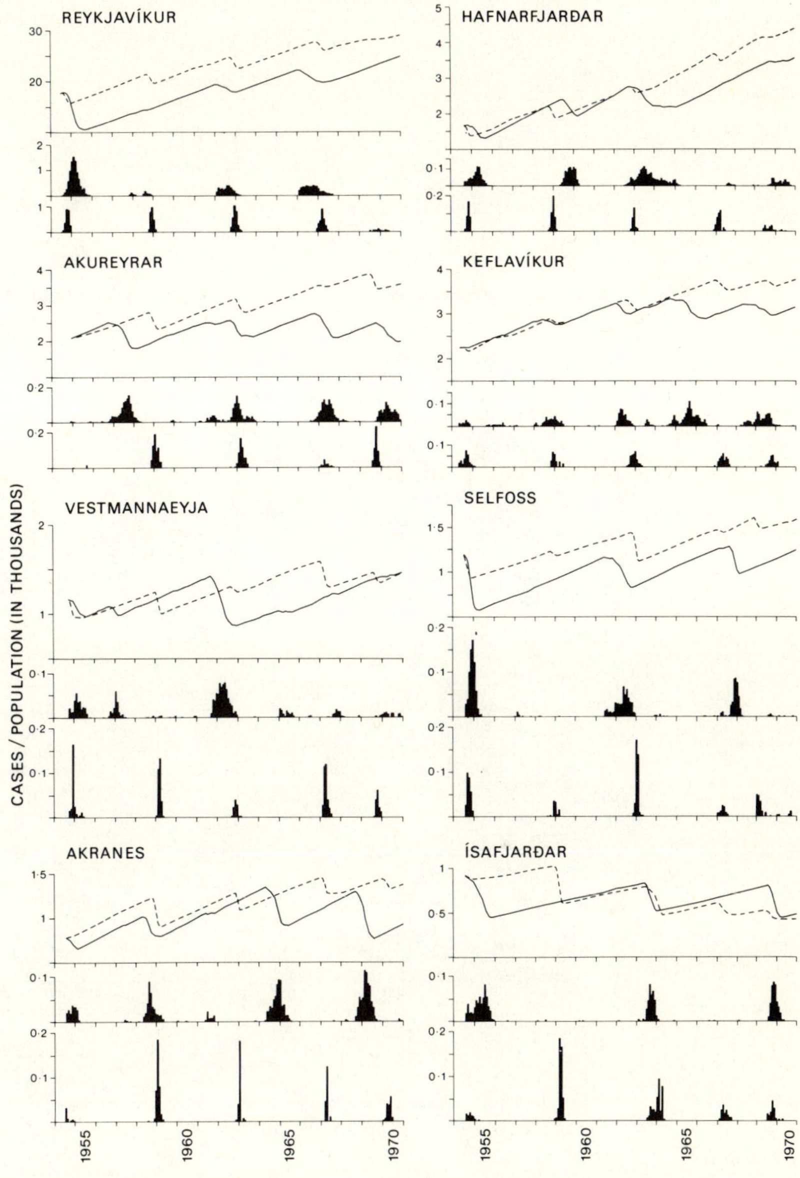

Fig. 7.5 Results of the Hamer–Soper model for selected Icelandic medical districts. For definitions, see text.

models sensitive to any hint of an epidemic as indicated by cases reported or a rapid build-up of S. Large epidemics then tend to be forecast.

The central importance of the threshold theorem in the Hamer–Soper model is evident in Figure 7.5 for medical districts such as Sauðárkróks, Siglufjarðar, Nes and Grenivíkur (districts 35, 37, 53 and 38 on Figure 4.1); isolated cases and perhaps only one or two major epidemics in 15 years are acceptably modelled.

A basic assumption of the model is that the average size of S is constant through time. Obviously, oscillations around this occur before and after epidemics. We know from section 3.4.2 that this assumption is

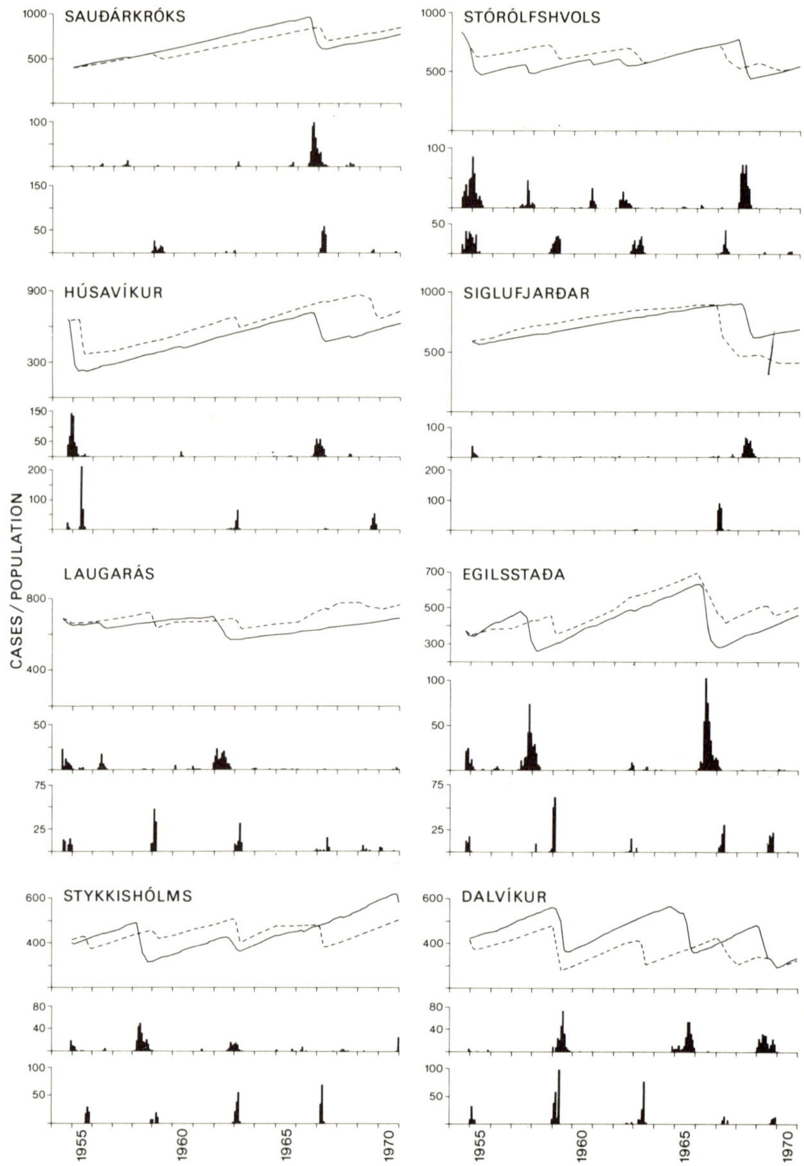

Fig. 7.5 (contd)

not tenable for Icelandic medical districts. In many, *S* has grown steadily (for example, Reykjavíkur in Figure 7.5). Others, such as Ísafjarðar (district 24 on Figure 4.1), have declining *S* populations. Only a few, like Stykkishólms (district 14 on Figure 4.1), have roughly constant *S* populations over time. The model seems to be able to cope reasonably well with all except declining populations. Thus, in Ísafjarðar, Figure 7.5 shows that too few epidemics are forecast because the *S* population does not reach the critical threshold.

7.3.3 Use in forecasting

Three main types of forecast are possible with the Hamer–Soper model:

(1) As in Figure 7.5, the model can be calibrated on data up to a

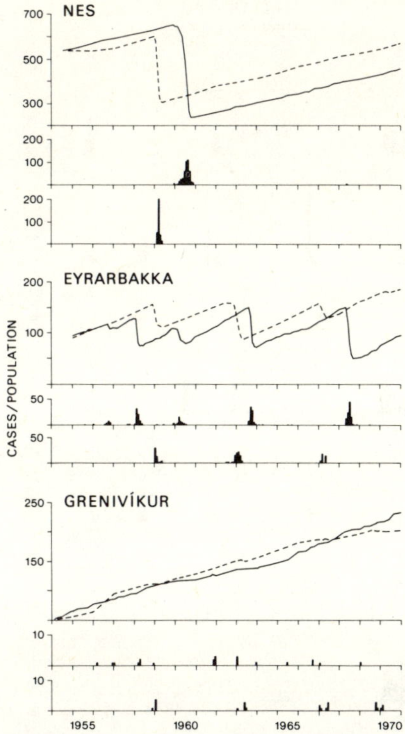

Fig. 7.5 (contd)

particular time period, t, and simply be allowed to run on from that point. We refer to this type of forecast as a *Hamer–Soper* forecast in Figure 7.6;

(2) *One-epidemic-ahead* forecasts can be constructed by running the model from t through to the end of the next *observed* epidemic (at time $t+k$, say). At this point, the end of the corresponding *forecast* epidemic is slid either forwards or backwards in time until it also ends at $t+k$. The next epidemic ahead is then forecast using the same parameter values, and the process is repeated. The effect of this procedure is to prevent phase errors accumulating in long runs of the model;

(3) At the end of each epidemic, we can *recalibrate* the model in several ways before forecasting further. We have chosen to retain the same parameter values, but to update the model by giving it new S population values as determined by the cohort model from demographic data. The updating points are indicated by the vertical steps on the solid line graphs of Figure 7.6. This change should help counteract failure by the model to forecast the total number of cases reported properly and help overcome difficulties arising from rising/falling populations in medical districts. We want, if at all possible, to avoid re-estimating model parameters. This is costly in expertise and computer time. To be used by health authorities, forecast procedures need to be kept as simple as possible, consistent with reliable results.

The three forecast strategies described have been applied to areas with rising, falling and roughly constant S populations. The results are

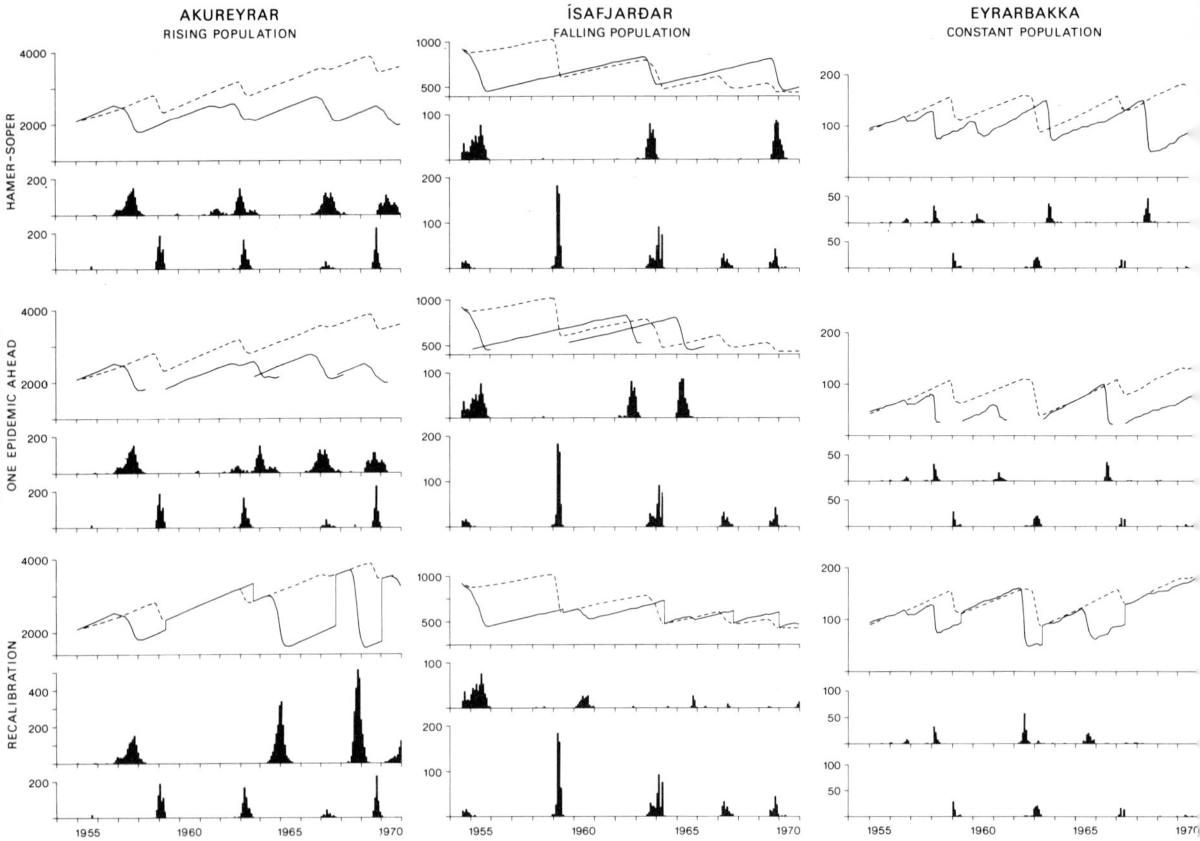

Fig. 7.6 Types of forecasts for places with rising, falling and constant populations. For definitions, see text. For a given medical district, the same parameter values were used for all three forecasts.

shown in Figure 7.6. The graphs and histograms are as defined in Figures 7.3 and 7.5. For areas with a falling *S* population, forecast (3) is preferred, producing better results both in terms of number of epidemics forecast and number of cases forecast. Somewhat surprisingly, forecast (3) is also substantially better than (1) and (2) for areas with constant *S* population; the spacing between epidemics for Eyrarbakka is clearly much improved. For areas with a rising *S* population (Akureyrar), methods (1) and (2) both produce reasonable forecasts for time of occurrence of epidemics (good phase agreement), but only mediocre estimates of number of cases; method (3) produces dreadful phase and amplitude agreement.

7.4 The chain binomial model: theory

We noted in section 7.1 that the chain binomial models, as originally developed, were designed to study intra-family transmission of infectious disease. Bailey (1975, chapter 14) gives a full account. Here, we develop adaptations of the models to provide forecasts at the aggregated-data level used in this book. The material is drawn from Cliff and Ord (1978).

7.4.1 The basic model for a single medical district

We suppose that it is possible to record the state of the system at times $t=0, 1, 2, \ldots$. Ideally, the time interval between recording points should correspond in length to the serial interval of the disease. This ensures that we do not witness multiple epidemic cycles in a single time period, provided that each infected individual is isolated after the appearance of symptoms. Given the measles chain outlined in section 3.3.4, this cannot be achieved with the monthly Icelandic data, and we return to this problem below. The total population in a given medical district at the beginning of time period t, which we denote by $N(t)$, will contain $S(t)$ susceptibles, $I(t)$ infectives who can transmit the disease to susceptibles, and $R(t)$ removals. During the tth time period, $N(t)$ may be modified by the addition of $A(t)$ arrivals (births and/or immigrants) and the loss of $D(t)$ departures (deaths and/or emigrants). Finally, let $X(t)$ denote the number of new cases which occur in time period t.

The following accounting identities may then be written down for each medical district (Figure 7.7):

$$N(t+1)=N(t)+A(t)-D(t),$$
$$N(t)=S(t)+I(t)+R(t). \tag{7.7}$$

If $\alpha_t A(t)$ denotes the number of individuals among the new arrivals who are infectives, while $\delta_t D(t)$ denotes the number of infectives among the departures, then

$$I(t+1)=I(t)+X(t)-[R(t+1)-R(t)]+\alpha_t A(t)-\delta_t D(t). \tag{7.8}$$

The arrivals term in (7.8) is vital in the Icelandic context, where we are considering a disease which has to be re-imported into an area after local fade-out; these arrivals are the individuals who trigger a recurrence of the disease when the number of susceptibles is high.

In common with Bailey (1964, p. 183), we say that there has been adequate contact by time t between the jth susceptible, S_j, and the infectives, $\{I_i\}$, if S_j contracts the disease during period t. The contact may have occurred one or more time periods earlier, depending upon the length of the serial interval and its relationship to the length of the data-recording interval.

We now define the probability that S_j is identified as an infective during the time period t as $\theta_{\bullet j}(t)$. One way of specifying $\theta_{\bullet j}(t)$ might be to assumed the following:

(a) the serial interval is relatively constant in length, and equal to the interval between observations, so that S_j is identified as being infected during period t if adequate contact was sustained during $(t-1)$;

(b) the disease is transmitted only by adequate contact between a susceptible and an infective;

(c) adequate contact with a single infective is sufficient to transmit the disease;

(d) contacts between S_j and the different infectives are independent events;

(e) there is homogeneous mixing between the susceptibles and infectives within a medical district at some standard rate of contacts per unit time.

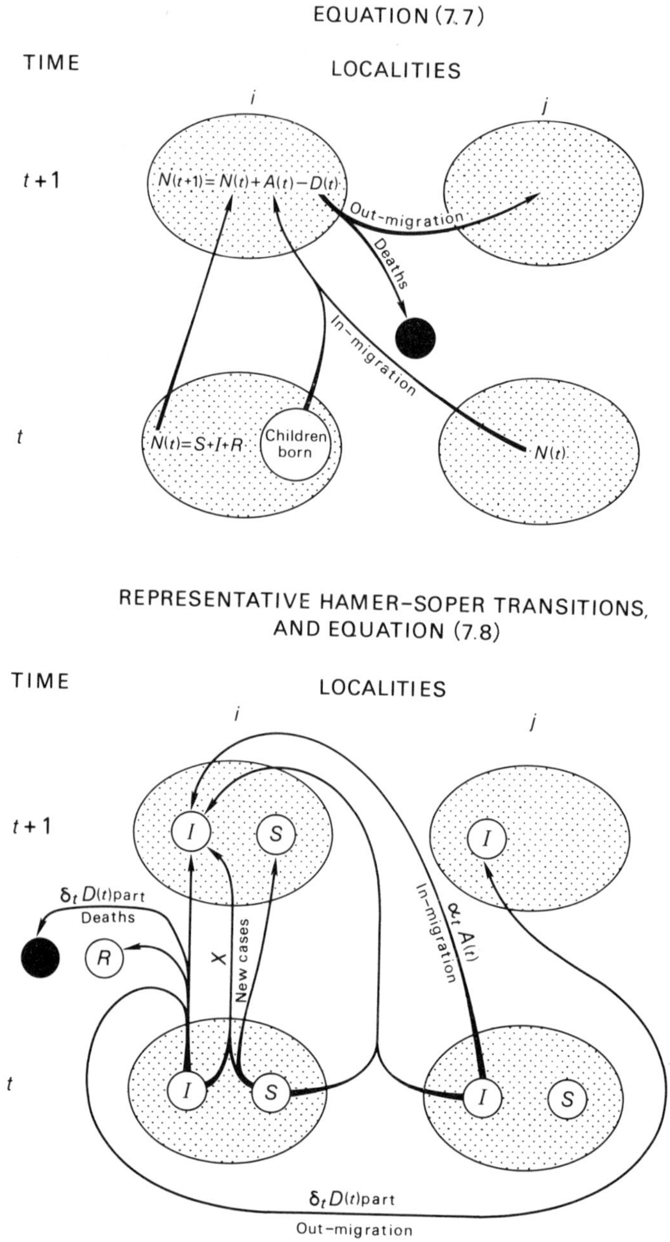

Fig. 7.7 Accounting identities for the typical medical district, *i*. For definitions, see text.

Then

$$\theta_{\bullet j}(t) = 1 - P(\text{no contact with any infectives})$$
$$= 1 - \prod_{i=1}^{I(t)} [1 - \theta_{ij}(t)], \qquad (7.9)$$

where $\theta_{ij}(t) = P$ (contact between I_i and S_j). Clearly, in equation (7.9), contacts between S_j and the different I_i are regarded as independent events (assumption (d)), and we need to consider only the infectives in circulation at time t (assumption (a)). The form of equation (7.9) is then given by assumption (c), with assumption (b) guaranteeing that the infection cannot arise from other courses. Finally, assumption (e) will allow simplification of equation (7.9) in particular cases.

It follows from equation (7.9) that the probability generating function (pgf) for the number of new cases, $X(t+1)$, during period $(t+1)$ is given by

$$G(z)=\prod_{j=1}^{S(t)}[1-\theta_{\bullet j}(t)+z\theta_{\bullet j}(t)]. \tag{7.10}$$

Equation (7.10) represents a more general version of the Reed–Frost chain binomial model. The assumptions underlying the model will vary in plausibility from one application to the next, although assumption (a) is likely to be the most difficult to meet. We now look at a few ways in which assumption (a) might be relaxed.

The length of the serial interval

If the serial interval is considerably shorter than the observation period, as in the case with measles in Iceland, we might modify function (7.10) by the inclusion of the pgf,

$$g(z)=\sum_{k=1}^{\infty}\alpha_k z^k, \tag{7.11}$$

where $\alpha_k = P$ (initial infected susceptible gives rise to a chain of k new cases in a single observation period, including himself); that is

$$G(z)=\prod_{j=1}^{S(t)}[1-\theta_{\bullet j}(t)+g(z)\theta_{\bullet j}(t)]. \tag{7.12}$$

For example, if the observation period is about m times the serial interval, a suitable form for α_k might be

$$\alpha_{k+1}=\binom{m}{k}\alpha^k(1-\alpha)^{m-k}$$

with

$$g(z)=z(1-\alpha+\alpha z)^m.$$

Then, the generalised version of function (7.10) is a chain binomial binomial (in the notation of Gurland, 1957), with the pgf

$$G(z)=\prod_{j=1}^{S(t)}[1-\theta_{\bullet j}(t)+z\theta_{\bullet j}(t)(1-\alpha+\alpha z)^m]. \tag{7.13}$$

Conversely, if the serial interval is longer than the observation period, we should consider

$$\theta_{\bullet j}(t,\tau)=P(S_j \text{ sustained contact during period } t-\tau),\ \tau>1.$$

A Poisson approximation

In the early stages of an epidemic, the number of new cases, as a proportion of the number of susceptibles, is likely to be small. Thus $\theta_{\bullet j}(t)$ is also likely to be small. If we take

$$\varphi(t) = \sum_{j=1}^{S(t)} \theta_{\bullet j}(t) \tag{7.14}$$

to be fixed as $S(t) \to \infty$, we obtain the limiting form

$$G(z) = exp[\varphi(t)(z-1)], \tag{7.15}$$

provided that

$$\sum_{j=1}^{S(t)} \theta^2_{\bullet j}(t) \to 0 \quad \text{as} \quad S(t) \to \infty .$$

Form (7.15) makes it easier to make probabilistic statements about $X(t+1)$ in the early stages of an outbreak. If $\theta_{\bullet j}(t)$ becomes larger so that the outbreak becomes extensive, we could use a normal approximation with

$$E[X(t+1)] = \varphi(t),$$

as before, and

$$\text{var}[X(t+1)] = \sum_{j=1}^{S(t)} \theta_{\bullet j}(t)[1-\theta_{\bullet j}(t)] .$$

In either case, the maximum-likelihood estimator, $\hat{\varphi}(t)$, will be the best predictor for $X(t)$. Successive forecasts will be generated from the estimated $\theta_{\bullet j}(t)$, with regular updating through the identities (7.7) and (7.8). For measles, it soon becomes fairly obvious when someone has contracted the disease (i.e., when the rash appears), and the individual concerned is then usually isolated (removed from circulation). It is thus reasonable to suppose, since the serial interval of the disease is shorter than the data-recording interval in Iceland, that all new cases observed during period t are removed by the end of that period, so that

$$I(t) = R(t+1) - R(t), \tag{7.16}$$

and identity (7.8) reduces to

$$I(t+1) = X(t) + \alpha_t A(t) - \delta_t D(t). \tag{7.8'}$$

7.4.2 Inter-regional model

We now suppose that data are recorded on a regional basis, with homogeneous mixing within medical districts. The $\theta_{ij}(t)$ then become special cases involving pairs of medical districts, rather than the pairs of individuals in a single medical district considered in section 7.4.1. Thus,

$$\theta_{ij}(t) = \theta(t,\ d_{km}),$$

where, for any infective, I_i, in medical district k and susceptible S_j in medical district m, d_{km} is a measure of 'distance' between districts k and m. The assumption of a common function form seems a convenient starting point, even if it ultimately proves unwarranted.

If, for any individual j in district m, the separate terms, $\theta_{ij}(t)$, are small, then for each individual in m, equation (7.9) reduces to

$$\theta_m(t) \approx \sum_i \theta_{ij}(t) = \sum_k I_k(t)\theta(t, d_{km}), \tag{7.17}$$

where $I_k(t)$ denotes the number of infectives in district k at time t. If $S_m(t)$ denotes the number of susceptibles in district m at time t, it follows from equation (7.14) that the expected number of new cases in district m at time $(t+1)$ is

$$E[X_m(t+1)] = \sum_{j=1}^{S(t)} \theta_m(t) = S_m(t) \sum_k I_k(t)\theta(t, d_{km}), \tag{7.18}$$

and

$$\text{var}\,[X_m(t+1)] = S_m(t)\theta_m(t)[1-\theta_m(t)]. \tag{7.19}$$

Equation (7.18) may be used as a basis for predictions using the GLIM methods described in section 6.4, and it is very similar in structure to the north-west Iceland regional models considered there (see end of this section). If we rewrite (7.18) as

$$\varphi_m(t) = \sum_k b_{km}(t) I_k(t), \tag{7.20}$$

where

$$b_{km}(t) = S_m(t)\theta(t, d_{km}),$$

it is apparent that a straighforward 'blind' autoregressive model (cf. section 6.2) for equation (7.20) would involve fixing b_{km} – by ignoring both the number of susceptibles, and by making θ a function of d_{km} only. An initial simplification would be to set

$$b_{km}(t) = S_m(t)h(d_{km}, \boldsymbol{\beta}_m), \tag{7.21}$$

where h is a known function except for the parameters $\boldsymbol{\beta}_m$. Using expression (7.21) we could estimate $\boldsymbol{\beta}_m$ by ordinary least squares for each region. Estimates of the initial value, $S_m(0)$, for the susceptibles are available from the procedures described in the book Appendix. The S population can then be updated using

$$S(t+1) = S(t) - X(t) - (1-\alpha_t)A(t) - (1-\delta_t)D(t). \tag{7.22}$$

This follows from equations (7.7), (7.8) and (7.16).

Specification of contact probabilities

The number of adequate contacts within a medical district will depend upon the level of both the S and I populations in the area. The threshold theorems suggest that, of these, the S population is more crucial. For interaction between districts, S population density and 'distance' between medical districts will be relevant. In this section, we assume time stationarity of the process; let ϱ_k denote the density of susceptible persons per unit area in k, and d_{km} denote the distance between the centroids of medical districts k and m. Then from equations (7.18) and (7.20), we specify

$$E[X_m(t+1)] = S_m(t)[\beta_0 + (\beta_1 \varrho_m^\alpha)I_m(t) + \beta_2 \sum_{k \neq m} \varrho_m^\alpha d_{km}^{-\gamma} I_k(t)], \quad (7.23)$$

where β_0, β_1, β_2, α and γ are parameters that will vary from one district to the next. The Paretian distance decay has been used as a convenient representation rather than a reflection of any strong beliefs on the subject. β_1 is the coefficient of the term generating new cases by *intra*-area mixing of susceptibles and infectives; β_2 is the coefficient of the term generating new cases by *inter*-area contact of infectives and susceptibles (cf. Figure 6.6). The term in β_0 is included to allow for (constant) sources of infection from areas other than $k \neq m$; that is, from 'the rest of the world'.

Comparison of equations (6.18) and (7.23) reveals that the GLIM and chain binomial eventually lead to rather similar structures. The inclusion of a density term in the chain binomial makes due allowance for population sparseness, while the GLIM model has a stronger emphasis on the lead area. However, it should be evident that neither of these factors is essential to the model actually used. Thus, the simplified chain binomial scheme could be fitted using the GLIM method, and the principal advantage of the chain binomial is that it introduces a proper model structure which an unaided GLIM approach cannot.

7.5 The chain binomial model: application to Iceland

7.5.1 Time-invariant parameters

As a first illustration of the model, we have taken a simplified version of (7.23), that is

$$E[X_m(t+1)] = S_m(t)[\beta_1 I_m(t)], \quad (7.24)$$

and applied it to Reykjavíkur for waves IX and XII. Direct comparison of the performance of the model with the AR(1) model used in section 6.2.3 is thus possible. Replicating the fitting procedure described there, and using S values from the cohort model, we obtained the one-month-ahead forecasts shown in Figure 7.8. We have reproduced there the results from the AR(1) model given in Figure 6.4 for comparison. The improvement obtained from the chain binomial is clear. Although, as with the AR(1) model, the forecasts have the one-month-lag feature initially, the chain binomial model locks on by the epidemic peaks; its forecasts then decay in much better harmony with the observed data than do those of the AR(1). The chain binomial also peaks more sharply than does AR(1).

7.5.2 Time-varying parameters[4]

Following the methods of section 6.3, we next fitted the model using the Kalman filter algorithm. The observation equation was based on (7.24), with the parameters being allowed to vary as described in section 6.3.2. As there, Reykjavíkur was taken as the test medical district, and the months of 1945–7 were used for calibration purposes. The following estimates were obtained from the calibration period.

$$m_0 = 1.796 \times 10^{-4}; \quad C_0 = 7 \times 10^{-9}; \quad \hat{\sigma}^2 = 2.868 \times 10^{-3}.$$

[4] See footnote to section 6.3.

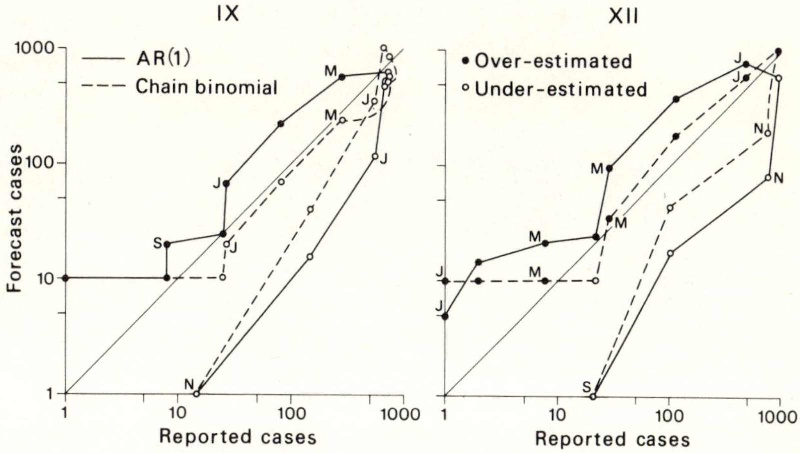

Fig. 7.8 Reported cases and one-month-ahead forecasts from the fixed-parameter chain binomial and AR(1) models applied to Reykjavíkur, waves IX and XII.

The model was then used to forecast the number of cases reported in Reykjavíkur in waves IX and XII. In Figure 7.9 the results are compared with those obtained from the AR model fitted in section 6.3.2 to the same wave using the Kalman algorithm. We give the case where $V=0$. Again, the chain binomial rapidly locks on the form of the epidemic, although both models miss the epidemic start. The model seems to have no marked advantage over the fixed-parameter version.

7.5.3 Multi-region model

We have seen in this section that, although the single-region chain binomial misses epidemic starts, it can rapidly pick up the course of an epidemic. We now consider whether the phase characteristics can be improved by using disease impulses from other areas to trigger epidemics, as we did in section 6.4. For comparability, the regional system considered is the same as in section 6.4 – namely the contiguous medical districts of Ísafjarðar, Bolungarvíkur, Flateyrar, Súðavíkur and Þingeyrar. Also as before, we have taken waves VIII, IX and XI (January 1947–March 1948; May 1951–February 1952; May 1954–March 1955) in north-west Iceland for calibration purposes and used the parameter estimates obtained to provide one-month-ahead forecasts for waves XII, XIII and XIV (December 1958–October 1959; July 1963–June 1964; January–December 1967). The time-invariant parameter model (7.23) was fitted. We arbitrarily set $\alpha=1$ and $\gamma=2$ throughout and estimated the remaining parameters using ordinary least squares. A stepwise regression program was employed to examine the order in which variables were entered. The $\{\varrho_k\}$ were the estimated S populations per square kilometre in each medical district in each month, and were based upon the susceptible population values from the cohort model given in the book Appendix. The $\{d_{km}\}$ were the distances between the geographical centroids of the medical districts. The following versions of model (7.23) were fitted:

(1) using all three regressors;
(2) omitting the term in β_2;
(3) using only the term in β_2.

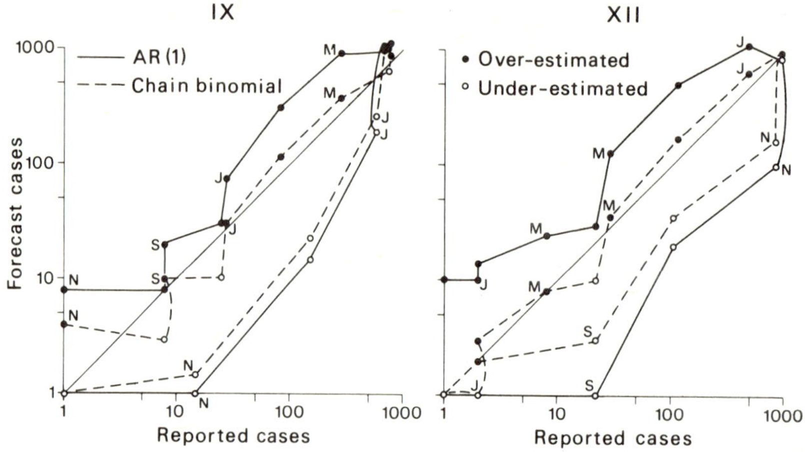

Fig. 7.9 Reported cases and one-month-ahead forecasts from the chain binomial and AR(1) models fitted to Reykjavíkur, waves IX and XII, using the Kalman filter algorithm. $V = 0$ (see text).

(2) and (3) were fitted to examine the importance of the inter-area transmission term. For all the medical districts except Ísafjarðar, the neighbours included Ísafjarðar. If the spread process is mainly from Ísafjarðar to other areas in the locality, we would expect to be able to model with (7.23) the phase characteristics of epidemics in other areas substantially better than in Ísafjarðar itself.

The results of the analysis for the calibration period are summarised in Table 7.3 and Figure 7.10. The following points are worth noting:

(1) Table 7.3 shows that the model is dominated by regressor two – that is, the within-area mixing of susceptibles and infectives in the previous time period. We would expect most cases in the following time period to arise in this fashion. However, as illustrated in Figure 7.10, results based on regressors one and two above produce the familiar 'one-month-in-arrears' effect, and epidemic starts are always missed by one month.

(2) Although regressor three (inter-area mixing of S and I) contributes trivially to R^2 once regressors one and two are entered, it is this term which improves our ability to detect epidemic starts in all areas except Ísafjarðar; indeed, the effect of this variable is to produce more activity in these medical districts than actually occurred (see Figure 7.10). The lag effect in numbers of cases is still present.

(3) The fact that inclusion of regressor three improves phase characteristics for all the medical districts *except Ísafjarðar* suggests a disease transmission process starting in Ísafjarðar and spreading to surrounding areas, with no real backwash of disease from other areas to Ísafjarðar.

(4) As the standard errors in Table 7.3 indicate, the term in β_0 is statistically insignificant at conventional significance levels for all areas except Ísafjarðar, where it is beginning to be quite important. Recall from section 7.4.2 that this term was included to allow introduction of infection from the rest of the world. The results therefore imply arrival of the disease in Ísafjarðar from outside the north-west region, followed by spread ((3) above) from Ísafjarðar to surrounding areas. The model

Table 7.3. *Regression results for chain binomial models, calibration period*

Medical district	Model (1) β_0	β_1	β_2	Order of entry	R^2	Model (2) β_0	β_1	Order of entry	R^2	Model (3) β_2	R^2
Ísafjarðar	0.65 (0.41)	0.01 (0.00)	−0.14 (0.31)	2, 1, 3	0.45	0.56 (0.35)	0.01 (0.00)	2, 1	0.45	0.47 (0.32)	0.07
Bolungarvíkur	1.00 (1.63)	0.28 (0.09)	4.68 (6.16)	3, 1, 2	0.43	1.81 (1.23)	0.27 (0.09)	2, 1	0.42	10.93 (5.50)	0.12
Flateyrar	0.47 (0.47)	0.15 (0.05)	0.80 (2.10)	2, 1, 3	0.49	0.60 (0.32)	0.15 (0.05)	2, 1	0.49	4.23 (1.62)	0.19
Þingeyrar	0.92 (0.94)	2.50 (0.63)	−9.52 (27.06)	2, 1, 3	0.54	0.70 (0.68)	2.55 (0.60)	2, 1	0.54	29.78 (27.37)	0.04
Súðavíkur	0.21 (0.22)	2.05 (0.57)	−55.89 (106.46)	2, 1, 3	0.39	0.12 (0.14)	2.09 (0.56)	2, 1	0.38	54.19 (82.92)	0.01

Notes. All coefficient values and standard errors (given in brackets under coefficient values) are × 10^2. Order of entry gives order in which variables referred to by β_0, β_1 and β_2 respectively were entered into regression equation. Thus, 2, 1, 3 means regressor 1 entered second, regressor 2 entered first and regressor 3 entered third. There are 31 months in the calibration period.

Form of model is:

$$E[X_m(t+1)] = S_m(t)[\beta_0 + (\beta_1 \varrho_m^{\alpha}) I_m(t) + \beta_2 \sum_{k \neq m} \varrho_m^{\alpha} d_{km}^{-\gamma} I_k(t)] .$$

is therefore consistent with the known spread patterns established in chapter 4.

(5) The time-stationary parameter form of the chain binomial used is responsible, in the three-variable model, for the smoothing of the one-month-ahead estimates of cases through the highs and lows of the numbers of cases actually reported. As we have noted in section 6.2.3, the epidemics are badly non-stationary between the build-up and fade-out phases, and any fixed-parameter model will average, to some extent, the peaks and troughs. As a result, model estimates of cases reported are consistently poor.

We conclude that inclusion of an inter-area transmission term is important as a binary switch to trigger epidemics, but that levels of cases cannot be estimated reliably.

In Figure 7.11, the one-month-ahead forecasts from model (1) for three post-1954 epidemics in Ísafjarðar, Bolungarvíkur and Flateyrar are given. For Ísafjarðar, the smoothing through highs and lows noted in (5) above, is evident; however, cases/no cases are correctly forecast as a binary variable in all months, except at the very end of the epidemics. For the smaller medical districts of Bolungarvíkur and Flateyrar, cases are always forecast when reported, but the model gives several false alerts in the form of forecast cases when none are reported. Forecasts of levels of cases are poor. We conclude that the best use of the model is as a predictor of the likelihood of an epidemic.

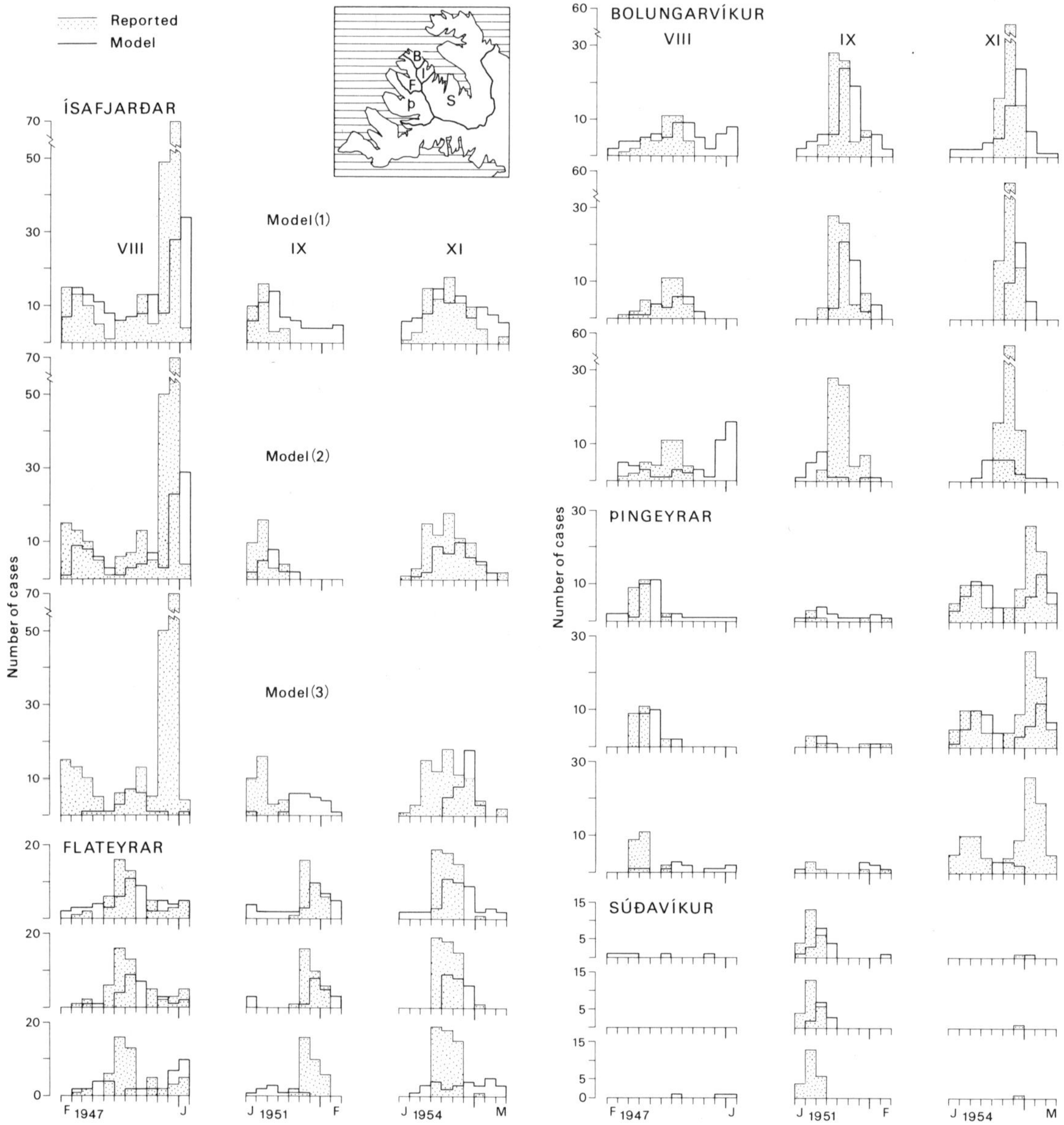

Fig. 7.10 One-month-ahead estimates of reported measles cases from chain binomial model calibrated on data for five medical districts in north-west Iceland, waves VIII, IX and XI. Definitions of models (1), (2) and (3) are given in text, and results from them are in the same order for other medical districts as for Ísafjarðar.

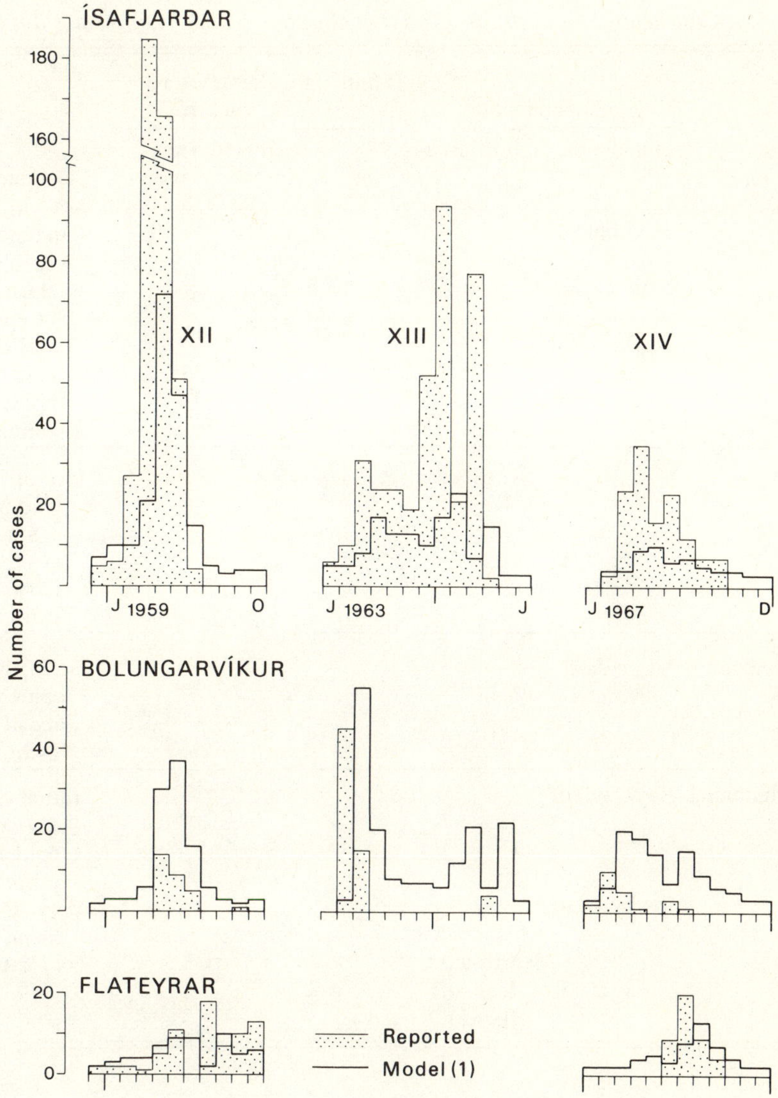

Fig. 7.11 One-month-ahead forecasts of reported measles cases from chain binomial model (1) (defined in text) for selected medical districts in north-west Iceland, waves XII–XIV. Forecasts are based upon parameter values estimated from data for the period, 1947–55.

7.6 Conclusion

In this and the previous chapter, an armada of different models has been applied to the Icelandic measles data. In Table 7.4, the models developed, and the medical districts to which they have been applied, are summarised. The main strengths and weaknesses of each model are also listed. On the basis of this table, several main conclusions can be reached:

(1) No 'Rosetta stone' model which gives reasonable projections of (a) epidemic recurrences, and (b) epidemic size has yet been found. Generally, if a model is devised which will forecast recurrences acceptably, epidemic size is over-estimated. This is because, to forecast recurrences properly, the model has to be made sensitive to changes signalling the approach of an epidemic with the result that it overshoots when the epidemic is in progress.

Table 7.4. *Characteristics of models fitted in chapters 6 and 7 to measles data for Iceland 1945–70*

Model type	Regional application		Main data inputs		Parameter structure		Comments
	Single-area	Multi-area	S	I	Fixed	Time-varying	
AR(1)	Reykjavíkur			×	×		One-month-lag effect; consistently misses epidemic starts; reasonable estimates of epidemic size.
	Reykjavíkur			×		×	Initial one-month-lag effect; able to adapt to changing phase characteristics; over-estimates of epidemic size.
GLIM		North-west Iceland ($n=5$)	×	×	×		Use of Ísafjarðar as epidemic lead indicator produces good estimates of epidemic starts in other medical districts in north-west Iceland. Poor estimates of epidemic size.
Hamer–Soper	All medical districts		×	×	×		Good ability to forecast epidemic recurrences years ahead; average to poor on estimates of epidemic size.
Chain binomial	Reykjavíkur		×	×	×		Initial one-month-lag effect; able to lock on to course of epidemic; reasonable estimates of epidemic size.
	Reykjavíkur		×	×		×	Very similar to fixed-parameter form.
		North-west Iceland ($n=5$)	×	×	×		As for GLIM.

(2) Models which are based only on the size of the infective population in previous time periods consistently fail to detect the approach of an epidemic. Instead, they provide reasonable estimates of cases reported, but tend to run in arrears.

(3) Models with parameters fixed through time have a tendency to smooth through the highs and lows of an epidemic because they are unable to adapt to the changes between build-up and fade-out phases of an epidemic. Time-varying parameter models are better at avoiding this problem.

(4) Epidemic recurrences can be reasonably anticipated only by incorporating into the model information on the size of the susceptible population and/or properly identifying the lead–lag structure among medical districts for disease transmission. Incorporation of spatial interaction information markedly improves our ability to forecast recurrences in lagging areas. Information on susceptible population

levels also serves to prime a model to the possibility of a recurrence, as is made clear by the various threshold theorems. Models based on susceptible populations, but which are single- rather than multi-region, tend to miss the start of epidemics but rapidly lock on to the course of an epidemic thereafter. Models which are dominated by spatial transmission information at the expense of information on the level of the susceptible population in the reference region, produce estimates of epidemic size which reflect the course of the epidemic in the triggering regions rather than in the reference region.

(5) Process models, such as those used in this chapter, can serve to strengthen the time series models of chapter 6 and identify a better scheme for forecasting.

These conclusions all highlight the fact that naïve models produce poor results. However, Table 7.4 indicates clearly the gains to be made for each extra element of complexity added to our models, namely:

(1) time-varying parameters to handle the non-stationary nature of within-epidemic structure, particularly the fundamentally different character of the build-up and fade-out phases of an epidemic;

(2) spatial lead–lag information to improve our ability to forecast epidemic recurrences;

(3) incorporation of data upon the susceptible population level to improve estimates both of epidemic size and likely recurrence intervals.

It is important to be able to identify the gains accrued by increasing model complexity, since it is all too easy to specify sophisticated models which often achieve little more than simple trend predictors.

As far as community medicine is concerned, the purpose of most forecasting is to allow more time for effective control programmes – whether by isolation and/or vaccination – to be instituted. Indeed, the historical record suggests that inhabitants of one geographical area have seen the approach of an epidemic from another area as a wave about to engulf their own population. Thus, in the United Kingdom, by the late nineteenth century, the pressures for some kind of early-warning system for the approach of such waves had become very strong. So we find that in 1888, Dr J. Tatham was arguing for a compulsory notification system for infectious diseases so that '. . . the sanitary authorities of one notification town may be warned in time of the approach of any infectious disease from other towns' (cited in Benjamin, 1968, p. 142). Iceland is no different from the United Kingdom in this respect, with its public-health reporting organised on a standard basis since 1896. If early warning is the goal, then, until better models become available, we feel it is proper, as we have done in this book, to measure the success of our models by their ability to predict recurrences (i.e., phase characteristics) of epidemics, even though this may produce erratic estimates of epidemic size.

8 Conclusion

8.1 Introduction

The history of geography is rich with examples of general concepts which emerged from the study of specific areas. Christaller's central-place theory, drawn from a detailed study of the settlements of south Germany and Ravenstein's ideas on gravity models developed from an analysis of migration between English cities, illustrate the case. In this book, therefore, we have had no apology to make for using a single geographical area, the island of Iceland, to explore further some central issues in spatial diffusion. Indeed, we have argued earlier (section 3.4) that Iceland is uniquely endowed for such a study.

In this final chapter, we review the findings of the research reported and try to set them in a broader context. Our starting point is with spatial diffusion studies. What have we been able to learn about the way in which spatial spread processes appear to work? Our second question is the more pragmatic one: What have such studies to contribute to population welfare, and in particular to public-health planning? Finally, we look back to the particular region that provided the arena for the research, and ask what further secrets its rich data sources may hold.

8.2 Implications for spatial diffusion studies

In the discussion of innovation diffusion in chapter 2, we indicated that spread tends to occur down the urban-size hierarchy, and also contagiously outwards from early adopting centres to other areas. It is clear from chapter 4 that this mixed hierarchical/contagious diffusion model summarises the main elements of the transmission process for measles epidemics in Iceland. The results we obtained in chapter 6 and 7 continue to suggest, as Hägerstrand found in 1953 (section 2.3.2), that it is extremely difficult to predict both the levels and the times and places of occurrence of diffusion phenomena. We have argued that modelling the latter successfully is more important than estimating ultimate size; this suggests that the development of good probability forecasts of 'where' and 'when' should be our aim. Models ranging from simple trend predictors based on the past history of reported case levels, to those which explicitly incorporate the stochastic structure of the birth/death process, have been tried. It is evident that the simple models are very unsatisfactory and that, while the stochastic process versions give reasonable estimates of occurrences in time and space, still greater accuracy needs to be obtained if they are to be used with certainty as a basis for policy decisions.

In chapter 3, we argued that the repeating nature of measles waves should aid model development by providing separate waves for calibration and testing purposes. This hope was borne out in practice. For example, this approach highlighted the deficiencies of the GLIM in section 6.4.3 in a way that would not have been apparent otherwise.

Part of the aim in chapters 6 and 7 was to increase model complexity in a systematic way and to try to identify the gains or otherwise each change produced. Thus, fixed- (in time) parameter trend predictors were replaced by models with time-varying parameters to handle the change between epidemic and non-epidemic phases more satisfactorily. Multi-region rather than single-region models were used to structure the lead–lag relationships between areas implied by a mixed hierarchical/contagious diffusion process. Finally, estimates of the population at risk (susceptibles, S) were included to enable threshold ideas to be incorporated. If forecasting where and when is the aim for diffusion studies, clear improvements can be detected when spatial components and estimates of S are employed. The use of time-varying parameters seems less crucial.

We would not claim to have exhausted all the spatial diffusion models currently available. The publication of Thom's book on catastrophe theory (1975) has excited interest in the application of algebraic topology to many areas of applied research, although, at the time of writing, few substantive gains can be reported. Holling (1978) has used a simple cusp-catastrophe model to formulate the epizootics of spruce budworm in New Brunswick, Canada, while Gatrell (1979) has placed Mollison's work on the velocity and stability of epidemic wavefronts (section 2.3.1) within the framework of a fold catastrophe. So far, the insights from these models have been qualitative rather than quantitative.

8.3 Demographic and public-health implications

As we saw in chapter 2, spatial diffusion as an academic study sometimes has consequences for certain practical fields. Thus, studies of the spread of hybrid corn on farms in the Middle Western states of the United States had direct implications for the improvement of agricultural productivity. In the case study reported here, any findings relate clearly to the demography and health of the susceptible population.

8.3.1 Measles epidemics and population mortality

Over the period covered by the 16 major measles waves (1896–1975), less than 1,000 deaths are listed in Table 4.1 as attributable to that disease in Iceland. Given that, over the same period, the total deaths from all causes was approximately 95,000, measles can be argued to be only a small factor shaping the mortality pattern of the Icelandic population, especially when we bear in mind from Table 4.1 that most of the measles deaths were associated with waves I–III.

Such a judgement must, however, be qualified in a number of ways. First, the records for deaths from measles are certainly an under-estimate and there is conflicting evidence in the published records for the period up to 1908. Second, since deaths from measles usually arise from secondary complications (particularly diseases of the respiratory system such as pneumonia and bronchitis), there is some risk of misdiagnosis and misreporting. Third, measles remains one of the world's important

Table 8.1 *Mortality due to measles in tropical Africa*

Date	Place	Class of patient	Case mortality (%)
1962	Nigeria	Hospital admission	22
1964	Gambia	Village, domestic	14–15
1967	Zambia	Hospital admission	30 (at peak, age 6–18 months)
1967	E. Africa	In-patients	6

Source: Fraser and Martin (1978).

killer diseases in isolated and undernourished communities. For example, in Iceland in the nineteenth century, the two major measles outbreaks were telling in their effects; the 1846 wave claimed 2,026 lives (35 per 1,000 inhabitants) and that of 1882, 1,700 (24 per 1,000 inhabitants). Similar figures have been reported in tropical Africa today, as indicated in Table 8.1. Fraser and Martin (1978, pp. 2–3) comment:

This is a high mortality associated with lack of food, especially protein starvation. In these circumstances the disease is as severe as it was 150 years ago in western European countries which are now prosperous and relatively unaffected by mortality due to measles. It is insufficient to say that this behaviour is solely a matter of undernourishment, for few virus infections have this particular effect. Working out the mechanism behind this pathogenic process will be of the greatest interest and consequence for its cure and prevention.

This view is supported by Pyle (1979, pp. 42–3) who reproduces lists of the leading causes of death in the world as given in United Nations' demographic year books at different dates. In 1947, measles ranked sixth (53 reporting countries), in 1956 eighth (88 countries), in 1965 eighth (99 countries) and in 1974 sixth (78 countries). The stark facts of Table 8.2 are often not appreciated when looking at causes of death through western eyes. On a more hopeful note, Burnet and White (1972, p. 17) have argued that total eradication of measles from the world should be possible in the same way as has recently been achieved for smallpox (which stood fifth on the 1974 list):

Measles cannot persist indefinitely in small isolated communities. That statement carries the very important implication that in principle vaccination against measles could allow the eradication of measles from the globe.

If deaths directly caused by measles are difficult to measure, then indirect deaths are still harder to establish. Increasing clinical evidence points to links between measles in childhood and the subsequent development of neurological diseases. The two most commonly linked to measles are subacute sclerosing panencephalitis (SSPE) and multiple sclerosis (MS). A. P. Ball (1977, p. 252) notes that the measles virus 'is

Table 8.2 *Leading causes of death in 78 countries, 1974*

1. Typhoid	11. Anaemias
2. Enteritis	12. Meningitis
3. Tuberculosis	13. Rheumatic heart disease
4. Whooping cough	14. Hypertensive disease
5. Smallpox	15. Ischaemic heart disease
6. MEASLES	16. Other heart disease
7. Cholera	17. Cerebrovascular disease
8. Malignant neoplasms	18. Influenza
9. Diabetes	19. Pneumonia
10. Avitaminosis	20. Bronchitis

Source: Pyle (1979, p. 43).

almost certainly responsible for SSPE, the risk being increased amongst those who develop measles in infancy.' It is generally assumed (Fraser and Martin, 1978, chapter 9) that the virus enters the brain during the childhood illness where it remains latent for up to five years. It may then reactivate, leading to convulsions, spastic paralysis, and death within a matter of months.

The relationship between measles and MS is more conjectural. Miller (in Ball, A.P., 1977, p. 252) has found that patients with MS have higher levels of measles antibody than control populations. It is suggested that, as with SSPE, virus infection of the brain occurs during childhood and that 'subsequent episodes of reactivation after many years are causally related to MS' (Ball, A. P., 1977, p. 253). This link is also suggested in Fraser and Martin (1978, chapter 12). The lag between brain infection and subsequent reactivation appears to be of the order of 20 years. Studies of the worldwide distribution of MS show an apparent latitudinal variation with rates of 5 per 100,000 in equatorial countries, rising to over 50 per 100,000 in high-latitude countries. A. P. Ball (1977) considers that such variation, if confirmed, may be an age-dependent host response to infection, with the low risk of MS in the tropics being related to measles' acquisition early in life, whereas in the temperate latitudes measles tends to attack older children (Table 8.3). Figure 8.1 shows that in Iceland, while the mean age of attack has decreased this century (probably reflecting measles' greater prevalence as links with the rest of the world increased), it is still a disease of older rather than younger children. Alter (1977) has reviewed MS incidence within immigrant groups and his findings support the idea of an adolescent or pre-adolescent factor in the subsequent development of MS. Any evidence which points to the measles virus as a possible pre-disposing agent in a disease like MS reinforces the case for its control with systematic vaccination programmes.

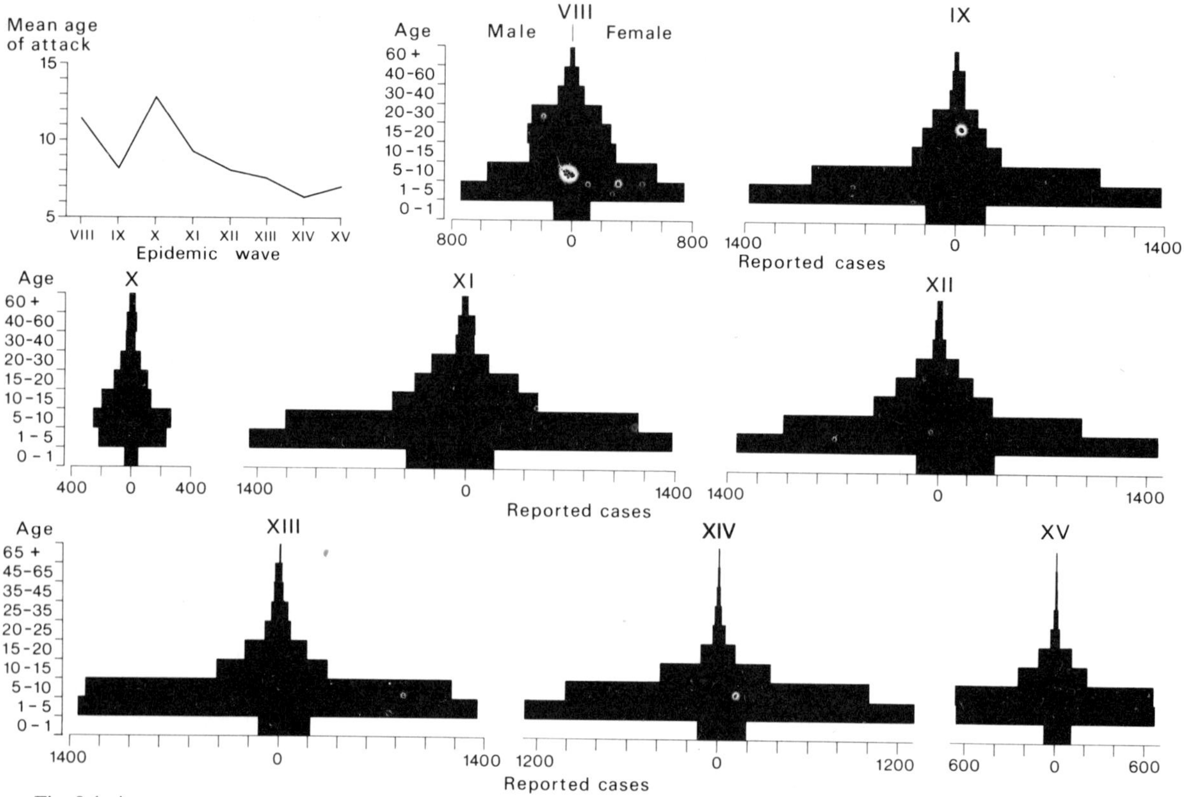

Fig. 8.1 Age–sex distribution of measles cases for waves VIII to XV, Iceland, 1945–70. *Sources:* As for Figures 4.10–4.17.

8.3.2 Measles epidemics and control measures

By choosing to study a series of diffusion waves which were inimical to the popuiation that received them, we have necessarily had to consider the defensive measures used by that population for self-protection; indeed, we stressed the need for control in identifying goodness-of-fit criteria for the models used in chapters 6 and 7. Three aspects of the defensive system merit further comment.

(a) Geographical isolation

Study of the individual reports from medical officers scattered around Iceland showed a population aware of the scourge of infectious disease and anxious to control it. For measles, the main method used was simply isolation: boats with an infected crew member were quarantined, carriers placed in fever hospitals (where available), assemblies banned, and infected farmsteads or villages avoided where possible. See, for example, the quotations cited in chapter 4 for waves I, II, III and V.

(b) Immunisation

Immunisation provides another line of defence against the disease. Two types of immunisation are used for measles. *Gammaglobulin* from a person who has had the disease may be injected into the person to be protected. If this is done early in the incubation period, measles may be prevented; if later in the incubation period, the severity of the disease

Table 8.3. *Age of measles attack in various countries*

Country	Median age in months
N. Nigeria	16.5
Jordan	18.0
E. Nigeria	21.5
Ghana	24.7
S. Africa, Zambia, Rhodesia	29.7
England and Wales	51.7

may be modified (McKhann, 1973, p. 26). *Live vaccine* from attenuated measles virus was developed and tested by J. F. Enders and his associates in 1958. This vaccine and a killed-virus vaccine were licensed for manufacture in the United States in 1963. The effect of widespread use of these vaccines from 1965 in the United States shows up in the time series of reported measles cases in Figure 3.1.

In Iceland, the discussion of wave VI in chapter 4 indicates that injections of convalescent serum were experimented with by doctors as a control procedure at irregular intervals from 1924. However, to this day, vaccination protection against measles in Iceland is at the initiative of local doctors, rather than being centrally directed. The first statistics of vaccination against measles in the tables of *Heilbrigðisskýrslur* are in 1951. The distribution of vaccinations since then is shown in Figure 8.2. As in the United States, the main use in Iceland dates from 1965 following the development there of a highly effective vaccine. There is little evidence of any distinctive spatial pattern – as we would expect in the absence of a centralised vaccination policy. The most consistent programme seems to have been developed in Dalvíkur (near Akureyrar), but recorded vaccinations are almost absent in north-west Iceland. The cost of prevention as well as local variations in clinical practice must go some way towards accounting for this uneven spatial pattern.

Where detailed studies of the cost effectiveness of measles vaccination have been carried out, results have generally been encouraging. In Austria, Ambrosch, Wiedermann, and Harasek (1978) calculated that, five years after the start of a measles vaccination programme of one-year-old children, the accumulated costs of vaccination are equalled by the profit gained by prevention of the disease. They compute a cost–benefit ratio of 3.95, where vaccination costs per case were estimated at around £10 (vaccine, plus physician and additional anti-pyretic) and the average costs of the therapy saved (home treatment, plus hospital treatment and residual cerebral damage for a small proportion of cases) are nearly four times as great.

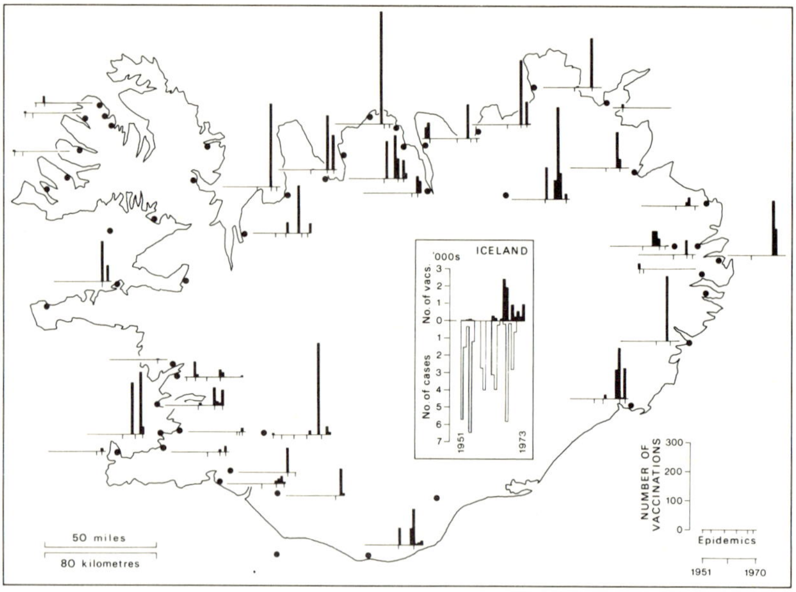

Fig. 8.2 Number of vaccinations against measles performed in Iceland by medical district, 1951–73. *Sources:* As for Figures 4.11–4.18.

(c) Early-warning systems

We have noted in section 7.6 and elsewhere (Cliff and Haggett, 1980) that one of the main reasons for establishing a compulsory notification system for infectious diseases in England in the 1880s was to create a warning system which allowed information to be passed between local sanitary authorities. Both the preceding defensive strategies, geographical isolation and immunisation, depend to some degree on advance knowledge of the presence of the measles virus in the population.

The problem of early warning is partially solved by prompt reporting. The early growth of the telephone network in Iceland (a link between Reykjavík and Seyðisfjörður was begun in 1906) is suggested in some doctors' reports as an important factor in the speedy reporting of infected cases and, therefore, improved containment of the disease. Attempts to use highly mobile epidemiological teams to stamp out the spread of measles in the United States (for example, the Seattle 'virus-watch program') depend on rapid toll-free telephone reporting by patients when first symptoms occur. But the reporting of existing infections, however soon, can be only part of the early-warning programme. The other essential is a forward estimate, in probabilistic terms, of the likelihood of infection occurring *ahead* of its arrival. We have stressed this aspect in the modelling chapters (chapters 6 and 7), and have assessed the progress made in section 8.2.

8.4 Iceland as a diffusion laboratory

We have set out in section 3.4 our reasons for selecting islands in general and Iceland in particular for special study. From the viewpoint of future work, it is important to note that the Icelandic morbidity record is of equal interest for many diseases other than measles. *Heilbrigðisskýrslur* currently records 32 diseases on the same basis as for measles (i.e., monthly, and by medical district). Figure 8.3 plots the monthly distribution for measles and three other infectious diseases for the period 1901 to 1974. The pattern for German measles is an irregular one, with four very small outbreaks up to World War II and four very large ones subsequently. That for whooping cough is for more regularly spaced epidemics to occur at about five-year intervals, with a substantial peak in 1935. The influenza pattern shows the highest frequency; there is a winter or spring peak in every year from 1918 onwards. The varied temporal pattern of these and other diseases clearly raises important questions for further research. How far do the significant differences in timing and amplitude relate to their geographical pattern of incidence and spread? Do the different virus strains in the case of influenza have different spread patterns related to the susceptibility of different age groups? Does the experience of measles give any guide to the behaviour of other epidemic diseases? Has the breakdown of Iceland's internal and external isolation, particularly from the early 1940s onwards, had equivalent effects on all infectious diseases?

5 Conclusion

Within the whole range of geographical research, the study of spatial diffusion occupies a central place. The dynamics by which a phenomenon originally located at one point becomes transferred to another is a question which is as difficult to answer as it is easy to pose. In this book, we have tried to outline the current state of research in spatial diffusion (chapter 2) and to identify some of the areas in which progress is possible. We consider that, for all the difficulties encountered and unsolved problems which remain, the study of multiple-wave diffusion in an insular context offers one of the most promising ways forward. It gives better prospects for formulating and testing hypotheses, of contributing to model building, and finally of using such models in a way which promises to increase our understanding of the spread of a disease which poses a continuing threat to public health, particularly in developing nations.

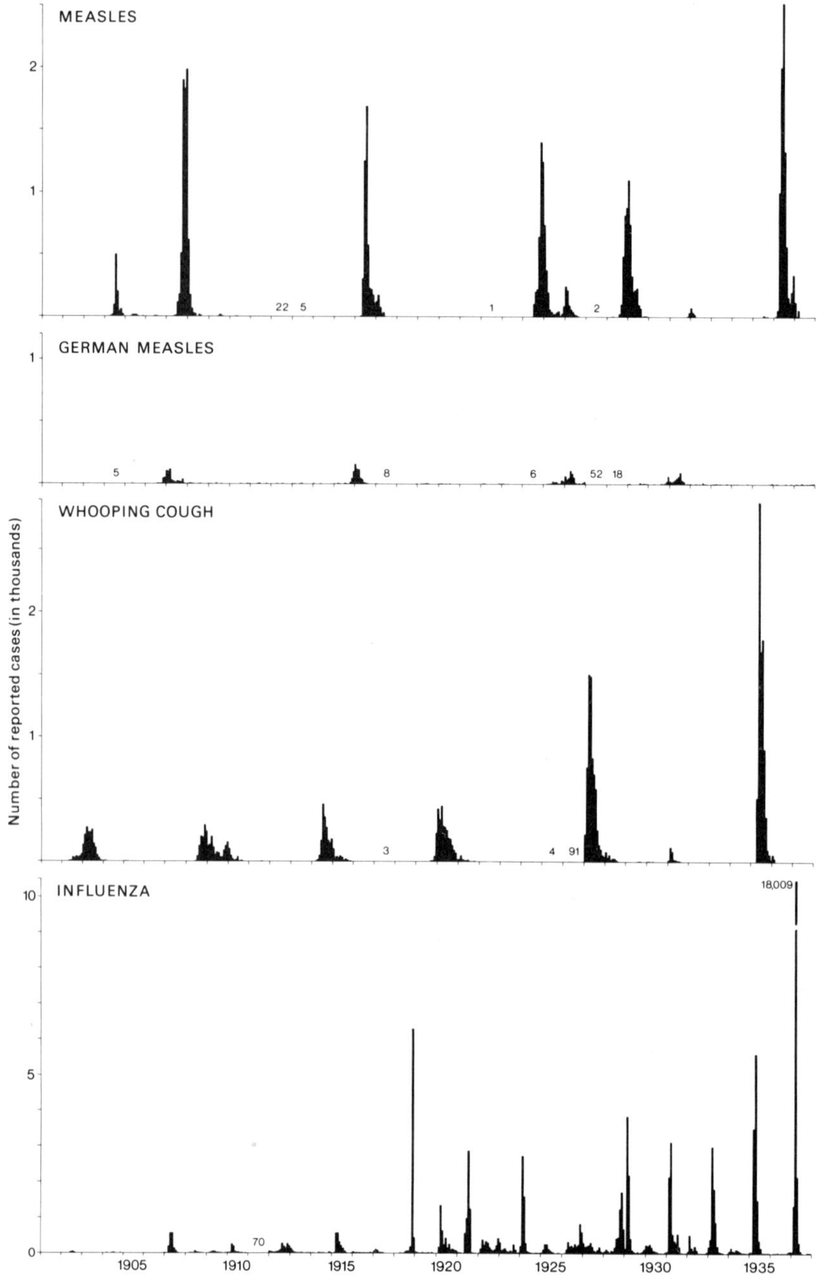

Fig. 8.3 Time series of reported cases of measles, German measles, whooping cough and influenza, Iceland, 1901–74. *Sources:* As for Figures 4.3–4.18.

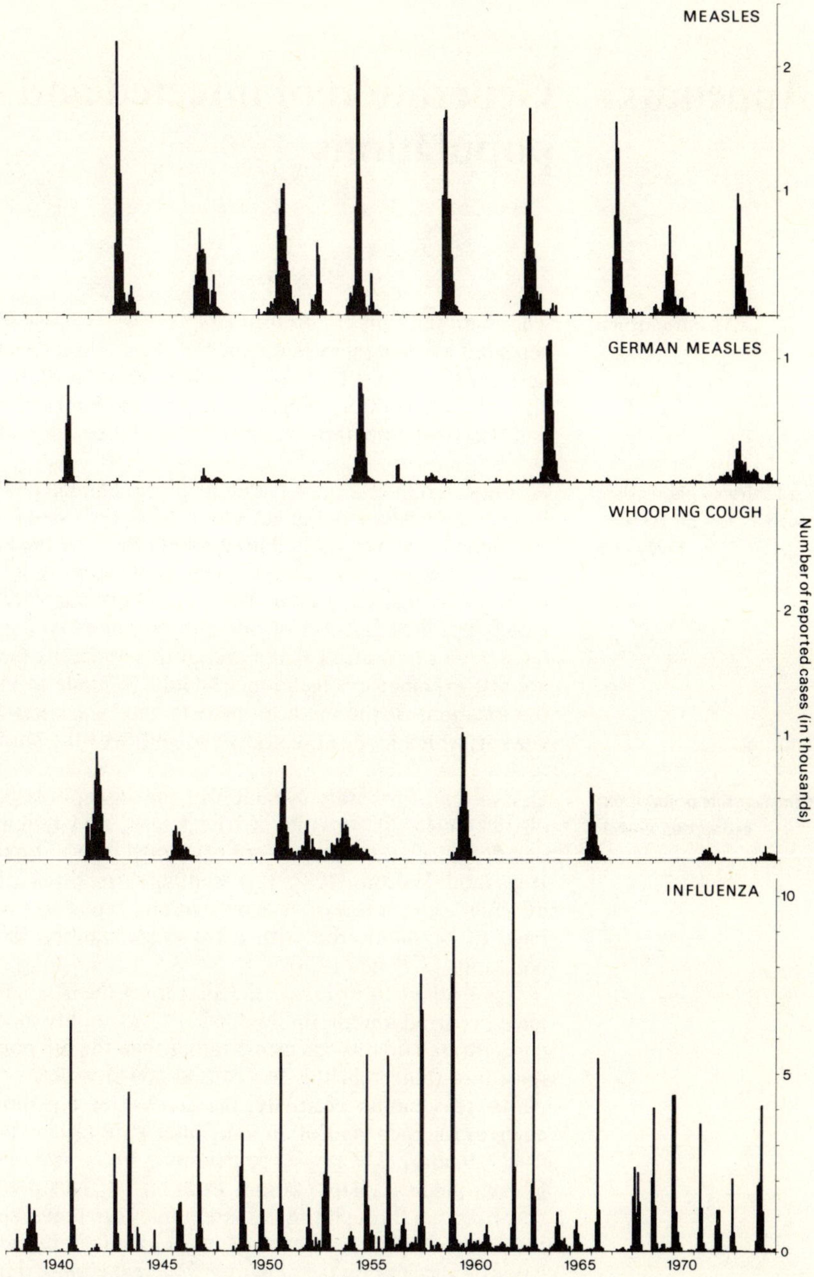
MEASLES
GERMAN MEASLES
WHOOPING COUGH
INFLUENZA
Number of reported cases (in thousands)
2
1
1
2
1
10
5
0
1940
1945
1950
1955
1960
1965
1970

Fig. 8.3 (contd)

Appendix: Generation of infected and susceptible populations

A1 Introduction

The main data inputs used in chapters 4–7 consist of the monthly numbers of reported cases of measles for each of the medical districts of Iceland, 1896–1975, and, for the period 1945–70, monthly estimates of the numbers of individuals at risk – the susceptible population. This appendix gives the data on case levels and describes how the susceptible population estimates were obtained.

A2 Infected population: reported cases for Iceland, 1896–1975

As indicated in section 4.1, details of the numbers of cases of measles reported in each medical district in each month are recorded in *Heilbrigðisskýrslur* for all the epidemic waves studied here except those of 1904 and 1907 (waves I and II). For these waves, figures are given only monthly for Iceland as a whole, and annually by district, rather than being both spatially and temporally disaggregated. The data matrices of case numbers employed in our analysis of each wave have been reproduced at the end of this appendix (see data tables). The tables are self-explanatory. Reference should be made to Figures 4.1–4.2 for maps of the locations of the medical districts and to section 4.2 for a discussion of the ways in which medical districts evolved over the study period.

A3 Susceptible population: estimating model[1]

Derivation of monthly estimates of the susceptible population in each medical district, 1945–70, was not a trivial task, and required the construction of a demographic accounting or cohort model (see, for example, Rogers (1968) and Rees and Wilson (1977)). Essentially, patterns of births, deaths, in- and out-migration, levels of vaccinations and reported cases in each medical district have to be monitored with a set of accounting identities in the manner of equations (7.7) and (7.8).

It is evident from Figure 8.1 that most measles cases in the post-war period have occurred among the under-20s. To simplify modelling, we have therefore concentrated on this age group rather than the full population range. There is no reason to think that this has caused any significant errors. To give the cohort model reasonable sensitivity, the accounting equations defined below monitor changes for each year of an individual's life rather than for blocks of years (say 0–4, 5–9, etc.). The largest contribution to the size of the susceptible population in each medical district comes from births. This pool of susceptibles has to be decremented through time as individuals are removed, primarily by contracting the disease (which confers lifelong immunity), but also, for example, in a few cases by vaccination (see Figure 8.2). At the same time, children are being born and added to the pool. Monthly estimates of the population of each medical district in one-year age classes, 0.5–19, were determined as shown in Figure A1.[2] The under-six-months category can be ignored because of mother-conferred immunity from measles. *Mannfjöldaskýrslur* gives the population annually for each medical district and we assumed linear growth between years to calculate monthly estimates of population totals. We can obtain from *Manntal á Íslandi* the percentage of the population in five-year age groups for each settlement at

[1] See footnote to section 5.3.5.
[2] We refer to children under one as being of age 0 years, and so on.

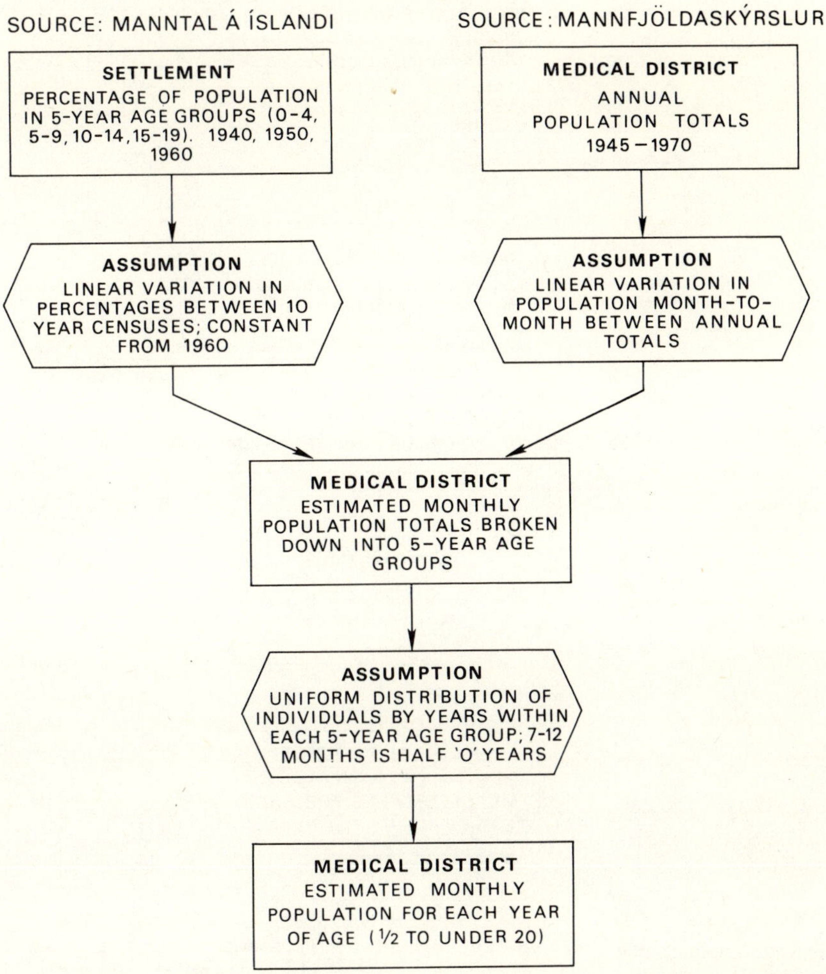

Fig. A1 Procedure adopted to obtain monthly estimates of the population of each medical district aged 0, 1, . . ., 19 years.

the decennial census dates (no census was conducted in 1970). Linear variation in these percentages between censuses is assumed up to 1960 and no change thereafter. As shown in Figure A1, these percentages were applied to the medical district totals to give monthly estimates of the population in five-year age groups. Finally, we took a uniform distribution of individuals by years within each five-year age group to produce the necessary estimated monthly population in each medical district for each year of age 0–19. A similar procedure yields estimates of the numbers of measles cases in each medical district on a comparable basis. The method is shown in Figure A2. A measles profile model (discussed below) was used to smooth the annual percentages of measles cases from age groups to single-year age categories. Alternatively, we could have assumed simply that cases were distributed uniformly among the years in each group.

A3.1 The measles profile model

The model to be outlined is illustrated in Figure A3. The histograms shown with the pecked lines give the percentages of reported measles cases in each age

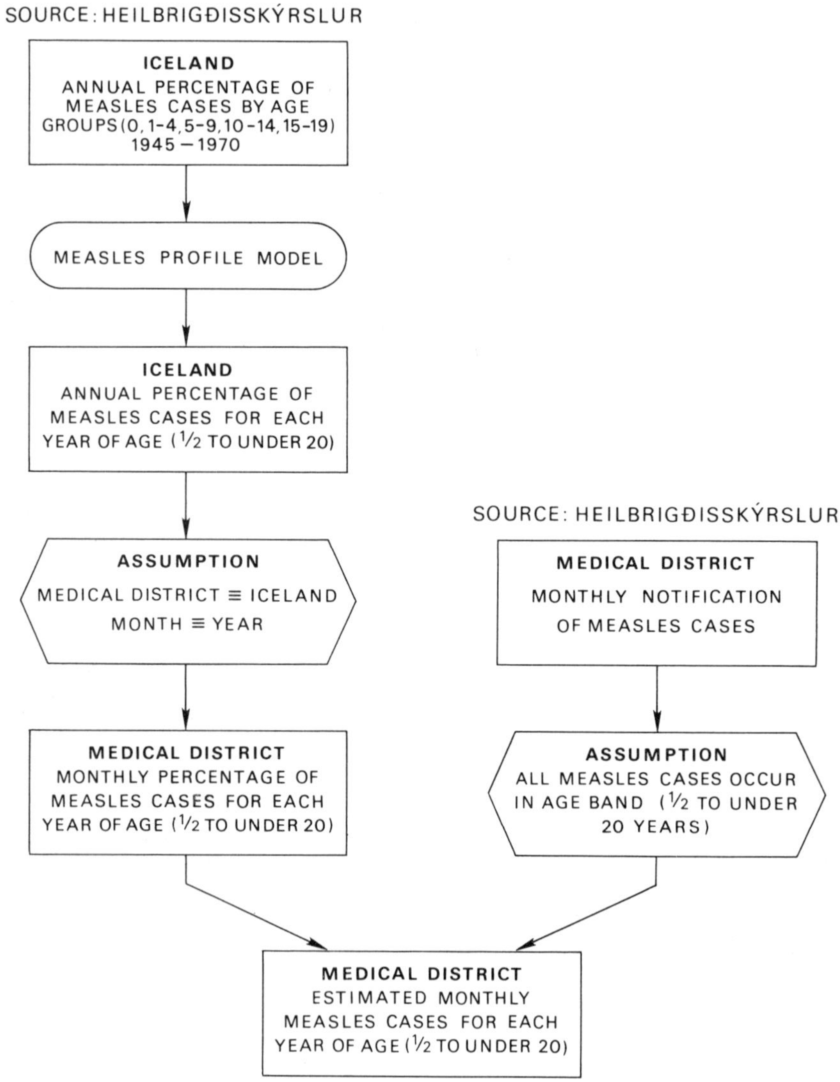

Fig. A2 Procedure adopted to obtain monthly estimates of the number of measles cases reported among persons aged 0, 1, . . ., 19 years in each medical district.

group 0–1, 1–5, etc. as shown in *Heilbrigðisskýrslur*; the solid line histograms represent the percentages by one-year divisions after smoothing. Let $a(i)$ denote the actual percentage of cases in each age group 0–1, 1–4, 5–9, 10–14, 15–19, and let $b(j)$, $j = 1, \ldots, 20$ be the percentages in each of the 20 one-year classes from the model (j increasing with age). We have $b(1)/2 = a(1)$, $b(2) + b(3) + b(4) + b(5) = a(2)$, etc. Suppose that $0 \leqslant x \leqslant 20$ denotes age x. The piecewise linear function, $f(x)$, defined on $[0.5, 20.5]$ is to be specified such that it has the value $c(k)$ at $x = d(k)$, $k = 1, 2, \ldots, 6$, and is linear elsewhere. Set $d(1), \ldots, d(6) = 0.5, 3.0, 7.5, 12.5, 17.5, 20.5$ respectively, corresponding to the midpoint of each age group of the raw data. Hence $b(j) = f(j - 0.5)$. We then take $c(6) = 0$ (which is consistent with the assumption that all cases occur

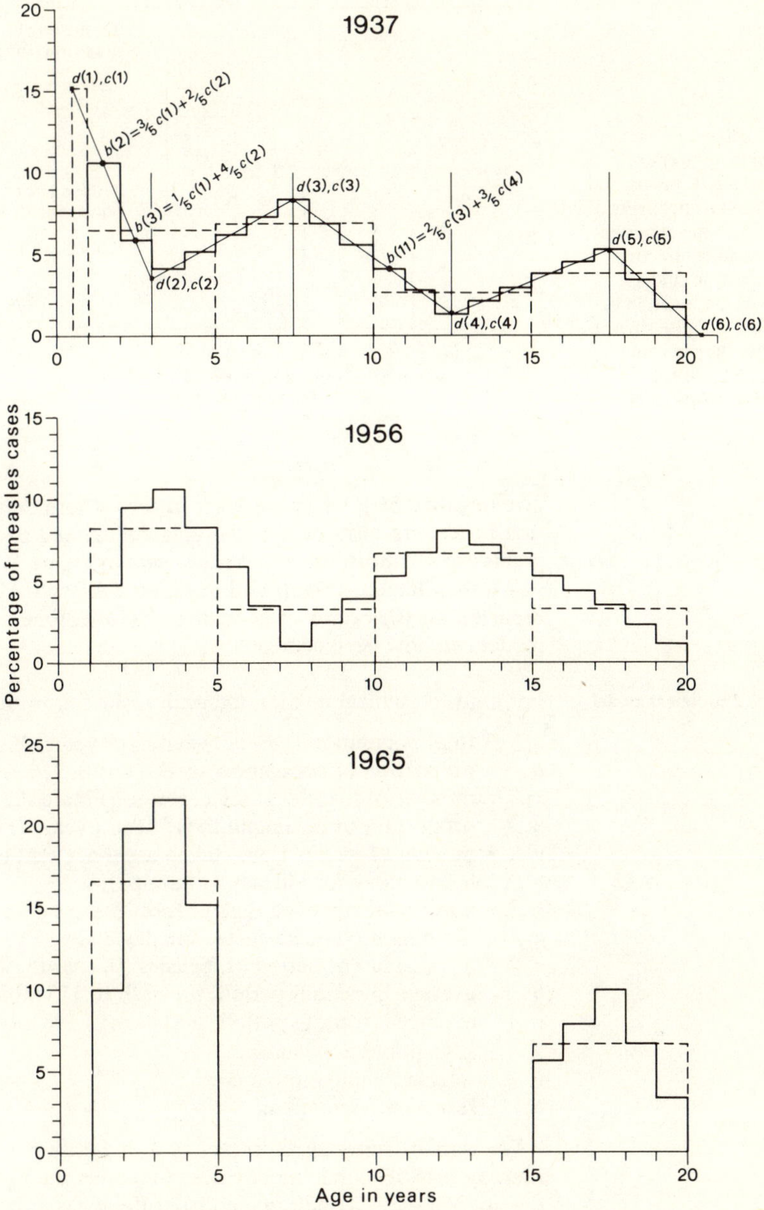

Fig. A3 The measles profile model. Terms are defined in text.

among the under-20s), and solve for $c(1), \ldots, c(5)$ and $b(1), \ldots, b(20)$. By linear interpolation,

$$\begin{bmatrix} a(1) \\ a(2) \\ a(3) \\ a(4) \\ a(5) \end{bmatrix} = \begin{bmatrix} 1/2 & 0 & 0 & 0 & 0 \\ 4/5 & 124/45 & 4/9 & 0 & 0 \\ 0 & 2/3 & 56/15 & 3/5 & 0 \\ 0 & 0 & 3/5 & 19/5 & 3/5 \\ 0 & 0 & 0 & 3/5 & 17/5 \end{bmatrix} \begin{bmatrix} c(1) \\ c(2) \\ c(3) \\ c(4) \\ c(5) \end{bmatrix}$$

is the necessary system of equations for the $c(k)$ and hence the $b(j)$ in terms of the $a(i)$. The equations are readily solved by matrix inversion. The method can

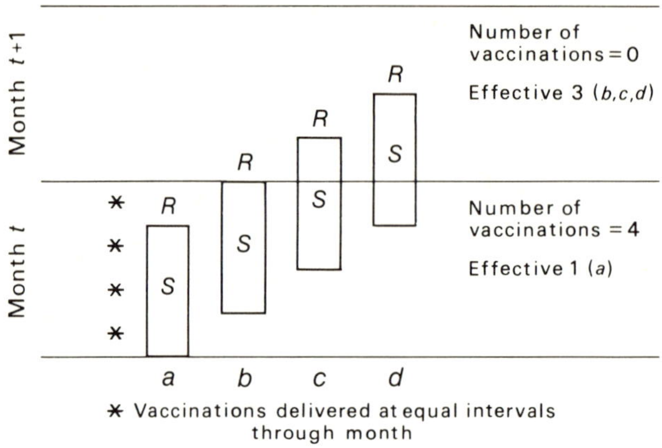

Fig. A4 Effect of vaccination upon four individuals, 1–4, vaccinated in weeks 1–4 respectively of month t. Vaccine assumed to become fully effective after 21 days, so that individuals are taken to be susceptible (S) until then. Thereafter they become immune and join the removed population, R.

give negative $b(j)$, which were set to zero where they occurred. The interpolation procedure ensures that the areas under the pecked- and solid-line histograms are identical. Examples are shown in Figure A3 for 1937, 1956 and 1965.

We then have, as illustrated in Figures A1 and A2, data for population and reported measles cases on a comparable age, time and area basis. The cohort model can now be specified.

A3.2 The cohort model

For a given medical district in month t, the following definitions are made:

- q_t total population aged between 0–19 years (Figure A1);
- $f_{i,t}$ proportion of population aged i, $i = 0, 1, \ldots, 19$ (Figure A1);
- m_t number of measles cases reported (Figure A2);
- $w_{i,t}$ proportion of m_t among those aged i years (Figure A2);
- v_t number of vaccinations (taken as 90 per cent of those reported in Figure 8.2 to allow for efficacy of vaccine);
- $r_{i,t}$ number of removeds aged i (post-rash and vaccinated individuals);
- $n_{i,t}$ net migration/death factor for those aged i years;
- a average latent period of measles (0.329 month – Figures 3.4 and A5);
- b average infectious period, pre-rash (0.115 month – Figures 3.4 and A5);
- c average infectious period, post-rash (0.148 month – Figures 3.4 and A5);
- S_t susceptible population;
- I_t infected population;
- R_t removed population.

We wish to generate estimates of S_t monthly for 1945–70; $t = 0$ is taken as January 1945. The number of cases of measles among individuals of age i in year y – say $N_{i,y}$ – can be determined from the measles profile model. We can then initialise $r_{i,t}$ at $t = 0$ as:

$$r_{i,t} = N_{i,1944} + N_{i-1,1943} + \ldots N_{i-19,1926},$$

where $N_{i,y} = 0$ for negative i. There were no vaccinations in the pre-war periods (see section 8.3.2). The assumption is made that, within a given one-year age group, birthdays are uniformly distributed throughout the year. Hence, at the end of a month, 1⁄12 (1⁄6 aged 0) move into the next age year. It follows that, without migration, $q_t f_{i,t}$ can be estimated as:

$$\widehat{q_t f_{i,t}} = \tfrac{11}{12} q_{t-1} f_{i,t-1} + \tfrac{1}{12} q_{t-1} f_{i-1,t-1}$$

for $y = 1, 2, \ldots$. The ratio,

$$n_{i,t} = q_t f_{i,t} / \widehat{q_t f_{i,t}},$$

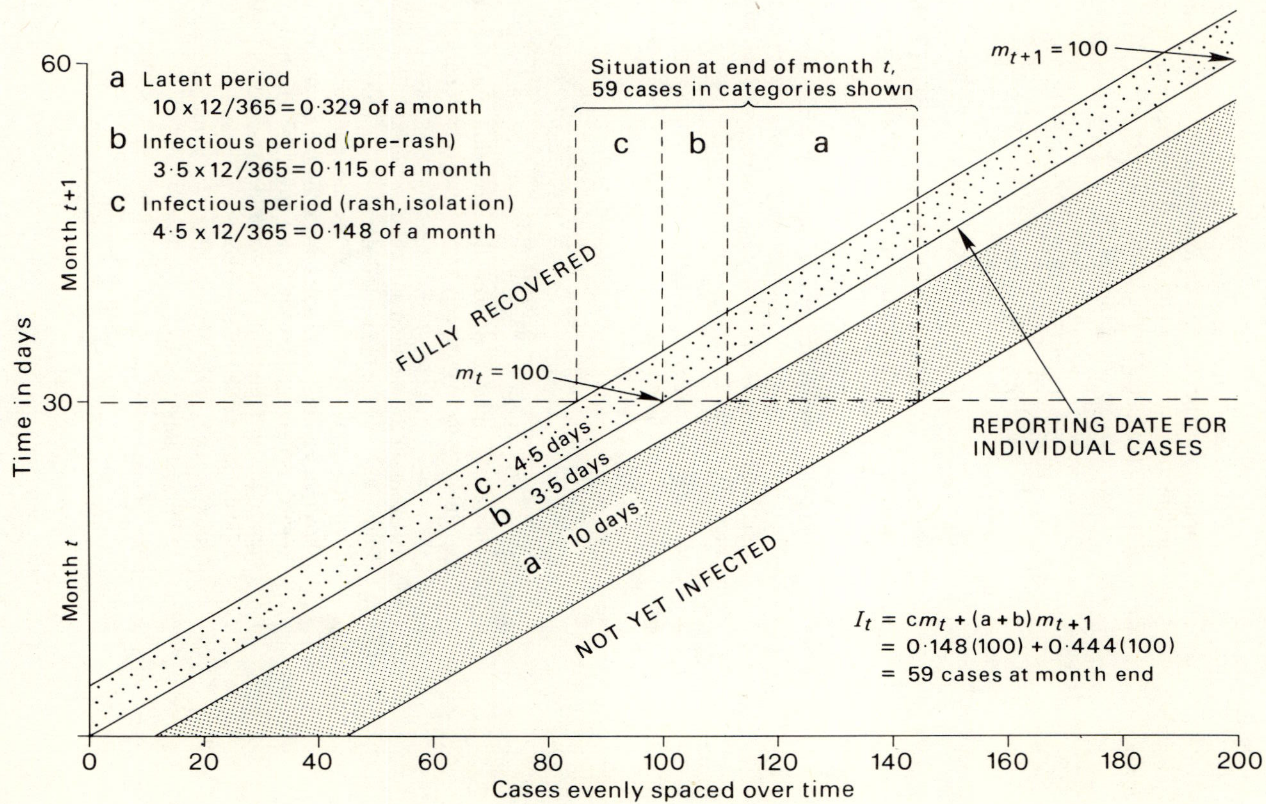

Fig. A5 Application of accounting identity for I_t in cohort model to 100 individuals infected at regular intervals in each of months t and $(t + 1)$. See text for definition of terms.

is a measure of net migration and death. We assume that all members of the population, whether S, I or R, are equally likely to migrate/die, and use $n_{i,t}$ to update items on a pro-rata basis. This is necessary because no usable migration data are published at the medical district level.

The recursive equations for the $\{r_{i,t}\}$ are:

$$r_{0,t} = n_{i,t}(m_t w_{0,t} + \tfrac{5}{6} r_{0,t-1} + v_t w_{0,t});$$

$$r_{1,t} = n_{i,t}(m_t w_{1,t} + \tfrac{11}{12} r_{1,t-1} + \tfrac{1}{6} r_{0,t-1} + v_t w_{1,t});$$

$$r_{i,t} = n_{i,t}(m_t w_{i,t} + \tfrac{11}{12} r_{i,t-1} + \tfrac{1}{12} r_{i-1,t-1} + v_t w_{i,t}),$$

for $i = 2, 3, \ldots, 19$. That is, appropriate parts of each age class are moved into the next class each month. Vaccinations are taken to be distributed among age categories in the same way as measles cases are.

It should be borne in mind that, when an individual is vaccinated, it takes about three weeks before full immunity is built up (Figure A4). In addition, by the end of a month, a proportion, c, of the measles cases occurring during that month will have reached the post-rash category and will have been removed. We then arrive, finally, at the accounting identities:

$$S_t = q_t + \tfrac{3}{4} v_t - [(a+b) m_{t+1} + r_{0,t} + r_{1,t} + \ldots + r_{19,t}];$$

$$I_t = c m_t + (a+b) m_{t+1};$$

$$R_t = r_{0,t} + r_{1,t} + \ldots + r_{19,t} - c m_t - \tfrac{3}{4} v_t;$$

$$S_t + I_t + R_t = q_t, \quad \text{as it should.}$$

Figure A5 illustrates how the equation for I_t works for 100 individuals contracting measles evenly over a one-month period (that is, at a rate of about three per day). The accounting equations have been evaluated monthly since 1945 but, in the modelling of chapters 6 and 7, the estimates of S_t have generally been used only for the period after 1954 to allow any initialisation errors to work themselves out. Examples of the susceptible population curves obtained are shown in Figure 7.5. (Tables are available on request from A.D.C.) Further, as regards I_t in chapter 6 and 7, we have, for simplicity, worked directly with the reported cases given in the accompanying tables, rather than introducing the adjustment implied by the accounting equation for I_t. Our aim here is to provide estimates of S_t of the appropriate order of magnitude, rather than figures correct to the last individual.

Wave I: *April 1904 to November 1904*

District	Reported cases
Dala (16)	11
Hesteyrar (27)	101
Ísafjarðar (24)	310
Nauteyrar (26)	114
Reykhóla (17)	113
Seyðisfjarðar (52)	1
Siglufjarðar (37)	8
Stranda (29)	109
Þingeyrar (21)	35
Iceland (Total)	802

Month	Reported cases
April	1
May	15
June	91
July	393
August	196
September	41
October	58
November	27
Iceland (Total)	822

Wave II: *May 1907 to August 1908*

District	Reported cases 1907	Reported cases 1908
Akureyrar (41)	346	6
Berufjarðar (56)	170	
Bíldudals (20)	111	
Blönduós (33)	68	28
Borgarfjarðar (12)	56	1
Borgarnes (13)	58	
Dala (16)	86	12
Eyrarbakka (7)	334	14
Fáskrúðsfjarðar (55)	206	101
Flateyjar (18)	93	
Fljótsdals (49)	65	7
Grímsnes (6)	46	4
Höfðahverfis (38)	120	
Hofsós (36)	54	60
Hornafjarðar (57)	324	
Hróarstungu (48)	133	
Húsavíkur (43)	240	27
Ísafjarðar (24)	43	30
Keflavíkur (10)	281	25
Miðfjarðar (32)		243
Mýrdals (59)	67	35
Ólafsvíkur (15)	227	2
Patreksfjarðar (19)	28	2
Rangár (60)	128	
Reyðarfjarðar (54)	121	44
Reykhóla (17)	33	
Reykjavíkur (1)	1604	12
Sauðárkróks (35)	30	9
Seyðisfjarðar (52)	148	21
Síðu (58)	44	
Siglufjarðar (37)	101	48
Skipaskaga (11)	302	
Stranda (29)	9	
Stykkishólms (14)	256	7
Svarfdæla (39)		16
Vestmannaeyja (63)	63	
Vopnafjarðar (47)	80	
Þingeyrar (21)	417	151
Iceland (Total)	6492	905

Month	Reported cases
May 1907	1
June	7
July	114
August	180
September	506
October	1894
November	1818
December	1973
Iceland (Total)	6493

Month	Reported cases
January 1908	616
February	166
March	60
April	25
May	19
June	0
July	13
August	6
Iceland (Total)	905

Wave III: *April 1916 to May 1917*

District	Month: 4/16	5/16	6/16	7/16	8/16	9/16	1
Akureyrar (41)		1	20	90	66	57	
Axarfjarðar (44)					2	3	
Berufjarðar (56)			1				
Bíldudals (20)			20	37	16		
Blönduós (33)			8	30	11	2	
Borgarfjarðar (12)		3	17	40	1	1	
Dala (16)			28	29	6		
Eyrarbakka (7)		2	10	33	36	11	
Fáskrúðsfjarðar (55)		1	62	67	13		
Flateyjar (18)				1			
Flateyrar (22)		27	60	7	3		
Fljótsdals (49)			35	14			
Grímsnes (6)		32	74	19	21		
Hafnarfjarðar (3)		1	10	27	21		
Hesteyrar (27)		8	42	17			
Höfðahverfis (38)				2	2		
Hofsós (36)				7	9	1	
Hróarstungu (48)			1	2			
Húsavíkur (43)			2	1			
Keflavíkur (10)			1	17	5	12	
Miðfjarðar (32)			1	15			
Mýrdals (59)			6	51	28	5	4
Nauteyrar (26)				19	2		
Norðfjarðar (53)			13	69	40	6	
Ólafsvíkur (15)			2	3	11	40	2
Patreksfjarðar (19)	1	24	13	8	7		
Rangár (60)		1		4	8	1	
Reyðarfjarðar (54)			4	74	47	4	
Reykdæla (42)		8			2	6	
Reykhóla (17)			24	11			
Reykjavíkur (1)		121	716	840	83	10	
Sauðárkróks (35)				2	11		
Seyðisfjarðar (52)		3	3	4	18	26	
Síðu (58)			3	6	30		
Siglufjarðar (37)	5	12	29	17	5	5	
Skipaskaga (11)		1	4	51	23	8	
Stranda (29)		50					
Stykkishólms (14)		10	27	31	3		
Svarfdæla (39)			5	14	16		
Vestmannaeyja (63)							
Vopnafjarðar (47)				3	4		
Þingeyrar (21)						12	
Þistilfjarðar (46)			3	17	28	16	
Iceland (Total)	6	305	1244	1679	578	226	21

11/16	12/16	1/17	2/17	3/17	4/17	5/17	Total	District
64	39	7					420	Akureyrar (41)
			73	16			94	Axarfjarðar (44)
10	4						15	Berufjarðar (56)
							73	Bíldudals (20)
8	5						92	Blönduós (33)
	1	11	1				75	Borgarfjarðar (12)
							63	Dala (16)
							92	Eyrarbakka (7)
1	1						145	Fáskrúðsfjarðar (55)
							1	Flateyjar (18)
							97	Flateyrar (22)
							49	Fljótsdals (49)
							146	Grímsnes (6)
							59	Hafnarfjarðar (3)
							67	Hesteyrar (27)
1	1						20	Höfðahverfis (38)
							19	Hofsós (36)
11	13	1					35	Hróarstungu (48)
		2	77	52	11		145	Húsavíkur (43)
							41	Keflavíkur (10)
							16	Miðfjarðar (32)
11	1						145	Mýrdals (59)
							21	Nauteyrar (26)
1	3						132	Norðfjarðar (53)
4	15	6					101	Ólafsvíkur (15)
							53	Patreksfjarðar (19)
1							15	Rangár (60)
29	7						174	Reyðarfjarðar (54)
	9	29	10	4	7	30	105	Reykdæla (42)
							35	Reykhóla (17)
9		5			2		1787	Reykjavíkur (1)
	3						20	Sauðárkróks (35)
1							58	Seyðisfjarðar (52)
17							56	Síðu (58)
							74	Siglufjarðar (37)
							87	Skipaskaga (11)
							50	Stranda (29)
							71	Stykkishólms (14)
7							44	Svarfdæla (39)
	3	59	7				69	Vestmannaeyja (63)
							7	Vopnafjarðar (47)
							12	Þingeyrar (21)
							64	Þistilfjarðar (46)
175	105	120	168	72	20	30	4944	Iceland (Total)

Wave IV: *June 1924 to August 1926*

District	Month: 7/24	8/24	9/24	10/24	11/24	12/24	1/25	2/25	3/25	4/25	5/25	6/25	7/25	8/2
Akureyrar (41)	2	2			17	26	64	17	13					4
Berufjarðar (56)					1									
Borgarfjarðar (12)	39	34		1		7	2							
Borgarnes (13)	11	13			3	5	1							
Dala (16)	8	16	1			6	2		5					
Eyrarbakka (7)		7	10	5	51	88	94	13	107	33				
Fáskrúðsfjarðar (55)											25	13		
Flateyjar (18)					2	1					7			
Flateyrar (22)			1			8	19	6						
Fljótsdals (49)													10	
Grímsnes (6)					14	9	13	5						
Hafnarfjarðar (3)				4	145	224	13	2						
Höfðahverfis (38)														
Hólmavíkur (31)					15	6								
Hóls (25)							14	44	11					
Hornafjarðar (57)														
Hróarstungu (48)														
Húsavíkur (43)					2	6								31
Ísafjarðar (24)	6	19	4	17	93	76	32	5	5			1		
Keflavíkur (10)				9	39	41	10		5					1
Miðfjarðar (32)														
Mýrdals (59)					6									
Nauteyrar (26)					1									
Norðfjarðar (53)														
Patreksfjarðar (19)					1	9								
Rangár (60)		1		5	11	15	1							
Reyðarfjarðar (54)												7	9	1
Reykdæla (42)					1	12								
Reykhóla (17)											10			
Reykjavíkur (1)	29	64	188	573	831	496	133	69	24	20				
Seyðisfjarðar (52)	1	7				7	1							
Síðu (58)								7						
Siglufjarðar (37)	4	8												
Skipaskaga (11)	1	23	4	14	127	158	35	1						
Stykkishólms (14)			2	3		3	16	21	20	6				
Svarfdæla (39)			11	13	30	20	1							
Vestmannaeyja (63)				2			250	148	5				1	
Vopnafjarðar (47)	1	7												
Þingeyrar (21)					1	18	35	36						
Iceland (Total)	102	201	221	646	1391	1241	736	374	195	59	42	21	20	37

9/25	10/25	11/25	12/25	1/26	2/26	3/26	4/26	5/26	6/26	7/26	8/26	Total	District
		21	79	203	152	25	27	5	3			660	Akureyrar (41)
												1	Berufjarðar (56)
												83	Borgarfjarðar (12)
												33	Borgarnes (13)
												38	Dala (16)
												408	Eyrarbakka (7)
												38	Fáskrúðsfjarðar (55)
												10	Flateyjar (18)
												34	Flateyrar (22)
												10	Fljótsdals (49)
												41	Grímsnes (6)
												388	Hafnarfjarðar (3)
			1	1	29	16	13	21				81	Höfðahverfis (38)
												21	Hólmavíkur (31)
												69	Hóls (25)
					1	2	4		1			8	Hornafjarðar (57)
									8			8	Hróarstungu (48)
36				15								90	Húsavíkur (43)
												258	Ísafjarðar (24)
												105	Keflavíkur (10)
				19	12	1						32	Miðfjarðar (32)
												6	Mýrdals (59)
												1	Nauteyrar (26)
				3	1	1						5	Norðfjarðar (53)
												10	Patreksfjarðar (19)
												33	Rangár (60)
3	1				9	7		1				38	Reyðarfjarðar (54)
												13	Reykdæla (42)
												10	Reykhóla (17)
	6	7	4									2444	Reykjavíkur (1)
					5	39	18	18	10	12	3	121	Seyðisfjarðar (52)
												7	Síðu (58)
												12	Siglufjarðar (37)
												363	Skipaskaga (11)
												71	Stykkishólms (14)
			1									76	Svarfdæla (39)
												406	Vestmannaeyja (63)
												8	Vopnafjarðar (47)
												90	Þingeyrar (21)
39	7	28	85	241	209	91	62	45	22	12	3	6130	Iceland (Total)

Wave V: *August 1928 to December 1929*

District	Month: 8/28	9/28	10/28	11/28	12/28	1/29	2/29	3/29	[illegible]
Akureyrar (41)		2	13	10	69	183	43	6	
Berufjarðar (56)									
Bíldudals (20)									
Blönduós (33)			16	37	66	11	4		
Borgarfjarðar (12)			1		4		1		
Borgarnes (13)						14			
Dala (16)			2	1		7	3	1	
Eyrarbakka (7)						38	7		
Fáskrúðsfjarðar (55)					7	56	13		
Fljótsdals (49)					5				
Grímsnes (6)				8		45	4		
Hafnarfjarðar (3)			3	1	4	25	33	59	[illegible]
Hesteyrar (27)									
Höfðahverfis (38)			35	14	13	3		3	
Hofsós (36)		3	27	29	14	3			
Hólmavíkur (31)			7	33	44	65	15	3	
Hóls (25)									
Hróarstungu (48)				63	8	7			
Húsavíkur (43)			2	1					
Ísafjarðar (24)			1	7	1			10	[illegible]
Keflavíkur (10)						2	6	12	1
Miðfjarðar (32)			9	100	50				
Mýrdals (59)						11	77	10	
Norðfjarðar (53)			3	35	61	1			
Ólafsvíkur (15)									
Patreksfjarðar (19)									[illegible]
Rangár (60)				8	8	6	17	2	[illegible]
Reyðarfjarðar (54)				7	30	34	25	6	
Reykdæla (42)			1	47	11				
Reykhóla (17)									
Reykjavíkur (1)		1	58	156	285	489	380	143	[illegible]
Sauðárkróks (35)		13	192	179	72				
Seyðisfjarðar (52)			7	11	19				[illegible]
Síðu (58)							1		
Siglufjarðar (37)	22	75	63	16	5				
Skipaskaga (11)		2	8	5		11	13	16	[illegible]
Stykkishólms (14)							14		
Svarfdæla (39)			27	41	88	60	25	8	
Vestmannaeyja (63)		1	9	1	5	27	80	51	[illegible]
Vopnafjarðar (47)					2	1			
Þingeyrar (21)				7					
Þistilfjarðar (46)									
Iceland (Total)	22	97	484	817	871	1099	761	330	205

[illegible]	6/29	7/29	8/29	9/29	10/29	11/29	12/29	Total	District
4	38							378	Akureyrar (41)
3	8	2						33	Berufjarðar (56)
7	13	9						29	Bíldudals (20)
2		9						145	Blönduós (33)
	3	3						12	Borgarfjarðar (12)
	2	1						17	Borgarnes (13)
	18	1	2					35	Dala (16)
								64	Eyrarbakka (7)
1	19	8	13					117	Fáskrúðsfjarðar (55)
								5	Fljótsdals (49)
1								58	Grímsnes (6)
6	1	1						191	Hafnarfjarðar (3)
	10	1						11	Hesteyrar (27)
								74	Höfðahverfis (38)
								76	Hofsós (36)
								167	Hólmavíkur (31)
			1					1	Hóls (25)
								78	Hróarstungu (48)
								3	Húsavíkur (43)
50	55	22	6					177	Ísafjarðar (24)
6								38	Keflavíkur (10)
30	30	3						222	Miðfjarðar (32)
1	1	4						104	Mýrdals (59)
3	2							105	Norðfjarðar (53)
				1				1	Ólafsvíkur (15)
19	16	9	14					74	Patreksfjarðar (19)
15								74	Rangár (60)
								102	Reyðarfjarðar (54)
		8	10					77	Reykdæla (42)
			1		4	2		7	Reykhóla (17)
15	7	3	7		3	6	2	1594	Reykjavíkur (1)
								456	Sauðárkróks (35)
1	2							41	Seyðisfjarðar (52)
								1	Síðu (58)
1	4							186	Siglufjarðar (37)
								76	Skipaskaga (11)
	1	12	12	2				41	Stykkishólms (14)
								249	Svarfdæla (39)
								184	Vestmannaeyja (63)
								3	Vopnafjarðar (47)
3								10	Þingeyrar (21)
1								1	Þistilfjarðar (46)
219	230	96	66	3	7	8	2	5317	Iceland (Total)

Wave VI: *February 1936 to March 1937*

District Month:	2/36	3/36	4/36	5/36	6/36	7/36	8/36	
Akureyrar (41)				2	30	100	69	
Axarfjarðar (44)				6	30	71	6	
Berufjarðar (56)				11	14			
Bíldudals (20)	4	10		2	3	3		
Blönduós (33)				5	38	27	7	
Borgarfjarðar (12)				4	17	22	4	
Borgarnes (13)				21	47	20	2	
Dala (16)				15	45	14	2	
Eyrarbakka (7)		1	19	79	208	71	10	
Fáskrúðsfjarðar (55)				35	103	20	1	
Flateyjar (18)				10	20	7	5	
Flateyrar (22)				5	15	6	3	
Fljótsdals (49)				12	39	21		
Grímsnes (6)				24	56	17	12	
Hafnarfjarðar (3)			6	118	319	62	5	
Hesteyrar (27)					5	29	10	
Höfðahverfis (38)								
Hofsós (36)				2	2	5	7	
Hólmavíkur (31)				3	5	25	20	
Hóls (25)					15	78	4	
Hornafjarðar (57)				8	14	1		
Hróarstungu (48)				6	36	42	4	
Húsavíkur (43)				16	31	12	21	
Ísafjarðar (24)			2	72	90	37	4	
Keflavíkur (10)		7	25	50	101	22	2	
Miðfjarðar (32)				8	26	22	10	
Mýrdals (59)				5	21	3	1	
Norðfjarðar (53)				7	16	9	14	
Ögur (26)				8	16	6	2	
Ólafsfjarðar (40)				11	61	6	6	
Olafsvíkur (15)			13	44	43	2		
Patreksfjarðar (19)				5	31	26	19	
Rangár (60)			2	38	42	20	23	
Reyðarfjarðar (54)				30	50	25	15	
Reykdæla (42)					1		8	
Reykhóla (17)			1	4	34	13	53	
Reykjarfjarðar (30)				2	23	14	2	
Reykjavíkur (1)		26	922	1102	292	38	5	
Sauðárkróks (35)				13	23	34	16	1
Seyðisfjarðar (52)				22	53	49	13	
Síðu (58)				3	75	38	4	
Siglufjarðar (37)				4	38	52	42	3
Skipaskaga (11)			2	23	86	108	44	
Stykkishólms (14)				6	42	36	34	1
Svarfdæla (39)				1	7	31	26	
Vestmannaeyja (63)		7	7	75	91	17	1	
Vopnafjarðar (47)				63	122	21	10	
Þingeyrar (21)				4	12	4		
Þistilfjarðar (46)				7	25	33	20	
Iceland (Total)	4	51	999	1991	2513	1319	566	15

10/36	11/36	12/36	1/37	2/37	3/37	Total	District
42	122	295	68			761	Akureyrar (41)
			3			116	Axarfjarðar (44)
						25	Berufjarðar (56)
						22	Bíldudals (20)
						77	Blönduós (33)
						49	Borgarfjarðar (12)
						90	Borgarnes (13)
		1				77	Dala (16)
						388	Eyrarbakka (7)
						159	Fáskrúðsfjarðar (55)
						55	Flateyjar (18)
						30	Flateyrar (22)
						72	Fljótsdals (49)
						109	Grímsnes (6)
						510	Hafnarfjarðar (3)
						47	Hesteyrar (27)
						6	Höfðahverfis (38)
2		11	24			54	Hofsós (36)
						57	Hólmavíkur (31)
						105	Hóls (25)
						23	Hornafjarðar (57)
						89	Hróarstungu (48)
		2				84	Húsavíkur (43)
						205	Ísafjarðar (24)
						207	Keflavíkur (10)
						66	Miðfjarðar (32)
						30	Mýrdals (59)
2	3					53	Norðfjarðar (53)
						32	Ögur (26)
						84	Ólafsfjarðar (40)
	1					103	Ólafsvíkur (15)
						82	Patreksfjarðar (19)
						125	Rangár (60)
						123	Reyðarfjarðar (54)
						9	Reykdæla (42)
						105	Reykhóla (17)
						41	Reykjarfjarðar (30)
	1	1				2390	Reykjavíkur (1)
						102	Sauðárkróks (35)
						138	Seyðisfjarðar (52)
						124	Síðu (58)
33	52	4	3	1		261	Siglufjarðar (37)
						265	Skipaskaga (11)
29	16	10	8			199	Stykkishólms (14)
	6	12	7	1	48	139	Svarfdæla (39)
						199	Vestmannaeyja (63)
						216	Vopnafjarðar (47)
						20	Þingeyrar (21)
						85	Þistilfjarðar (46)
108	201	336	113	2	48	8408	Iceland (Total)

Wave VII: *February 1943 to May 1944*

District Month:	2/43	3/43	4/43	5/43	6/43	7/43	8/43	9/
Akureyrar (41)			4	15	118	175	216	7
Álafoss (5)			24	31	5	1		
Axarfjarðar (44)			2	20	21	17	3	
Berufjarðar (56)								
Bíldudals (20)			2	41	55	18	5	
Blönduós (33)				10	20	25	27	
Borgarfjarðar (12)			1	17	28	3		
Borgarnes (13)			4	41	17	3		
Dala (16)				16	5	4		
Eyrarbakka (7)			7	17	12	11		
Fáskrúðsfjarðar (55)					29	11	5	
Flateyrar (22)				4	16	14	3	
Fljótsdals (49)			1	9	16	46	19	[illegible]
Grímsnes (6)			5	27	17	15	4	
Hafnarfjarðar (3)		1	30	123	94	28	12	[illegible]
Hesteyrar (27)				1	1			
Höfðahverfis (38)				4	10	5		
Hofsós (36)					6	99	6	3
Hólmavíkur (31)				18	32	17	21	
Hóls (25)				3	36	10	9	6
Hornafjarðar (57)					8	3		
Húsavíkur (43)			4	30	107	58	8	6
Ísafjarðar (24)				19	170	137	27	7
Keflavíkur (10)		21	65	36	28			
Miðfjarðar (32)			6	6	16	26	1	
Mýrdals (59)						6		
Norðfjarðar (53)				3	3	1	1	4
Ögur (26)				14	12	3		
Ólafsfjarðar (40)						6	5	
Ólafsvíkur (15)				7	5	3		
Patreksfjarðar (19)				24	51	11		
Rangár (60)			3		18	32		
Reyðarfjarðar (54)				3	23	14		
Reykdæla (42)			2	4	1	4	4	
Reykjarfjarðar (30)						12	16	
Reykjavíkur (1)	3	54	412	1280	190	8	17	2
Sauðárkróks (35)				9	52	112	15	7
Seyðisfjarðar (52)					1			
Síðu (58)					6			
Siglufjarðar (37)			2	59	79	56	42	
Skipaskaga (11)				114	162	17	3	
Stykkishólms (14)			1	65	14	8	3	
Svarfdæla (39)					2	22	19	5
Vestmannaeyja (63)				4	19	28	8	32
Vopnafjarðar (47)			1	17	7	3	3	
Þingeyrar (21)				4	66	39		8
Þistilfjarðar (46)			1	92	22	21	5	10
Iceland (Total)	3	76	577	2187	1600	1132	507	178

3	11/43	12/43	1/44	2/44	3/44	4/44	5/44	Total	District
[illegible]	47	80	215	132	100	12		1260	Akureyrar (41)
								61	Álafoss (5)
[illegible]								69	Axarfjarðar (44)
							22	22	Berufjarðar (56)
								121	Bíldudals (20)
								82	Blönduós (33)
								49	Borgarfjarðar (12)
								65	Borgarnes (13)
								25	Dala (16)
								47	Eyrarbakka (7)
								45	Fáskrúðsfjarðar (55)
								37	Flateyrar (22)
								99	Fljótsdals (49)
								68	Grímsnes (6)
								289	Hafnarfjarðar (3)
								2	Hesteyrar (27)
					2			21	Höfðahverfis (38)
								114	Hofsós (36)
								88	Hólmavíkur (31)
1								65	Hóls (25)
								11	Hornafjarðar (57)
						1		214	Húsavíkur (43)
3								363	Ísafjarðar (24)
								150	Keflavíkur (10)
								55	Miðfjarðar (32)
								6	Mýrdals (59)
	36	72	15					135	Norðfjarðar (53)
								29	Ögur (26)
								11	Ólafsfjarðar (40)
								15	Ólafsvíkur (15)
								86	Patreksfjarðar (19)
								53	Rangár (60)
1								41	Reyðarfjarðar (54)
			1	3		2	14	35	Reykdæla (42)
								28	Reykjarfjarðar (30)
				1		1		1968	Reykjavíkur (1)
								195	Sauðárkróks (35)
		5	10	2				18	Seyðisfjarðar (52)
								6	Síðu (58)
								238	Siglufjarðar (37)
								296	Skipaskaga (11)
								91	Stykkishólms (14)
2				3	3			56	Svarfdæla (39)
16	7	3						117	Vestmannaeyja (63)
								31	Vopnafjarðar (47)
7	3							127	Þingeyrar (21)
								151	Þistilfjarðar (46)
03	93	160	241	141	105	16	36	7155	Iceland (Total)

Wave VIII: *November 1946 to August 1948*

District	Month: 11/46	12/46	1/47	2/47	3/47	4/47	5/47	6/47	7/47	8/47	
Akranes (11)			1	2	3	25	50	53	20		
Akureyrar (41)		3			4	4	18	77	75	66	
Álafoss (5)				2	9	3	1				
Bakkagerðis (48)		3	3					4			
Bíldudals (20)					6	3					
Blönduós (33)						2	1	7	1	1	
Bolungarvíkur (25)					1	2	5	4	11	11	
Borgarnes (13)				3	3	2	5	16	9	12	
Breiðumýrar (42)							2	20	14	8	
Búða (55)							11	4			
Búðardals (16)							11	7			
Dalvíkur (39)						3	21	31	48	14	
Djúpavíkur (30)										1	
Djúpavogs (56)									14		
Egilsstaða (49)		6	10				10	18			
Eskifjarðar (54)								1	2		
Eyrarbakka (7)					5	4	18	34	13		
Flateyrar (22)					1	2		6	16	13	
Grenivíkur (38)				1			5	5	6	3	
Hafnar (57)			1	3			6	4			
Hafnarfjarðar (3)			4	26	72	92	50			1	
Hofsós (36)							3	7		8	
Hólmavíkur (31)								2			
Húsavíkur (43)								9	30	19	
Hvammstanga (32)					2	5	4	4		1	
Ísafjarðar (24)			1	15	13	10	5	1	6	7	
Keflavíkur (10)				8	32	51	28	10	6		
Kirkjubæjar (58)						5	22	3	5	1	
Kleppjárnsreykja (12)			1	2			4	2	4		
Kópaskers (44)					4		9	31	20	6	
Laugarás (6)						7			1		
Nes (53)							6				
Ólafsfjarðar (40)					1		1	18	12	7	
Ólafsvíkur (15)									8	3	
Patreksfjarðar (19)											
Reykhóla (17)								8			
Reykjavíkur (1)	5		221	244	270	311	79	15	13		
Sauðárkróks (35)							3	4	2	6	
Selfoss (8)					4	18					
Seyðisfjarðar (52)							1	6	3	6	
Siglufjarðar (37)					11	77	73	4	2	2	
Stórólfshvols (60)				6	12	20	42	57	27	10	
Stykkishólms (14)						1	2	2			
Súðavíkur (28)											
Vestmannaeyja (63)		1	1	4	1	5	11	35	98	89	
Víkur (59)			1	3	44	36	11				
Vopnafjarðar (47)							3	8	25	5	
Þingeyrar (21)						9	11		2		
Þórshafnar (46)									1		10
Iceland (Total)	5	13	244	319	498	697	532	517	494	300	20

10/47	11/47	12/47	1/48	2/48	3/48	4/48	5/48	6/48	7/48	8/48	Total	District
											154	Akranes (11)
5	75	154	102	28	12						643	Akureyrar (41)
											15	Álafoss (5)
											10	Bakkagerðis (48)
											9	Bíldudals (20)
		2	4								19	Blönduós (33)
											38	Bolungarvíkur (25)
			2								52	Borgarnes (13)
		1	5								51	Breiðumýrar (42)
											15	Búða (55)
											18	Búðardals (16)
		4	5	4	37	30	17	9	11	5	239	Dalvíkur (39)
											2	Djúpavíkur (30)
											14	Djúpavogs (56)
											44	Egilsstaða (49)
											3	Eskifjarðar (54)
		1									75	Eyrarbakka (7)
5	2	3	5								53	Flateyrar (22)
8		2	3	1		5					40	Grenivíkur (38)
											14	Hafnar (57)
3				3							254	Hafnarfjarðar (3)
		1	10	6							35	Hofsós (36)
											2	Hólmavíkur (31)
				2							60	Húsavíkur (43)
											16	Hvammstanga (32)
5	50	70	4								200	Ísafjarðar (24)
											135	Keflavíkur (10)
											36	Kirkjubæjar (58)
											13	Kleppjárnsreykja (12)
14	2	1									98	Kópaskers (44)
		2	8								18	Laugarás (6)
											6	Nes (53)
32	56	9									160	Ólafsfjarðar (40)
											11	Ólafsvíkur (15)
	1										1	Patreksfjarðar (19)
											8	Reykhóla (17)
6	6	2									1172	Reykjavíkur (1)
	1	64	27	10							122	Sauðárkróks (35)
											22	Selfoss (8)
											16	Seyðisfjarðar (52)
			1								170	Siglufjarðar (37)
		1	11	4							193	Stórólfshvols (60)
											5	Stykkishólms (14)
						4					4	Súðavíkur (28)
1						2					256	Vestmannaeyja (63)
		1									96	Víkur (59)
											42	Vopnafjarðar (47)
											22	Þingeyrar (21)
											110	Þórshafnar (46)
79	193	318	187	58	49	41	17	9	11	5	4791	Iceland (Total)

Wave IX: *January 1950 to March 1952*

District	Month: 1/50	2/50	3/50	4/50	5/50	6/50	7/50	8/50	9/50	10/50	11/50	12/50	1/51	
Akranes (11)														
Akureyrar (41)												1	6	
Álafoss (5)					6						4	7	2	
Bíldudals (20)														
Blönduós (33)						1	15	27	73	20	11	15	34	
Bolungarvíkur (25)														
Borgarnes (13)						4								
Breiðumýrar (42)												1	15	
Búða (55)														
Búðardals (16)							1							
Dalvíkur (39)					1									
Djúpavíkur (30)														
Djúpavogs (56)												10	1	
Egilsstaða (49)												1	7	
Eskifjarðar (54)														
Eyrarbakka (7)						1						1		
Flateyjar (18)														
Flateyrar (22)														
Hafnar (57)												7		
Hafnarfjarðar (3)						2	13	8	5		3	2	15	
Hofsós (36)									2	6	20	38	6	
Hólmavíkur (31)									2	43	35	7		
Húsavíkur (43)												31	3	
Hvammstanga (32)					1	3	3		2	4	29	15		
Ísafjarðar (24)					1									
Keflavíkur (10)			1					1	21	14	9	3	4	
Kirkjubæjar (58)														
Kleppjárnsreykja (12)														
Kópaskers (44)												6	6	
Laugarás (6)														
Nes (53)														
Ólafsvíkur (15)							11							
Patreksfjarðar (19)														
Reykhóla (17)											8	12		
Reykjavíkur (1)		47	1		10	7	5			1	15	152	569	68
Sauðárkróks (35)												1	1	
Selfoss (8)							5	9				1		
Seyðisfjarðar (52)													1	
Siglufjarðar (37)							1	1						
Stórólfshvols (60)				5	10							7		
Stykkishólms (14)						1								
Súðavíkur (28)				1	3									
Vestmannaeyja (63)						4	7	10				5	6	5
Víkur (59)														
Vopnafjarðar (47)												1	3	
Þingeyrar (21)	1										1	2		
Iceland (Total)	1	47	2	6	32	23	61	56	105	88	135	326	679	85

51	4/51	5/51	6/51	7/51	8/51	9/51	10/51	11/51	12/51	1/52	2/52	3/52	Total	District
8	44	33	22	27	8								143	Akranes (11)
4	1	1	6	5	1		2	1					34	Akureyrar (41)
0	7	14	5	1									58	Álafoss (5)
4	1		2										7	Bíldudals (20)
				1	11	2							211	Blönduós (33)
				3	28	26	4	7					68	Bolungarvíkur (25)
			7										11	Borgarnes (13)
				1									86	Breiðumýrar (42)
				22	28	12	10	6	4				82	Búða (55)
			6	45	1								53	Búðardals (16)
													1	Dalvíkur (39)
			3	3	1								7	Djúpavíkur (30)
				5	1	2							19	Djúpavogs (56)
			1	1									10	Egilsstaða (49)
			5	4	7	5	17	40	102				180	Eskifjarðar (54)
		2											4	Eyrarbakka (7)
				19	5								24	Flateyjar (18)
						1	16	10	6	9	12	2	56	Flateyrar (22)
1		4	5										17	Hafnar (57)
77	28	112	137	37	1								458	Hafnarfjarðar (3)
		10		18	18				7				125	Hofsós (36)
													87	Hólmavíkur (31)
													34	Húsavíkur (43)
													57	Hvammstanga (32)
		10	16	3	4								34	Ísafjarðar (24)
30	31	35	22	30	17	10	12	2					255	Keflavíkur (10)
			30	4	1								35	Kirkjubæjar (58)
		1	7		2								10	Kleppjárnsreykja (12)
				1									13	Kópaskers (44)
7	2	5	9										25	Laugarás (6)
			2	30	19	5							56	Nes (53)
5	100	37			3								156	Ólafsvíkur (15)
			4	7	7	18	8	5					49	Patreksfjarðar (19)
		10	2	7	11								50	Reykhóla (17)
752	720	284	80	27	25	8	8						3395	Reykjavíkur (1)
				25	5	5							37	Sauðárkróks (35)
10	7	45	34	17									128	Selfoss (8)
35	54	22	1										113	Seyðisfjarðar (52)
				7	8	8	9	4	14				52	Siglufjarðar (37)
1	3	1	8	4	8								47	Stórólfshvols (60)
			6	10	23	11			8	3			62	Stykkishólms (14)
		4	13	6									27	Súðavíkur (28)
77	53	9											226	Vestmannaeyja (63)
				1	10	18							29	Víkur (59)
			1										5	Vopnafjarðar (47)
			3	1				1					9	Þingeyrar (21)
021	1051	639	437	372	253	131	86	76	141	12	12	2	6645	Iceland (Total)

Wave X: *July 1952 to April 1953*

District	Month:	7/52	8/52	9/52	10/52
Akranes (11)			2		
Akureyrar (41)				2	39
Blönduós (33)					
Breiðumýrar (42)					1
Búða (55)					4
Dalvíkur (39)					
Djúpavogs (56)					1
Egilsstaða (49)		15	41	55	26
Eskifjarðar (54)		1	9	33	33
Grenivíkur (38)					
Hafnar (57)				4	94
Hofsós (36)					
Húsavíkur (43)					
Ísafjarðar (24)					
Kópaskers (44)		1	4		41
Nes (53)		1			
Ólafsfjarðar (40)					
Reykjavíkur (1)			3	2	2
Sauðárkróks (35)					
Selfoss (8)					2
Seyðisfjarðar (52)		14	66	21	5
Siglufjarðar (37)					
Stórólfshvols (60)					2
Iceland (Total)		32	125	117	250

/52	1/53	2/53	3/53	4/53	Total	District
					2	Akranes (11)
8	117	32	15	20	792	Akureyrar (41)
1					1	Blönduós (33)
					1	Breiðumýrar (42)
					4	Búða (55)
6	66	26			98	Dalvíkur (39)
					4	Djúpavogs (56)
18					328	Egilsstaða (49)
					94	Eskifjarðar (54)
12	27	10	10	28	87	Grenivíkur (38)
4					236	Hafnar (57)
6					6	Hofsós (36)
	21	1			22	Húsavíkur (43)
1	4				5	Ísafjarðar (24)
	3				49	Kópaskers (44)
5	3				9	Nes (53)
1	1				2	Ólafsfjarðar (40)
3	1				12	Reykjavíkur (1)
1	5				6	Sauðárkróks (35)
			1		3	Selfoss (8)
					107	Seyðisfjarðar (52)
1					2	Siglufjarðar (37)
					2	Stórólfshvols (60)
347	248	69	26	48	1872	Iceland (Total)

Wave XI: *March 1954 to November 1955*

District	Month:	3/54	4/54	5/54	6/54	7/54	8/54	9/54	10/54	11/54	12/54	
Akranes (11)		3	71	66	89	33	8	2	4	7	3	
Akureyrar (41)						1	2		5		10	
Álafoss (5)							5	9	14	11	6	
Bakkagerðis (48)								1	9			
Blönduós (33)						7	3	5	57	17	4	
Bolungarvíkur (25)									16	57	14	
Borgarnes (13)					3	5	2	10	67	8		
Breiðumýrar (42)								1	2			
Búða (55)									2			
Búðardals (16)									2	5		
Dalvíkur (39)										1	5	
Djúpavogs (56)												
Egilsstaða (49)									13	11	18	
Eskifjarðar (54)							1					
Eyrarbakka (7)							4	16	85	54	5	
Flateyjar (18)									4	1		
Flateyrar (22)							19	18	5		1	
Hafnar (57)											2	
Hafnarfjarðar (3)				8	11	9	7	18	90	172	86	
Hofsós (36)								16	18	11	8	
Hólmavíkur (31)								33	24	18	5	
Húsavíkur (43)							1	2	24	9		
Hvammstanga (32)						5		6	30	9	2	
Ísafjarðar (24)					1	3	15	12	18	11	10	
Keflavíkur (10)				19	29	13	37	75	56	21	13	
Kirkjubæjar (58)										7	4	
Kleppjárnsreykja (12)								4	27	48	6	
Kópaskers (44)								7	56	19	3	
Laugarás (6)						14	12		8	15	8	
Nes (53)							1					
Ólafsfjarðar (40)										1	10	10
Ólafsvíkur (15)					1	1	1	1	68	6	8	
Patreksfjarðar (19)						2		11	12			
Reykhóla (17)									1	3		
Reykjavíkur (1)				3	26	28	91	380	917	878	290	2
Sauðárkróks (35)								80	120	71	4	
Selfoss (8)							28	100	90	58	15	
Seyðisfjarðar (52)										1	1	
Siglufjarðar (37)								2	5	197	109	
Stórólfshvols (60)						16	7	38	24	37	33	2
Stykkishólms (14)								5	78	79	10	
Súðavíkur (28)											1	
Vestmannaeyja (63)								4	17	21	165	2
Víkur (59)									12	38	65	3
Vopnafjarðar (47)					5	2	3			1	46	1
Þingeyrar (21)				1	5	10	10	4		4	9	2
Þórshafnar (46)								1	9	57	33	
Iceland (Total)		3	71	97	170	149	257	861	1989	1964	1012	30

5	3/55	4/55	5/55	6/55	7/55	8/55	9/55	10/55	11/55	Total	District
										286	Akranes (11)
3				3			19	2	1	52	Akureyrar (41)
										45	Álafoss (5)
			3	23	5	4	4			49	Bakkagerðis (48)
										93	Blönduós (33)
										87	Bolungarvíkur (25)
										95	Borgarnes (13)
			7	28	8	6	2			54	Breiðumýrar (42)
			16	28	18	7				71	Búða (55)
										7	Búðardals (16)
3	9	9								66	Dalvíkur (39)
			11	16						27	Djúpavogs (56)
										44	Egilsstaða (49)
						5				6	Eskifjarðar (54)
										164	Eyrarbakka (7)
										5	Flateyjar (18)
										43	Flateyrar (22)
										2	Hafnar (57)
										403	Hafnarfjarðar (3)
										64	Hofsós (36)
										80	Hólmavíkur (31)
			11	216	69	11				343	Húsavíkur (43)
					1					54	Hvammstanga (32)
	2									76	Ísafjarðar (24)
5										274	Keflavíkur (10)
										11	Kirkjubæjar (58)
										86	Kleppjárnsreykja (12)
				2	1					88	Kópaskers (44)
										57	Laugarás (6)
										1	Nes (53)
24										137	Ólafsfjarðar (40)
										92	Ólafsvíkur (15)
										25	Patreksfjarðar (19)
										4	Reykhóla (17)
13	1		6	2	1	3				2663	Reykjavíkur (1)
					1					276	Sauðárkróks (35)
3										295	Selfoss (8)
										2	Seyðisfjarðar (52)
										314	Siglufjarðar (37)
16	32	2	3							235	Stórólfshvols (60)
							18	30	21	241	Stykkishólms (14)
										1	Súðavíkur (28)
9	3	5	13	3						266	Vestmannaeyja (63)
61										215	Víkur (59)
9	9	4								94	Vopnafjarðar (47)
19	5									93	Þingeyrar (21)
				1						101	Þórshafnar (46)
195	61	20	70	322	104	36	43	32	22	7787	Iceland (Total)

Wave XII: *March 1958 to December 1959*

District	Month: 3/58	4/58	5/58	6/58	7/58	8/58	9/58	10/58	11/58	12/58
Akranes (11)					3	1			8	71
Akureyrar (41)								1	46	127
Álafoss (5)										20
Bíldudals (20)										8
Blönduós (33)										17
Bolungarvíkur (25)										
Borgarnes (13)										12
Breiðumýrar (42)										1
Búða (55)										1
Búðardals (16)					11	9			5	9
Dalvíkur (39)										1
Djúpavíkur (30)										
Djúpavogs (56)										
Egilsstaða (49)	10								1	4
Eskifjarðar (54)										
Eyrarbakka (7)										
Flateyjar (18)										
Flateyrar (22)										2
Grenivíkur (38)									1	
Hafnar (57)										1
Hafnarfjarðar (3)								8	22	107
Hofsós (36)										11
Hólmavíkur (31)									4	1
Húsavíkur (43)										1
Hvammstanga (32)										12
Ísafjarðar (24)										5
Keflavíkur (10)								2	27	68
Kirkjubæjar (58)										2
Kleppjárnsreykja (12)				1	10	1	3		37	7
Kópaskers (44)										
Laugarás (6)									8	9
Nes (53)										2
Ólafsfjarðar (40)									1	
Ólafsvíkur (15)									3	2
Patreksfjarðar (19)										3
Reykhóla (17)										1
Reykjavíkur (1)		1	1		1	2	22	104	774	981
Sauðárkróks (35)										5
Selfoss (8)						2		4		36
Seyðisfjarðar (52)										
Siglufjarðar (37)										
Stórólfshvols (60)							1	2	9	17
Stykkishólms (14)										6
Súðavíkur (28)										1
Vestmannaeyja (63)										
Víkur (59)										4
Þingeyrar (21)										
Þórshafnar (46)										
Iceland (Total)	10	1	1	1	25	15	26	121	946	1555

2/59	3/59	4/59	5/59	6/59	7/59	8/59	9/59	10/59	11/59	12/59	Total	District
81	18	6									374	Akranes (11)
95	116	34									610	Akureyrar (41)
3	2										36	Álafoss (5)
50											111	Bíldudals (20)
	2	10									49	Blönduós (33)
		14	9	5			1				29	Bolungarvíkur (25)
											12	Borgarnes (13)
1	3	1									10	Breiðumýrar (42)
2	2										12	Búða (55)
											45	Búðardals (16)
38	58	11									117	Dalvíkur (39)
		2									2	Djúpavíkur (30)
1											1	Djúpavogs (56)
62											128	Egilsstaða (49)
		1	19	32	30	17	1				100	Eskifjarðar (54)
14	2	3	4								53	Eyrarbakka (7)
					10	7					17	Flateyjar (18)
2	1	5	11		18	7	10	13			71	Flateyrar (22)
											5	Grenivíkur (38)
	7	8	11								29	Hafnar (57)
82	11	1									451	Hafnarfjarðar (3)
1				1	1						21	Hofsós (36)
3			7								16	Hólmavíkur (31)
	3					1					9	Húsavíkur (43)
53	62	19	1								205	Hvammstanga (32)
27	185	166	51	4							444	Ísafjarðar (24)
25	24		16				1	1			221	Keflavíkur (10)
1											3	Kirkjubæjar (58)
8	3										80	Kleppjárnsreykja (12)
7											10	Kópaskers (44)
33											98	Laugarás (6)
51	203	43	13								312	Nes (53)
											1	Ólafsfjarðar (40)
36	8	9	10								85	Ólafsvíkur (15)
		2									20	Patreksfjarðar (19)
											7	Reykhóla (17)
114	29	22	8	2	2	1	1	2		2	2551	Reykjavíkur (1)
13	8	10	16	14	4						98	Sauðárkróks (35)
4	16										96	Selfoss (8)
											2	Seyðisfjarðar (52)
	1		1								2	Siglufjarðar (37)
29	30	25									134	Stórólfshvols (60)
	20	12									46	Stykkishólms (14)
	2	10	19	5							41	Súðavíkur (28)
110	134	38	3			1					291	Vestmannaeyja (63)
8	3										26	Víkur (59)
1											12	Þingeyrar (21)
						1	4	4			9	Þórshafnar (46)
955	953	452	199	63	65	35	18	20		2	7102	Iceland (Total)

Wave XIII: *April 1962 to May 1964*

District	Month: 4/62	5/62	6/62	7/62	8/62	9/62	10/62	11/62	12/62	1/63	2/63	3/63	4[illegible]
Akranes (11)								4	40	182		7	
Akureyrar (41)						5		2	5	24	85	169	1
Álafoss (5)						4	14	30	37	27	14	6	
Bakkagerðis (48)									1	12			
Blönduós (33)				1	6	22	91	4	2	4			
Bolungarvíkur (25)													
Borgarnes (13)								3	2	2			
Breiðumýrar (42)					6				1	69	11		
Búða (55)								4				14	2
Búðardals (16)								7	7	15	1	8	
Dalvíkur (39)						3	2		4			1	
Djúpavogs (56)												6	1
Egilsstaða (49)					1		2	15			5		
Eskifjarðar (54)					2	5	14	34	1	2		2	
Eyrarbakka (7)				2	2	1	2	2	16	20	22	15	
Flateyrar (22)									1				
Grenivíkur (38)										1			
Hafnar (57)						1	2		2				
Hafnarfjarðar (3)		1		2				14	78	134	23	18	
Hofsós (36)						4	21	8	15	23			
Hólmavíkur (31)					7				1				
Húsavíkur (43)					5		6	2	3	33	67	3	
Hvammstanga (32)			1						2				
Ísafjarðar (24)													
Keflavíkur (10)					4	9	49	53	57	70	32	15	1
Kirkjubæjar (58)									3	1			
Kleppjárnsreykja (12)				6	3					6	13		
Kópaskers (44)				1	58	74	35	21	4		1	2	
Laugarás (6)									9	7	12	32	1
Ólafsvíkur (15)								5		1	16	41	25
Patreksfjarðar (19)									1	1	2	2	2
Reykhóla (17)		1	8	3	4								
Reykjavíkur (1)	1	12	3	11	17	17	191	557	1043	813	269	92	53
Sauðárkróks (35)				4					6				
Selfoss (8)								8	30	171	139	9	3
Seyðisfjarðar (52)													115
Siglufjarðar (37)									2	3	3		
Stórólfshvols (60)							5	16	23	9	15	24	30
Stykkishólms (14)									2	22	39	56	4
Vestmannaeyja (63)			1	1	2	3	24	42	29	3	3		
Víkur (59)							1	38	6	3	13	10	
Vopnafjarðar (47)						3						1	5
Þórshafnar (46)					16	7							3
Iceland (Total)	1	14	13	31	133	158	459	869	1433	1658	785	533	445

/63	6/63	7/63	8/63	9/63	10/63	11/63	12/63	1/64	2/64	3/64	4/64	5/64	Total	District
													236	Akranes (11)
55	55	23	4										542	Akureyrar (41)
													132	Álafoss (5)
													13	Bakkagerðis (48)
													131	Blönduós (33)
		45	15								4		64	Bolungarvíkur (25)
													7	Borgarnes (13)
													87	Breiðumýrar (42)
16	7												67	Búða (55)
													43	Búðardals (16)
8	27	77	3										134	Dalvíkur (39)
9													27	Djúpavogs (56)
	1												24	Egilsstaða (49)
													64	Eskifjarðar (54)
													87	Eyrarbakka (7)
													1	Flateyrar (22)
3	1												5	Grenivíkur (38)
													5	Hafnar (57)
													271	Hafnarfjarðar (3)
													71	Hofsós (36)
													8	Hólmavíkur (31)
													119	Húsavíkur (43)
													3	Hvammstanga (32)
		6	10	31	24	24	19	52	94	21	77	2	360	Ísafjarðar (24)
6													309	Keflavíkur (10)
													4	Kirkjubæjar (58)
													28	Kleppjárnsreykja (12)
1													197	Kópaskers (44)
													70	Laugarás (6)
													88	Ólafsvíkur (15)
													8	Patreksfjarðar (19)
													16	Reykhóla (17)
5			1	4		2		1		2	1		3095	Reykjavíkur (1)
				1									11	Sauðárkróks (35)
2													362	Selfoss (8)
38	1												154	Seyðisfjarðar (52)
1													9	Siglufjarðar (37)
14	2	1											139	Stórólfshvols (60)
													123	Stykkishólms (14)
													108	Vestmannaeyja (63)
													71	Víkur (59)
													9	Vopnafjarðar (47)
27	26	20	4										103	Þórshafnar (46)
185	120	172	37	36	24	26	19	53	94	23	82	2	7405	Iceland (Total)

Wave XIV: *November 1966 to August 1968*

District	Month: 11/66	12/66	1/67	2/67	3/67	4/67	5/67	6/67	7/67	8/67	9/
Akranes (11)		2	2	1	45	125		11			
Akureyrar (41)			5	16	12	45	20	22	7	11	
Álafoss (5)		2	2	1	26	22	4	4	1		
Bíldudals (20)							1				
Blönduós (33)					17	53	51	4			
Bolungarvíkur (25)			2	10	5	1		3	1		
Borgarnes (13)				9	6	15	31	39		2	
Búða (55)			1	4							
Búðardals (16)			9	9	5						
Dalvíkur (39)						1	7	14		8	
Djúpavogs (56)				4		1					
Egilsstaða (49)				6	8	21	31				
Eskifjarðar (54)								1			
Eyrarbakka (7)				4	17		15				
Flateyrar (22)								9	20	9	
Grenivíkur (38)			2	1			1	3			
Hafnar (57)	3	14				1					
Hafnarfjarðar (3)		7	36	79	103	118		20	8	1	
Hofsós (36)				24	3	4	8	1	1		
Hólmavíkur (31)			1	2			2				
Húsavíkur (43)							6	5	2		
Hvammstanga (32)		1	2			1		5			
Ísafjarðar (24)				3	24	35	16	23	12	7	7
Keflavíkur (10)		5		24	38	46	62	27	43	34	12
Kirkjubæjar (58)			1	15	14			8			
Kleppjárnsreykja (12)			1	3			4				
Kópaskers (44)								2			
Laugarás (6)	1	3	1	2		2		16	5		
Ólafsfjarðar (40)								19	7	6	
Ólafsvíkur (15)						3	14	18	47	20	8
Patreksfjarðar (19)					1	2	26	8	2		
Reykhóla (17)				2	13						
Reykjavíkur (1)	6	124	328	433	899	507	244	81	12	5	7
Sauðárkróks (35)				10	49	60	41				
Selfoss (8)			8	8	12	25	23	8	5		
Seyðisfjarðar (52)					2	11	11	16	17		
Siglufjarðar (37)		2	67	194	77	5			4	2	
Stórólfshvols (60)		2		3	4	17	41	10	5	1	
Stykkishólms (14)					35	71	4	1			
Súðavíkur (28)					1	3	9	2	3	2	
Vestmannaeyja (63)				28	115	120	41	22	9	1	
Víkur (59)			1			3	15	12			
Vopnafjarðar (47)							11	11	5	27	13
Þingeyrar (21)					13	28	10				
Þórshafnar (46)					2						
Iceland (Total)	10	162	469	895	1546	1346	749	425	216	136	55

/67	11/67	12/67	1/68	2/68	3/68	4/68	5/68	6/68	7/68	8/68	Total	District
											186	Akranes (11)
2											143	Akureyrar (41)
						19		20			101	Álafoss (5)
											1	Bíldudals (20)
											125	Blönduós (33)
											22	Bolungarvíkur (25)
											102	Borgarnes (13)
											5	Búða (55)
									1		24	Búðardals (16)
											30	Dalvíkur (39)
											5	Djúpavogs (56)
											66	Egilsstaða (49)
											1	Eskifjarðar (54)
											36	Eyrarbakka (7)
											42	Flateyrar (22)
											7	Grenivíkur (38)
											18	Hafnar (57)
		5		3						1	381	Hafnarfjarðar (3)
											42	Hofsós (36)
											5	Hólmavíkur (31)
											13	Húsavíkur (43)
											9	Hvammstanga (32)
											127	Ísafjarðar (24)
											291	Keflavíkur (10)
											38	Kirkjubæjar (58)
							5				13	Kleppjárnsreykja (12)
											2	Kópaskers (44)
											30	Laugarás (6)
											32	Ólafsfjarðar (40)
	11										121	Ólafsvíkur (15)
											39	Patreksfjarðar (19)
											15	Reykhóla (17)
1	6	7	42	14	1					2	2719	Reykjavíkur (1)
											160	Sauðárkróks (35)
											89	Selfoss (8)
											57	Seyðisfjarðar (52)
											351	Siglufjarðar (37)
											83	Stórólfshvols (60)
											111	Stykkishólms (14)
											20	Súðavíkur (28)
											336	Vestmannaeyja (63)
											31	Víkur (59)
3											70	Vopnafjarðar (47)
											51	Þingeyrar (21)
											2	Þórshafnar (46)
6	17	12	42	17	1	19	5	20	1	3	6152	Iceland (Total)

Wave XV: *October 1968 to December 1970*

District	Month: 10/68	11/68	12/68	1/69	2/69	3/69	4/69	5/69	6/69	7/69	8/69	9/69	10/69	11/69
Akranes (11)											1			
Akureyrar (41)										3	38	108	232	[illegible]
Álafoss (5)			2	6	1					4	3			
Bakkagerðis (48)												13		
Blönduós (33)										2		14	1	
Bolungarvíkur (25)										3	7	9	15	[illegible]
Borgarnes (13)												1		
Breiðumýrar (42)					27						18	25	20	[illegible]
Búða (55)										2	12			
Búðardals (16)														
Dalvíkur (39)											1	3	10	[illegible]
Djúpavíkur (30)														
Djúpavogs (56)														
Egilsstaða (49)										9	19	17	22	
Eskifjarðar (54)									37	35	83	43	49	[illegible]
Eyrarbakka (7)						2		1						
Flateyrar (22)									14	8			17	
Grenivíkur (38)													3	
Hafnar (57)							3			1	10	35	5	
Hafnarfjarðar (3)							1		17	34	13	14	25	3
Hofsós (36)		1												
Hólmavíkur (31)														1
Húsavíkur (43)										1	17	38	58	[illegible]
Hvammstanga (32)										1	5			
Ísafjarðar (24)										15	12	18	45	[illegible]
Keflavíkur (10)							4	2	2	10	13	28	50	[illegible]
Kleppjárnsreykja (12)										1	2			
Laugarás (6)					1	7	2	3		2				
Ólafsfjarðar (40)										1	3	6	14	[illegible]
Patreksfjarðar (19)														
Reykhóla (17)								9						
Reykjavíkur (1)	4	14	12	16	10	2	4	24	17	58	29	55	57	[illegible]
Sauðárkróks (35)											5	7	1	
Selfoss (8)				50	48	35	11		8			2		
Seyðisfjarðar (52)											15	14	11	6
Siglufjarðar (37)								1	1		1	2	1	
Stórólfshvols (60)							4							
Stykkishólms (14)									1					
Súðavíkur (28)													10	
Vestmannaeyja (63)										1	3	41	63	23
Vopnafjarðar (47)												1	2	
Þingeyrar (21)												1		
Þórshafnar (46)										1	11	5	22	18
Iceland (Total)	4	15	14	72	87	46	29	40	97	192	321	500	733	452

/69	1/70	2/70	3/70	4/70	5/70	6/70	7/70	8/70	9/70	10/70	11/70	12/70	Total	District
1	2	6	39	37	56	9							151	Akranes (11)
32	7												512	Akureyrar (41)
17	7	1	1	7		6							62	Álafoss (5)
													13	Bakkagerðis (48)
													22	Blönduós (33)
6	22			7	6								98	Bolungarvíkur (25)
				3		2							6	Borgarnes (13)
													109	Breiðumýrar (42)
													14	Búða (55)
1				1	4	3							9	Búðardals (16)
13													38	Dalvíkur (39)
						1	6						7	Djúpavíkur (30)
						2							2	Djúpavogs (56)
							1						68	Egilsstaða (49)
29													301	Eskifjarðar (54)
2					4	2	1		2				14	Eyrarbakka (7)
							7	4					57	Flateyrar (22)
	1	2											7	Grenivíkur (38)
								1					55	Hafnar (57)
7	7		1	7	11	2	4		2	1			180	Hafnarfjarðar (3)
													1	Hofsós (36)
11									1	12			39	Hólmavíkur (31)
													134	Húsavíkur (43)
	3				3								12	Hvammstanga (32)
5		3	1	4			1						131	Ísafjarðar (24)
20	16	22			1	2					2		224	Keflavíkur (10)
													3	Kleppjárnsreykja (12)
	5	4							1				25	Laugarás (6)
													29	Ólafsfjarðar (40)
					3	2							5	Patreksfjarðar (19)
													9	Reykhóla (17)
116	66	28	23	67	52	26	21	4	3	1	3	2	776	Reykjavíkur (1)
			1	1						3			18	Sauðárkróks (35)
	3	3						5	11				176	Selfoss (8)
													46	Seyðisfjarðar (52)
													6	Siglufjarðar (37)
		1				4	5	5					19	Stórólfshvols (60)
													1	Stykkishólms (14)
2	6	10	8	2									38	Súðavíkur (28)
14													145	Vestmannaeyja (63)
													3	Vopnafjarðar (47)
			2										3	Þingeyrar (21)
													57	Þórshafnar (46)
276	145	80	76	136	140	61	46	19	20	17	5	2	3625	Iceland (Total)

Wave XVI: *October 1972 to January 1974*

District Month:	10/72	11/72	12/72	1/73	2/73	3/73	4/73	5/73
Akranes (11)				4	4	12		[illegible]
Akureyrar (41)					37	45	50	[illegible]
Álafoss (5)	2		4	2	26	57	29	
Bakkagerðis (48)							1	
Bíldudals (20)						8		
Blönduós (33)						4	5	
Bolungarvíkur (25)				1				
Borgarnes (13)		1		1	17	50	21	
Breiðumýrar (42)				1	6			
Búða (55)				2	2			1
Dalvíkur (39)							1	2
Egilsstaða (49)						12	65	1
Eskifjarðar (54)							1	
Eyrarbakka (7)				3	6	26	15	
Grenivíkur (38)					6	7	3	
Hafnar (57)								
Hafnarfjarðar (3)			20	96	163	79	5	[illegible]
Hellu (62)				12	9	1		
Höfða (34)							15	[illegible]
Hofsós (36)					5		8	[illegible]
Hólmavíkur (31)					2			
Húsavíkur (43)					12	11	4	
Hvammstanga (32)					3	4		[illegible]
Hveragerðis (9)				13	14	43	19	[illegible]
Hvols (61)					4	4	16	13
Ísafjarðar (24)				4	10	7	8	
Keflavíkur (10)				12	39	50	40	25
Kleppjárnsreykja (12)				7	72	76		
Kópaskers (44)					6			
Kópavogs (2)			10	29	42	13		1
Laugarás (6)			7	2	12	11	2	4
Ólafsfjarðar (40)								
Ólafsvíkur (15)					30	36	14	8
Patreksfjarðar (19)					9	21		18
Reykjavíkur (1)			27	333	362	144	50	10
Sauðárkróks (35)					3	8	41	31
Selfoss (8)				34	43	46	35	5
Seyðisfjarðar (52)					1	28	25	8
Siglufjarðar (37)								1
Stykkishólms (14)				2	32	73	14	5
Súðavíkur (28)							4	2
Suðureyrar (23)					1			
Víkur (59)			1	1				8
Vopnafjarðar (47)					1	12	12	
Þórshafnar (46)								17
Iceland (Total)	2	1	69	559	979	888	503	331

3	7/73	8/73	9/73	10/73	11/73	12/73	1/74	Total	District
3	3							83	Akranes (11)
8	15	9				1		189	Akureyrar (41)
1				3			1	131	Álafoss (5)
								1	Bakkagerðis (48)
	3	1						12	Bíldudals (20)
7				9	19	14		63	Blönduós (33)
								1	Bolungarvíkur (25)
2						1		95	Borgarnes (13)
								7	Breiðumýrar (42)
								18	Búða (55)
25	25	3	3					84	Dalvíkur (39)
2								97	Egilsstaða (49)
								1	Eskifjarðar (54)
								50	Eyrarbakka (7)
								16	Grenivíkur (38)
2	7							9	Hafnar (57)
		2		3	1			376	Hafnarfjarðar (3)
		1						23	Hellu (62)
3					3	5		31	Höfða (34)
	6				2	3		32	Hofsós (36)
			59	8				69	Hólmavíkur (31)
			3				1	31	Húsavíkur (43)
39	6		8	18	2			97	Hvammstanga (32)
								94	Hveragerðis (9)
2	1		1	1				42	Hvols (61)
		10						39	Ísafjarðar (24)
9					4			179	Keflavíkur (10)
								155	Kleppjárnsreykja (12)
								6	Kópaskers (44)
2								97	Kópavogs (2)
								38	Laugarás (6)
34	15	6						55	Ólafsfjarðar (40)
								88	Ólafsvíkur (15)
		1						49	Patreksfjarðar (19)
7	1		2					936	Reykjavíkur (1)
5	2			7	8			105	Sauðárkróks (35)
								163	Selfoss (8)
								62	Seyðisfjarðar (52)
21	31	1			14			68	Siglufjarðar (37)
						5	2	133	Stykkishólms (14)
			1					6	Súðavíkur (28)
								2	Suðureyrar (23)
								10	Víkur (59)
								25	Vopnafjarðar (47)
30	38							85	Þórshafnar (46)
222	153	34	77	49	53	29	4	3953	Iceland (Total)

Printed Data Sources, References and Author Index

The list which follows is divided into two parts, A – printed data sources, and B – references and author index. In B, the surnames of Icelandic authors have been given in both the Icelandic and Anglicised forms, and Christian names of these authors have been spelled out in full. This convention has been followed to allow works to be traced in Icelandic libraries, where the card indexes list Christian names first. Numbers in brackets after names refer to sections of the book in which the author is cited.

A Printed data sources

Epidemiological

Skýslur um heilbrigði manna á Íslandi árin
1881–90 (Report on public health in Iceland, 1881–90). Reykjavík, reprinted 1965, 132 pp; *1891–5* (with supplementary tables for 1896–1900) (reprinted, 1961), 115 pp; *1896* (1897), 10 pp; *1897* (1899), 15 pp; *1898* (1900), 9 pp; *1899* (1901), 12 pp; *1900* (1903), 7 pp.

Skýrslur um heilsufar og heilbrigðismálefni á Íslandi
1901 og 1904 (Report on the state of sanitation and public health in Iceland for the years 1901 to 1904). Reykjavík, 1941, 111 pp; *1905–6* (no date), 69 pp; *1907–8* (no date), 42 pp; *1909–10* (no date), 39 pp.

Heilbrigðisskýrslur 1911–20 (Public health in Iceland, 1911–20).
Reykjavík, 1922 486 pp (I–CVI, 1–200, 1*–180*); *1921–5* (1927), 351 pp (1*–XII*, I–LXIX, 1–106, 1*–164*); *1926* (1928), 90 pp; *1927* (1928), 92 pp; *1928* (1929), 110 pp; *1929* (1931), 138 pp; *1930* (1932), 131 pp; *1931* (1933), 146 pp; *1932* (1934), 153 pp; *1933* (1935), 187 pp; *1934* (1936), 153 pp; *1935* (1938), 219 pp; *1936* (1939), 187 pp; *1937* (1940), 175 pp; *1938* (1940), 196 pp; *1939* (1941), 196 pp; *1940* (1943), 216 pp; *1941* (1945), 200 pp; *1942* (1946), 258 pp; *1943* (1947), 214 pp; *1944* (1947), 215 pp; *1945* (1949), 270 pp; *1946* (1950), 243 pp; *1947* (1951), 259 pp; *1948* (1952), 261 pp; *1949* (1953), 303 pp; *1950* (1954), 303 pp; *1951* (1955), 248 pp; *1952* (1955), 213 pp; *1953* (1956), 218 pp; *1954* (1957), 224 pp; *1955* (1958), 228 pp; *1956* (1959), 225 pp; *1957* (1960), 183 pp; *1958* (1962), 197 pp; *1959* (1963), 240 pp; *1960* (1964), 186 pp; *1961* (1965), 181 pp; *1962* (1965), 204 pp; *1963* (1966), 227 pp; *1964* (1967), 171 pp; *1965* (1968), 182 pp; *1966* (1969), 190 pp; *1967* (1970), 180 pp; *1968* (1971), 168 pp; *1969* (1972), 171 pp; *1970* (1973), 172 pp; *1971* (1974), 150 pp; *1972* (1976), 139 pp; *1973* (1977), 202 pp; *1974* (1978), 154 pp.

Demographic

Manntal á Íslandi árið 1703 (Population census of Iceland, 1703). Reykjavík, 1923–47; *1 nóvember 1901* (1904), 102 pp; *1 desember 1910* (1913), 17 + 198 pp; *1 desember 1920* (1926–8), 68 + 158 pp; *2 desember 1930* (1937), 67 + 169 pp; *2 desember 1940* (1949), 53 + 181 pp; *1 desember 1950* (1958), 77 + 196 pp;

Mannfjöldaskýrslur árin 1911–15 (Population and vital statistics, 1911–15). Reykjavík, 1921, 39 + 71 pp; *1916–20* (1928), 72 pp; *1921–5* (1929),

38 + 64 pp; *1926–30* (1933), 36 + 64 pp; *1931–5* (1938), 35 + 60 pp; *1936–40* (1946), 57 pp; *1941–50* (1952), 46 + 132 pp; *1951–60* (1963), 41 + 92 pp; *1961–70* (1975), 60 + 140 pp.

Other

Barnafræðsla árin 1909–14 (Primary education, 1909–14). Reykjavík 1922, 33 pp; *1914–15* (1918), 44 pp; *1916–20* (1920–3), 71 pp.

Barnafræðsluskýrslur árin 1920–66 (Primary education, 1920–66). Reykjavík, 1967, 81 pp.

Tölfræðihandbók (Statistical abstract of Iceland). Reykjavík, 1967, 16 + 367 pp; 1974, 12 + 253 pp.

B References and author index

Abbey, J. (1952). 'An examination of the Reed–Frost theory of Epidemics.' *Human Biology*, **24,** 201–33. (1.3.2, 7.1)

Abler, R., Adams, J. S. & Gould, P. R. (1972). *Spatial Organisation: the Geographer's View of the World.* Englewood Cliffs: Prentice-Hall. (2.2.5)

Alter, M. (1977). 'Is multiple sclerosis an age-dependent host response to measles?' *Neuologia-Neuocirugia-Psiquiatria,* **18,** 341–55. (8.3.1)

Alves, W. R. (1974). 'Comment on Hudson's 'Diffusion in a central place system'.' *Geographical Analysis,* **6,** 303–8. (2.3.3)

Ambrosch, F., Wiedermann, G. & Harasek, G. (1978). Costs and benefits of measles vaccination. *Fortschritte der Medizin,* **96,** 409–14. (8.3.2)

Bacharach, M. (1970). *Biproportional Matrices and Input–Output Change.* Cambridge: The University Press. (5.4.2)

Bailey, N. T. J. (1957). *The Mathematical Theory of Epidemics.* London: Griffin. (1.2)

Bailey, N. T. J. (1964). *The Elements of Stochastic Processes.* New York: Wiley. (7.4.1)

Bailey, N. T. J. (1967). 'The simulation of stochastic epidemics in two dimensions.' *Proceedings of the Fifth Berkeley Symposium on Mathematical Statistics and Probability*, **4,** 237–57. (2.4.1)

Bailey, N. T. J. (1975). *The Mathematical Theory of Infectious Diseases.* London: Griffin. (3.1, 3.3, 6.1, 7.4)

Baldursson, Guðni. (1975). 'Population.' In Jóhannes Nordal & Valdimar Kristinsson (eds.), *Iceland 874–1974.* Reykjavík: Central Bank of Iceland, 22–32. (3.4.2)

Ball, A. P. (1977). 'Measles.' In G. M. Howe (ed.), *A World Geography of Human Diseases.* London: Academic Press, 237–54. (3.3.1, 3.3.4, 5.5.4, 8.3.1)

Ball, F. (1977). 'Measles outbreaks in Iceland.' Unpublished project, Diploma in Mathematical Statistics, Statistical Laboratory, University of Cambridge, England. (6.3)

Bartholomew, D. J. (1973). *Stochastic Models for Social Processes.* New York: Wiley. (2.4.1)

Bartlett, M. S. (1956). 'Deterministic and stochastic models for recurrent epidemics.' *Proceedings of the Third Berkeley Symposium on Mathematical Statistics and Probability,* **4,** 81–100. (7.2.1)

Bartlett, M. S. (1957). 'Measles periodicity and community size.' *Journal of the Royal Statistical Society A, 120,* 48–70. (3.3.2, 3.4.1, 5.5.1, 6.2.3)

Bartlett, M. S. (1960). *Stochastic Population Models in Ecology and Epidemiology*. London: Methuen. (3.4.1)

Bartlett, M. S. (1972). 'Epidemics.' In J. M. Tanur (ed.), *Statistics: a Guide to the Unknown.* San Francisco: Holden-Day, 66–76. (3.3.2)

Bassett, K. & Haggett, P. (1971). 'Towards short-term forecasting for cyclic behaviour in a regional system of cities.' In M. D. I. Chisholm, A. E. Frey & P. Haggett (eds.), *Regional Forecasting*. London: Butterworth, 389–413. (3.2)

Benjamin, B. (1968). *Health and Vital Statistics*. London: Allen and Unwin. (7.6)

Bennett, R. J. (1979). *Spatial Time Series*. London: Pion. (6.1, 6.2.1, 6.2.2, 6.3.1)

Berry, B. J. L. (1972). 'Hierarchical diffusion – the basis of developmental filtering and spread in a system of growth centres.' In N. M. Hansen (ed.), *Growth Centres in Regional and Economic Development*. New York: The Free Press, 108–38. (2.3.3)

Black, F. L. (1966). 'Measles endemicity in insular populations: critical community size and its evolutionary implication.' *Journal of Theoretical Biology*, **11**, 207–11. (3.3.3, 3.4.1, 5.5.1, 6.4.3)

Bowman, I. (1931). *The Pioneer Fringe*. New York: American Geographical Society. (2.2.1)

Box, G. E. P. & Jenkins, G. M. (1970). *Time Series Analysis, Forecasting and Control*. San Francisco: Holden-Day. (6.1)

Brown, L. A. (1968). *Diffusion Processes and Location: a Conceptual Framework and Bibliography*. Philadelphia: Regional Science Research Association, Bibliography Series, **4.** (2.2.5)

Brown, L. A. & Moore, E. G. (1969). 'Diffusion research in geography: a perspective.' *Progress in Geography*, **1**, 119–57. (2.2.5)

Burnet, Sir Macfarlane & White, D. O. (1972). *Natural History of Infectious Disease*, (fourth edition). Cambridge: The University Press. (3.3.4, 8.3.1)

Casetti, E. (1969). 'Why do diffusion processes conform to logistic trends?' *Geographical Analysis*, **1**, 101–5. (2.3.1)

Casetti, E. & Semple, R. K. (1969). 'Concerning the testing of spatial diffusion hypotheses.' *Geographical Analysis*, **1**, 154–9. (2.3.1)

Chapin, C. V. (1925). 'Measles in Providence, R. I.' *American Journal of Hygiene*, **5**, 635–55. (3.3.3, 3.3.4)

Clark, A. (1954). 'Historical geography.' In P. E. James & C. F. Jones (eds.), *American Geography: Inventory and Prospect*, 70–105. Syracuse, Syracuse University Press. (2.2.1)

Cliff, A. D., Haggett, P., Ord, J. K., Bassett, K. & Davies, R. B. (1975). *Elements of Spatial Structure: a Quantitative Approach*. London: Cambridge University Press. (2.4.2, 3.2, 3.4.1, 5.3.5, 6.1, 6.2.1, 6.4.3)

Cliff, A. D. & Haggett, P. (1980). 'Geographical aspects of epidemic diffusion in closed communities.' In N. Wrigley, (ed.), *Statistical Applications in the Spatial Sciences*. London: Pion, 5–44. (5.3.3, 8.3.2)

Cliff, A. D. & Murray, G. D. (1977). 'A stochastic model for measles epidemics in a multi-region setting.' *Institute of British Geographers, Transactions New Series*, **2**, 158–74. (7.2.1)

Cliff, A. D. & Ord, J. K. (1971). 'A regression approach to unvariate spatial forecasting.' In M. D. I. Chisholm, A. E. Frey & P. Haggett (eds.), *Regional Forecasting*. London: Butterworth, 46–70. (6.3.2)

Cliff, A. D. & Ord, J. K. (1973). *Spatial Autocorrelation*. London: Pion. (5.3.3)

Cliff, A. D. & Ord, J. K. (1975a). 'Space–time modelling with an application to regional forecasting.' *Institute of British Geographers, Publications*, **64**, 119–28. (2.3.1)

Cliff, A. D. & Ord, J. K. (1975b). 'Model building and the analysis of spatial pattern in human geography.' *Journal of the Royal Statistical Society, B*, **37**, 297–348. (2.3.1)

Cliff, A. D. & Ord, J. K. (1978). 'Forecasting the progress of an epidemic.' In R. L. Martin, N. J. Thrift & R. J. Bennett (eds.), *Towards the Dynamic Analysis of Spatial Systems*. London: Pion, 191–204. (7.4)

Cox, K. R. & Demko, G. J. (1967). 'Agrarian structure and peasant discontent in the Russian revolution of 1905.' *East Lakes Geographer,* **3,** 3–20. (2.2.5)

Crowley, W. K. (1978). 'Old order Amish settlement: diffusion and growth.' *Annals of the Association of American Geographers,* **68,** 249–64. (2.2.1)

Curry, L. (1976). 'Fluctuations in the random spatial economy and the control of inflation.' *Geographical Analysis*, **8,** 339–53. (2.2.2)

Edgell, M. C. R. (1973). *Monash Publications in Geography,* **5,** 7. (2.1)

Edmondson, M. S. (1961). 'Neolithic diffusion rates.' *Current Anthropology,* **2,** 71–102. (2.2.3)

Elíasson, Helgi. (1967). Education. In Jóhannes Nordal & Valdimar Kristinsson (eds.), *Iceland 1966*. Reykjavík: Central Bank of Iceland, 289–97. (5.5.3)

Eythorsson, Jón & Sigtryggsson, Hlynur. (1971). 'The climate and weather of Iceland.' *The Zoology of Iceland,* **1, 3,** 62 pp. (5.5.4)

Farmer, B. H. (1957). *Pioneer Peasant Colonisation in Ceylon: a Study in Asian Agrarian Problems*. London: Oxford University Press. (2.2.1)

Farmer, B. H. (ed.) (1977). *Green Revolution? Technology and Change in Rice Growing Areas of Tamil Nadu and Sri Lanka.* London: Macmillan. (2.1)

Fox, J. P., Elveback, L., Scott, W., Gatewood, L. & Ackerman, E. (1971). 'Herd immunity: basic concept and relevance to public health immunization practices.' *American Journal of Epidemiology,* **94,** 179–89. (5.5.3)

Fraser, K. B. & Martin, S. J. (1978). *Measles Virus and its Biology*. London: Academic Press. (3.3.4, 8.3.1)

Gatrell, A. C. (1979). 'Spatial diffusion and catastrophe theory: some preliminary speculations.' University of Salford. To appear. (8.2)

Gilg, A. W. (1973). 'A study in agricultural disease diffusion.' *Institute of British Geographers, Publications,* **59,** 77–97.

Goodall, C. (1978). 'Measles in Iceland.' Unpublished project, Diploma in Mathematical Statistics, Statistical Laboratory, University of Cambridge, England. (3.3.3, 5.3.5, 7.3.1)

Gould, K. L., Hermann, K. L. & Witte, J. J. (1971). 'The epidemiology of measles in the US Trust Territory of the Pacific Islands.' *American Journal of Public Health,* **61,** 1602–13. (3.4.1)

Greenwood, M. (1931). 'On the statistical measure of infectiousness.' *Journal of Hygiene,* **31,** 336–51. (7.1)

Griffiths, D. A. (1973). 'The effect of measles vaccination on the incidence of measles in the community.' *Journal of the Royal Statistical Society, A,* **136,** 441–9. (3.3.4)

Griliches, Z. (1957). 'Hybrid corn: an exploration in the economics of technological change.' *Econometrica,* **25,** 501–22. (2.3.1)

Gulley, J. L. M. (1959). 'The Turnerian frontier: a study in the migration of ideas.' *Tijdschrift voor Economische en Sociale Geografie,* **50,** 65–72, 81–91. (2.2.1)

Gurland, J. (1957). 'Some interrelations among compound and generalized distributions.' *Biometrika,* **44,** 265–8. (7.4.1)

Hägerstrand, T. (1952). 'The propagation of innovation waves.' *Lund Studies in Geography, B,* **4,** 3–19. (2.3.1)

Hägerstrand, T. (1953, 1969). *Innovationsförloppet ur korologisk synpunkt.* Lund: Gleerup. *Innovation Diffusion as a Spatial Process.* Translated by A. Pred. Chicago: University of Chicago Press. (2.3.1, 2.3.2)

Hägerstrand, T. (1967). 'On Monte Carlo simulation of diffusion.' In W. L. Garrison & D. F. Marble (eds.), *Quantitative Geography, Part I: Economic and Cultural Topics.* Northwestern University Studies in Geography, **13,** 1–32. (2.3.2, 2.3.3)

Haggett, P. (1972). 'Contagious processes in a planar graph: an epidemiological application.' In N. D. McGlashan (ed.), *Medical Geography.* London: Methuen, 307–24. (3.4.1, 7.2.1)

Haggett, P. (1975). 'Simple epidemics in human populations: some geographical aspects of the Hamer–Soper diffusion models.' In R. F. Peel, M. Chisholm & P. Haggett (eds.), *Processes in Physical and Human Geography: Bristol Essays*. London: Heinemann, 373–91. (2.4.2, 5.5.1, 7.2.1)

Haggett, P. (1976). 'Hybridizing alternative models of an epidemic diffusion process.' *Economic Geography,* **52,** 136–46. (5.3.3)

Haggett, P. (1978). 'Regional and local components in elementary space–time models of contagious processes.' In T. Carlstein, D. N. Parkes & N. J. Thrift (eds.), *Timing Space and Spacing Time*, vol. 3. London: Arnold, 19–34. (7.2.1)

Haggett, P. (1979). *Geography: a Modern Synthesis* (third edition). New York: Harper and Row. (2.1)

Haggett, P., Cliff, A. D. & Frey, A. E. (1977). *Locational Analysis in Human Geography* (second edition). London: Arnold. (2.3.3, 5.3.2, 5.3.3, 6.2.1)

Hamer, W. H. (1906). 'Epidemic diseases in England.' *Lancet,* **1,** 733–9. (1.3.2, 7.1, 7.2.1)

Harrison, P. J. & Stevens, C. F. (1976). 'Bayesian forecasting.' *Journal of the Royal Statistical Society, B,* **38,** 205–47. (6.3.1)

Hepple, L. W. (1978a). 'The econometric specification and estimation of spatio-temporal models.' In T. Carlstein, D. N. Parkes & N. J. Thrift (eds.), *Timing Space and Spacing Time.* London: Arnold, 66–80. (6.1, 6.2.1)

Hepple, L. W. (1978b). 'Forecasting the economic recession in Britain's depressed regions.' In R. L. Martin, N. J. Thrift & R. J. Bennett (eds.), *Towards the Dynamic Analysis of Spatial Systems.* London: Pion, 172–90. (6.3.1)

Holling, C. S. (ed.) (1978). *Adaptive Environmental Assessment and Management.* London: Academic Press. (8.2)

Hudson, J. C. (1969). 'Diffusion in a central place system.' *Geographical Analysis,* **1,** 456–8. (2.3.3)

Hudson, J. C. (1972). *Geographical Diffusion Theory.* Northwestern University Studies in Geography, **19,** (2.2.3, 3.1)

Hudson, J. C. (1973). 'Two Dakota homestead frontiers.' *Annals of the Association of American Geographers,* **63,** 442–62. (2.2.1, 2.4.1)

Hunter, J. M. & Young, J. C. (1971). 'Diffusion of influenza in England and Wales.' *Annals of the Association of American Geographers,* **61,** 637–53. (2.2.4)

Iowa State Planning Board (1935). Second Report. (2.2.2)

Jaynes, E. T. (1957). Information theory and statistical mechanics. *Physics Review,* **106,** 620–30. (6.5.1)

Joerg, W. L. G. (ed.) (1932). *Pioneer Settlement: Co-operative Studies.* New York: American Geographical Society. (2.2.1)

Jónsson, Vilmundur. (1940). 'Health in Iceland. A survey of public health organization and health conditions in Iceland.' Reykjavík: *Heilbrigðisskýrslur,* 1938, 161–87. (5.2)

Kalman, R. E. (1960). 'A new approach to linear filtering and prediction problems.' *Transactions of the ASME Journal of Basic Engineering,* **82,** 34–45. (6.3)

Kendall, D. G. (1957). 'La propagation d'une épidémie au d'un bruit dans une population limitée.' *Publications of the Institute of Statistics, University of Paris,* **6,** 307–11. (7.2.1, 7.3.1)

King, L. J. & Forster, J. (1973). 'Wage rate changes in urban labour markets.' *Regional Science Association, Papers,* **30,** 183–96. (2.2.2)

Kristinsson, Valdimar. (1975). 'Communication and tourism.' In Jóhannes Nordal & Valdimar Kristinsson (eds.), *Iceland 874–1974.* Reykjavík: Central Bank of Iceland, 231–7. (5.5.2)

Levison, M., Ward, R. G. & Webb, J. W. (1973). *The Settlement of Polynesia: a Computer Simulation.* Minneapolis: University of Minnesota Press. (2.3.3)

Lindley, D. V. (1965). *Introduction to Probability and Statistics from a Bayesian Viewpoint.* Cambridge: The University Press. (6.3.2, 6.7)

Lösch, A. (1940). *Die räumliche Ordnung der Wirtschaft.* Jena. (1954). *The Economics of Location.* New Haven: Yale University Press. (2.2.2)

MacArthur, R. H. & Wilson, E. O. (1967). *The Theory of Island Biogeography.* Princeton: Princeton University Press, Monographs in Population Biology, **1,** (3.4.1)

Mc. A. Sayers, B., Mansourian, B. G., Tan, T. P. & Bögel, K. (1977). 'A pattern-analysis study of a wild-life rabies epizootic.' *Medical Information,* **2,** 11–34. (2.1)

McKhann, C. F. (1973). 'Measles and German measles.' *Encyclopaedia Brittanica,* **15,** 25–6. (3.3.4, 8.3.2)

Mansfield, E. (1961). 'Technical change and the rate of innovation.' *Econometrica,* **29,** 741–66. (2.3.1)

Martin, R. L. (1978). 'Kalman filter modelling of time-varying processes in urban and regional analysis.' In R. L. Martin, N. J. Thrift & R. J. Bennett (eds.), *Towards the Dynamic Analysis of Spatial Systems.* London: Pion, 104–26. (6.3.1)

Martin, R. L. & Oeppen, J. E. (1975). 'The identification of regional forecasting models using space–time correlation functions.' *Institute of British Geographers, Publications,* **66,** 95–118. (6.2.2)

Mikesell, M. W. (1960). 'Comparative studies in frontier history.' *Annals of the Association of American Geographers,* **50,** 62–74. (2.2.1)

Mollison, D. (1977). 'Spatial contact models for ecological and epidemic spread.' *Journal of the Royal Statistical Society, B,* **39,** 283–326. (2.3.1, 3.1, 5.4.1)

Morrill, R. L. (1968). 'Waves of spatial diffusion.' *Journal of Regional Science,* **8,** 1–18. (2.3.3)

Morrill, R. L. (1970). 'The shape of diffusion in space and time.' *Economic Geography,* **46,** 259–68. (2.3.3)

Nelder, J. A. & Wedderburn, R. W. M. (1972). 'Generalised linear models.' *Journal of the Royal Statistical Society, A,* **135,** 370–84. (6.4.1)

Nystuen, J. D. & Kolars, J. F. (1974). *Geography.* New York: McGraw-Hill. (2.1)

Panum, P. L. (1940). 'Measles in the Faroe islands.' *Delta Omega Society, American Public Health Association,* being a translation of *Virchows Archiv für Pathologie und Medizin,* **1,** 1847, 492–512. (3.3.4, 3.4.1)

Parsons, J. J. (1949). 'Antioqueño colonisation in Western Columbia: an historical geography.' *Ibero-Americana,* **32,** 1–225. (2.2.1)

Pedersen, P. O. (1970). 'Innovation diffusion within and between national urban systems.' *Geographical Analysis,* **2,** 203–54. (2.3.3)

Preusser, H. (1976). *The Landscapes of Iceland: Types and Regions.* The Hague: Junk. (3.4.2, 5.4)

Pyle, G. F. (1969). 'Diffusion of cholera in the United States.' *Geographical Analysis,* **1,** 59–75. (2.3.3)

Pyle, G. F. (1979). *Applied Medical Geography.* New York: Wiley. (8.3.1)

Rapoport, A. (1951). 'Nets with distance bias.' *Bulletin of Mathematical Biophysics,* **13,** 85–92. (2.3.1)

Rees, P. H. & Wilson, A. G. (1977). *Spatial Population Analysis.* London: Arnold. (A3)

Riley, R. L. & O'Grady, F. (1961). *Airborne Infection: Transmission and Control.* New York: Macmillan. (3.3.4)

Rogers, A. (1968). *Matrix Analysis of Interregional Population Growth and Distribution.* California: University of California Press. (A3)

Rogers, E. M. (1962). *Diffusion of Innovations.* New York: The Free Press. (2.2.3)

Sauer, C. O. (1952). 'Agricultural origins and dispersals.' *American Geographical Society, Bowman Memorial Lectures,* **2,** (2.2.1)

Sauer, C. O. & Brand, D. (1930). 'Pueblo sites in south-eastern Arizona.' *University of California, Publications in Geography,* **3,** 415–48. (2.2.1)

Schutzbach, W. (1976). *Island. Feuerinsel am Polarkreis.* Bonn: Ferd Dummlers Verlag. (5.4)

Sigurjónsson, Július: (1975). 'Public health.' In Jóhannes Nordal & Valdimar Kristinsson (eds.), *Iceland, 874–1974.* Reykjavík: Central Bank of Iceland, 295–9. (5.2)

Soper, H. E. (1929). 'Interpretation of periodicity in disease prevalence.' *Journal of the Royal Statistical Society, A,* **92,** 34–73. (1.3.2, 7.1, 7.2.1)

Souza, R. C. (1978). 'A Bayesian entropy approach to forecasting.' Unpublished PhD thesis, Department of Statistics, University of Warwick, Coventry, England. (6.5.1, 6.5.3)

Souza, R. C. (1980). 'The forecasting of epidemics' progress using a Bayesian-entropy framework.' *Environment and Planning* (forthcoming). (6.5.1, 6.5.3)

Stanislawski, D. (1946). 'The origin and spread of the grid-pattern town.' *Geographical Review,* **36,** 105–20. (2.2.1)

Stokes, H. H., Jones, D. W. & Neuburger, H. M. (1975). 'Unemployment and adjustment in the labour market: a comparison between the regional and national responses.' *University of Chicago, Department of Geography, Research Paper,* No. 177. (2.2.2)

Stuart-Harris, C. H. (1965). *Influenza and Other Virus Infections of the Respiratory Tract,* (second edition). London: Arnold. (2.2.4)

Sutherland, A. (1979). 'Measles in Iceland.' Unpublished project, Diploma in Mathematical Statistics, Statistical Laboratory, University of Cambridge, England. (6.4)

Thom, R. (1975). *Structural Stability and Morphogeneous: an Outline of a General Theory of Models* (translated by D. H. Fowler). Reading, Mass.: Benjamin. (8.2)

Thorarinsson, Sigúrður. (1961). 'Populations changes in Iceland.' *Geographical Review,* **51,** 519–33. (3.4.2, 5.5.4)

Tornqvist, G. (1967). *Growth of TV Ownership in Sweden, 1956–65.* Uppsala: Uppsala University Press. (2.3.1)

Turner, F. J. (1920). *The Frontier in American History.* New York: Holt. (2.2.1)

United States, Secretary of State. (1831). *Census of Population, 1830.* Washington: U.S. Census Office. (2.3.3)

United States, Bureau of Census. (1851). *Population Census of 1850.* Washington: U.S. Census Office. (2.3.3)

United States, Bureau of Census. (1871). *Population Census of 1870.* Washington: U.S. Census Office. (2.3.3)

United States Surgeon-General's Office. (1875). 'The cholera epidemic of 1873 in the United States.' *Executive Document No. 95.* Washington: Government Printing Office. (2.3.3)

Waterman, A. M. C. (1972). *Economic Fluctuations in Australia, 1948 to 1964.* Canberra: Australian National University Press. (3.2)

Webb, W. P. (1927). *The Great Plains.* New York: Ginn. (2.2.1)

Weissbrod, R. (1976). *Diffusion of Relative Wage Inflation in Southeast Pennsylvania.* Northwestern University Studies in Geography, **23,** (2.2.2)

Wells, W. F. (1955). *Airborne Contagion and Air Hygiene.* Cambridge, Mass.: Harvard University Press. (3.3.4)

Yuill, R. S. (1965). 'A simulation study of barrier effects in spatial diffusion studies.' *Michigan Inter-University Community of Mathematical Geographers, Discussion Papers,* **5.** (2.2.3)

Þórarinsson, Sigúrður. See Thorarinsson, Sigúrður (1961).

Index